Differential Diagnosis
in Primary Eye Care

DEBRA J. BEZAN, O.D., FAAO

*Adjunct Professor, Northeastern State University
College of Optometry, Tahlequah, Oklahoma;
Staff Optometrist, Optometry Clinic,
W. W. Hastings Hospital, Tahlequah*

FRANK P. LARUSSA, O.D.

Private Practice and Omega Eye Associates, Birmingham, Alabama

JOHN H. NISHIMOTO, O.D., M.B.A., FAAO

*Associate Professor and Assistant Dean for External Programs,
Southern California College of Optometry, Fullerton*

DAVID P. SENDROWSKI, O.D., FAAO

*Associate Professor and Chief, Ophthalmology Consultation Service,
Ocular Disease and Special Testing Service,
Southern California College of Optometry, Fullerton;
Staff Optometrist, Family Practice Service,
California State University at Fullerton Health Clinic*

CARL H. SPEAR, O.D.

*Adjunct Assistant Professor, Northeastern State University,
College of Optometry, Tahlequah, Oklahoma;
Navarre Family Eye Care, Navarre, Florida*

DAVID K. TALLEY, O.D., FAAO

*Assistant Professor, Southern College of Optometry, Memphis;
Center Director, Southern Eye Associates, Memphis*

TAMMY P. THAN, M.S., O.D., FAAO

Consultative Optometry, McDonnell Eye Center, Magnolia, Arkansas

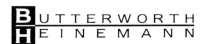

Boston • Oxford • Auckland • Johannesburg • Melbourne • New Delhi

Butterworth–Heinemann supports the efforts of American Forests and the Global ReLeaf program in its campaign for the betterment of trees, forests, and our environment.

Library of Congress Cataloging-in-Publication Data

Differential diagnosis in primary eye care / Debra J. Bezan ... [et al.].
    p. cm.
    Includes bibliographical references and index.
    ISBN 0-7506-9462-9
    1. Eye--Diseases--Diagnosis. 2. Diagnosis, Differential.
I. Bezan, Debra.
    [DNLM: 1. Eye Diseases--diagnosis. 2. Diagnosis, Differential.
3. Primary Health Care. WW 141 D569 1999]
RE75.D 1999
617.7'15--dc21
DNLM/DLC
for Library of Congress   98-46554
                                                          CIP

British Library Cataloguing-in-Publication Data
A catalogue record for this book is available from the British Library.

The publisher offers special discounts on bulk orders of this book.
For information, please contact:
Manager of Special Sales
Butterworth–Heinemann
225 Wildwood Avenue
Woburn, MA 01801-2041
Tel: 781-904-2500
Fax: 781-904-2620

For information on all Butterworth–Heinemann publications available,
contact our World Wide Web home page at: http://www.bh.com

10 9 8 7 6 5 4 3 2 1

Printed in the United States of America

Contents

Preface

As the old saying goes, "If you hear hoofbeats, think horses, not zebras." In the clinical diagnostic process, however, if you hear hoofbeats, think horses first but consider zebras. Based on the patient's chief complaint, history, and initial presentation, the clinician immediately develops a list of hypotheses (the differential diagnosis) to consider. Some of these hypotheses have a high probability of being the correct diagnosis (i.e., "horses") and some have a low probability of being correct (i.e., "zebras"). As the clinician gains experience, the list of possible diagnoses becomes longer and the probability of likelihood assigned to each possible diagnosis becomes more accurate.

During the course of a problem-focused examination, more information is obtained to help the clinician rule out diagnoses on the hypothesis list. In some cases, information beyond that typically obtained during the primary eye care practitioner's examination is necessary in the differential diagnostic process. Such information includes laboratory testing, electrodiagnostic evaluation, and diagnostic imaging. In many cases, a multidisciplinary approach to both the diagnosis and management of the patient's condition is needed.

This text is designed to help both the student and the experienced primary eye care practitioner in the process of differential diagnosis of most ocular conditions. Each chapter covers a commonly encountered clinical symptom or sign. At the beginning of each chapter is an "at a glance" list of diagnoses to consider for the particular symptom or sign. This list contains most, if not all, of the "horses" and some of the "zebras." Following the list is a series of SOP (subjective, objective, and plan) notes for some of the differential diagnosis. The authors have selected the most common, significant, and interesting diagnoses to include in this section. The notes are followed by a list of suggested reading. At the end of each chapter is a flowchart that summarizes the differential diagnostic process for the conditions covered in the SOP notes. In addition, the appendices at the end of the book provide information about laboratory tests and some of the pharmaceutical agents available to treat the conditions mentioned throughout the book.

Clinical diagnosis is often straightforward, but it can be quite difficult and complex. Our goal with this book is to help primary eye care practitioners efficiently track down both the "horses" and "zebras" and provide the best possible care to their patients.

Debra J. Bezan

Acknowledgements

We would like to thank Ken, Lori, "Doc," Barbara, and Karen for their patience, encouragement, and support. We would also like to thank Pat Humphres, Judy Badstuebner, Judy Higgins, Annie Greene, Olga Trammel, and Drs. Michelle Welch, Audry Brodie, and Lee Browning for their technical assistance.

I

Symptoms

1

Blurred Vision

Frank P. LaRussa

BLURRED VISION AT A GLANCE

Monocular blurred vision, usually normal pupils
  Age-related macular degeneration
  Cataract
  Branch retinal vein occlusion
  Diabetic retinopathy
  Macular hole
  Retinal detachment
  Toxoplasmosis
  Idiopathic central serous choroidopathy
  Postsurgical cystoid macular edema
  Keratitis
  Corneal edema
Monocular blurred vision, usually positive afferent
    pupillary defect
  Optic neuritis
  Anterior ischemic optic neuropathy
  Optic nerve tumor
Binocular blurred vision, pinhole improves vision
  Refractive error
Binocular blurred vision, pinhole does not improve vision
  Macular degeneration
  Cataract
  Diabetic retinopathy
  Open-angle glaucoma
  Corneal dystrophy
  Migraine
  Keratitis
  Binocular optic nerve disease

Blurred vision is probably the most common complaint an eye care practitioner hears. The complaint may be caused by a great number of eye conditions. The practitioner must use a systematic approach to determine the etiology of a given complaint of blurred vision.

The first step in narrowing the likely diagnosis is to determine whether the complaint is monocular or binocular. If the complaint is monocular, the next step is to determine if an afferent pupillary defect is present. If the pupils are normal, one can usually eliminate optic nerve conditions as the cause. If the blurred eye has an afferent pupillary defect, the etiology probably involves the optic nerve. Severe monocular retinal disease may cause a very mild afferent pupillary defect. If the complaint is binocular, the first step is to determine if a pinhole improves visual acuity. If a pinhole improves vision to 20/25 or better, the condition is usually refractive in nature. If a pinhole does not improve vision, the condition is probably pathologic.

MONOCULAR, USUALLY NORMAL PUPILS

Wet (Exudative) Age-Related Macular Degeneration

Subjective
Patients with wet age-related macular degeneration (ARMD) are generally over the age of 50. ARMD is more common in individuals with fair complexions. Patients with wet ARMD usually complain of a sudden drop in visual acuity and often state that their vision is distorted. They may also complain of a fuzzy area in the center of vision.

Objective
Refraction of these patients is difficult, and vision will not be improved. Amsler grid testing reveals distortion. Dilated fundus examination reveals an elevated macular region. Within the elevated portion, a gray-green area may be noted, which indicates the location of the bleed.

Fluorescein angiography helps with both the diagnosis and treatment of wet ARMD.

Plan

Patients with suspected wet ARMD should have a fluorescein angiogram taken as soon as possible and should be referred to a retinologist. The retinologist may elect to perform focal laser treatment if the foveal area is not involved. Surgical extraction of a subfoveal neovascular membrane may be attempted, but this procedure tends to be less successful in patients with ARMD than in patients with neovascularization from certain other conditions.

Branch Retinal Vein Occlusion

Subjective

Patients with branch retinal vein occlusion (BRVO) usually are over 50 years of age. Affected patients often have a history of hypertension or diabetes. Patients with BRVO often complain of a sudden loss of vision in one eye. They sometimes describe the area of blur as red. They also may complain of metamorphopsia.

Objective

Refraction is difficult, and vision will not improve to 20/20 if the macular region is involved. Dilated fundus examination reveals a wedge-shaped area of flame hemorrhages, usually adjacent to the superior or inferior temporal arcade. Cotton-wool spots and retinal edema may also be present. Often, the artery/vein crossing that led to the occlusion can be seen just proximal to the hemorrhaging.

Plan

In many cases, patients with BRVO should be referred to a retinologist. This step is indicated if there are signs of ischemia (cotton-wool spots) or if there is clinically significant macular edema. Fluorescein angiography performed after the hemorrhage has resolved enough to allow adequate viewing is the only way to rule out ischemia. The retinologist should perform scatter photocoagulation if the patient has neovascularization or if the ischemia indicates a high likelihood of future neovascularization. Grid laser photocoagulation may also be performed on patients with clinically significant macular edema. Patients with a small BRVO with no macular edema or ischemic signs often recover fully with no treatment. Patients with BRVO should also be referred to their family physician for systemic evaluation for underlying conditions such as diabetes or hypertension.

Diabetic Retinopathy

Subjective

Patients who have diabetic retinopathy may complain of vision problems if they have macular edema. These patients often complain of blurred vision and metamorphopsia. Some diabetic patients have blurred vision secondary to dramatic shifts in refractive error. Other patients may have large central hemorrhages, neovascularization with retinal traction, or vitreal hemorrhages that significantly reduce visual function.

Objective

Refraction is difficult and will not improve vision to 20/20 if macular edema or vitreal hemorrhage is present. The iris should be inspected for neovascularization before dilation. A dilated fundus examination should be performed to look for signs of diabetic retinopathy such as dot and blot hemorrhages, hard exudates, cotton-wool spots, venous beading, intraretinal microvascular anomalies, neovascularization, vitreal hemorrhage, and retinal detachment.

Plan

Retinologists have varying philosophies about when to initiate panretinal photocoagulation. Some treat patients with very severe nonproliferative retinopathy; others wait until the patient exhibits neovascularization; still others wait until the neovascularization is classified as "high risk." The primary eye care practitioner should establish his or her referral criteria accordingly. All cases of clinically significant macular edema should be referred to a retinologist. Clinically significant macular edema is defined as edema or hard exudates with adjacent edema within one-third disc diameter of the fovea, or an area of edema greater than one disc diameter in size, any portion of which is within a disc diameter of the fovea. The retinologist will perform fluorescein angiography to determine the leakage sites and will perform local or grid laser photocoagulation if indicated.

Macular Hole

Subjective

Patients with macular holes often complain of an area of missing vision in the center of sight. They often state that they see better if they look to the side of letters rather than directly at them. The condition is more common in women over the age of 40.

Objective

Refraction does not improve visual acuity. Dilated fundus examination will reveal a red area at the fovea, often with yellow spots within. This area represents a full-thickness macular hole. A Watzke-Allen test may be performed to confirm the presence of a full-thickness hole. In this test, a vertical light beam is passed over the suspected area, and the patient is asked to describe its appearance. If the patient reports a gap in the beam, a full-thickness hole is suggested.

Plan

Many patients with macular holes can now be treated with retinal surgery. Patients with macular holes should be referred to a retinologist with experience in macular hole repair. If an impending macular hole is noted, the patient should be referred to a retinologist for a vitrectomy evaluation.

Retinal Detachment

Subjective

The three main types of retinal detachment are rhegmatogenous, tractional, and exudative. Patients with retinal detachment often complain of a sudden loss of vision. They may complain of flashes of light or a dramatic onset of floaters. They may also complain of having a curtain or shadow over their vision.

Objective

Pupil testing may show a positive afferent pupillary defect if extensive retinal damage is present. Dilated fundus examination will reveal an area of detached retina. This area is usually corrugated, appears milky white, and undulates in the vitreous cavity with eye movements. With rhegmatogenous retinal detachments, pigment in the anterior vitreous and an associated retinal tear are often visible.

Plan

Patients with retinal detachments, particularly detachments involving the macula, should be referred to a retinologist as soon as possible for surgical repair.

Active Toxoplasmosis

Subjective

Toxoplasmosis is caused by congenital or acquired infection by the protozoan *Toxoplasma gondii*. Patients with active toxoplasmosis complain of foggy or smoky vision. They often complain of dramatic halos around lights. An underlying immunosuppressive condition should be considered in patients with active toxoplasmosis.

Objective

Dilated fundus examination reveals a vitritis. Often the vitritis does not allow an adequate view of the fundus.

The posterior pole, if visible, reveals a white or yellow elevated lesion, often in the macular region. This lesion may be adjacent to a pigmented scar designating the previous site of another active lesion.

Plan

Topical cycloplegics and topical steroids can be used to treat anterior uveitis associated with active toxoplasmosis lesions that are not a threat to vision due to their peripheral location and small size. Active toxoplasmosis lesions that are in the posterior pole region may be treated with a number of agents, including sulfadiazine, clindamycin, pyrimethamine, and folic acid, to prevent bone marrow depression. Oral prednisone may be prescribed to control inflammation, but should be used only in combination with one or more antimicrobial agents. A referral to a retinologist is highly recommended in the management of active toxoplasmosis.

Idiopathic Central Serous Retinopathy

Subjective

Idiopathic central serous retinopathy (ICSC) occurs 10 times more often in males than in females. Patients with ICSC are usually aged 25–50, and typically complain of a sudden onset of blurred vision or metamorphopsia.

Objective

Refraction is difficult, but vision may improve slightly. This slight improvement in vision is usually achieved with a correction for a hyperopic shift in refractive error. Amsler grid testing reveals distortion. Dilated fundus examination reveals a dome-shaped, elevated area involving the macula. No associated hemorrhaging or exudation is present.

Plan

Fluorescein angiography is strongly recommended for any patient with an elevated macula. The angiogram will rule out the existence of a subretinal neovascular membrane and help pinpoint the area of leakage. In most cases, ICSC improves without treatment. In cases that are persistent (lasting 4 months or longer), recurrent, or bilateral, or in which the patient cannot tolerate prolonged reduced vision, laser therapy should be considered.

Cystoid Macular Edema (Postsurgical)

Subjective

A few weeks after intraocular surgery, the patient who has developed cystoid macular edema usually complains of a blurring of vision. The blurring is often slow in onset.

Objective

Dilated fundus examination may reveal a slightly elevated area in the macular that indicates cystoid edema. The edema is often difficult to detect with ophthalmoscopy, and a fluorescein angiogram may be needed to confirm the diagnosis.

Plan

Treatment of cystoid macular edema is controversial. Many cases recover spontaneously. Nonsteroidal anti-inflammatory agents, corticosteroids, and vitrectomy also have been used to treat postsurgical cystoid macular edema, with variable degrees of success. In most cases, the surgeon who performed the initial surgery or a retinologist should be consulted concerning further evaluation and management.

Keratitis

Subjective

Keratitis can cause either binocular or monocular blurred vision depending on its etiology. Common causes of keratitis include dry eye, infection, and trauma (including mechanical, chemical, and radiation-induced trauma).

Objective

Refraction is difficult in these cases and does not improve acuity. Slit-lamp examination and sodium fluorescein staining reveal epithelial disruption. Corneal edema may also be present. Tear break-up time, other dry-eye evaluation tests, and ocular smears or cultures can provide additional diagnostic information.

Plan

Treatment of keratitis is determined by the underlying cause. Lubricants are typically the initial therapy for dry eye, whereas topical anti-infective agents are used to manage infective and traumatic keratitis. Punctal plugs are recommended for moderate to severe dry-eye cases.

Macular Degeneration (Dry, Atrophic)

Subjective

Macular degeneration is a common cause of vision loss among the elderly. Patients with macular degeneration often complain of blurred vision in the center of the visual field. Recognizing faces and reading are often difficult due to the central blur.

Objective

Refraction or pinhole testing does not improve visual acuity. In dry macular degeneration, dilated fundus examination reveals drusen and changes in the retinal pigment epithelium (RPE) in the macular region. Large confluent drusen with indistinct borders or focal RPE detachments indicate that the patient has an increased risk of developing exudative (wet) ARMD.

Plan

If the retina has RPE changes and drusen but no signs of wet macular degeneration, the patient should be educated about the condition and taught how to monitor for signs of wet degeneration with a home Amsler grid or similar technique. Low vision devices may be quite beneficial in helping patients best use their existing vision. The benefit of vitamin therapy is controversial and is currently under investigation; nevertheless, vitamins are often prescribed. If wet age-related degeneration is noted, the patient should be referred to a retinologist as soon as possible for further evaluation and treatment.

Cataract

Subjective

Cataract is a common cause of vision loss that is found primarily in the elderly population. Patients with cataracts often complain of blurred vision. The onset of blur is usually gradual. Patients often describe their vision as foggy or report the impression of looking through a film over their eyes. Sensitivity to glare is another symptom associated with certain types of cataract.

Objective

Refraction often reveals a myopic shift. Dilated examination reveals lens opacification. Nuclear, sclerotic, cortical, and posterior subcapsular cataracts are the most common types seen in older patients.

Plan

The practitioner should ascertain the degree of debilitation caused by the cataracts. If cataracts and signs of macular pathology are present, the practitioner should perform a potential acuity test (Potential Acuity Meter, interferometer, or super pinhole test) to estimate the postsurgical visual outcome. The patient with cataracts should be referred to a cataract surgeon if the patient can no longer perform desired tasks due to the opacity.

MONOCULAR, SUDDEN ONSET, POSITIVE AFFERENT PUPILLARY DEFECT

Optic Neuritis

Subjective

The patient with optic neuritis usually complains of rapid reduction in vision in the involved eye. The patient may complain of pain on eye movements and may note a reduction in vision during exercise or after taking a hot bath (Uhthoff symptom). When the medical history is taken, the patient should be questioned about past systemic viral infections, inflammatory diseases, and multiple sclerosis.

Objective
There is an afferent pupillary defect, decreased color vision grossly detectable with the red cap test, and reduced perception of light intensity in the involved eye. Perimetry usually reveals a central or cecocentral scotoma. The fundus examination may reveal a unilateral swollen disc with associated flame hemorrhages; however, it should be noted that, in retrobulbar cases, the disc often has a normal appearance. Later the disc may show pallor. Laboratory and radiologic testing—including erythrocyte sedimentation rate (ESR), complete blood count, fluorescent treponemal antibody absorption test, and magnetic resonance imaging—may be used when an underlying systemic cause is suspected.

Plan
Use of oral steroids is controversial and is no longer recommended as a primary treatment for optic neuritis. Observation is often recommended in cases where visual acuity is only mildly affected (acuity of 20/40 or better), and vision usually returns partially or fully with time. In more severe cases, intravenous steroids followed by oral steroids are often prescribed.

Anterior Ischemic Optic Neuropathy

Subjective
Patients with anterior ischemic optic neuropathy are usually 40 years old or older. They generally complain of a rapid, painless reduction of vision or visual field in one eye.

Objective
Reduced acuity and a relative afferent pupillary defect will be noted in the involved eye. The patient will have a visual field defect in the affected eye only. The most common field defect is altitudinal. The patient may have reduced color perception in the involved eye. The optic nerve is swollen if the condition is acute and appears pale if the condition is long-standing.

Plan
The patient should have an ESR test immediately to rule out giant cell arteritis. If the ESR is elevated, intravenous or oral steroid therapy should be initiated. A temporal artery biopsy may be needed in equivocal cases. If the ESR or temporal artery biopsy is normal and the vision loss is not progressive, the condition is assumed to be

nonarteritic ischemic optic neuropathy, and no further treatment is indicated except to refer the patient to an internal medicine specialist for evaluation for underlying systemic disease.

BINOCULAR BLURRED VISION

Refractive Error

Subjective
Patients who have a refractive error or changes in refractive error complain of blurred vision. The largest group of blurred vision complaints falls into the category of refractive error. Patients usually describe this blurred vision as having a gradual onset.

Objective
In most cases, refraction results in 20/20 visual acuity and a resolution of the blurred vision complaint. Pinhole testing of visual acuity can confirm a refractive cause for blurred vision when the clinician is unable to improve a patient's visual acuity via refraction. If the use of a pinhole improves visual acuity, there is a refractive component to the patient's blurred vision complaint.

Plan
Glasses or contact lenses traditionally have been the treatment for refractive errors. If the patient has irregular astigmatism, such as in keratoconus, a rigid contact lens should be considered as the initial therapy. Refractive surgery should also be discussed as an option when appropriate.

Macular Degeneration (Dry, Atrophic)

Subjective
Macular degeneration is a common cause of vision loss among the elderly. Patients with macular degeneration often complain of blurred vision in the center of the visual field. Recognizing faces and reading are often difficult due to the central blur.

Objective
Refraction or pinhole testing does not improve visual acuity. In dry macular degeneration, dilated fundus examination reveals drusen and changes in the RPE in the macular region. Large confluent drusen with indistinct borders or focal RPE detachments indicate that the patient has an increased risk of developing exudative (wet) ARMD.

Plan
If the retina has RPE changes and drusen but no signs of wet macular degeneration, the patient should be educated

about the condition and taught how to monitor for signs of wet degeneration with a home Amsler grid or similar technique. Low vision devices may be quite beneficial in helping patients best use their existing vision. The benefit of vitamin therapy is controversial and is currently under investigation; nevertheless, vitamins are often prescribed. If wet ARMD is noted, the patient should be referred to a retinologist as soon as possible for further evaluation and treatment.

Cataract

Subjective
Cataract is a common cause of vision loss that is found primarily in the elderly population. Patients with cataracts often complain of blurred vision. The onset of blur is usually gradual. Patients often describe their vision as foggy or report the impression of looking through a film over their eyes. Sensitivity to glare is another symptom associated with certain types of cataract.

Objective
Refraction often reveals a myopic shift. Dilated examination reveals lens opacification. Nuclear, sclerotic, cortical, and posterior subcapsular cataracts are the most common types seen in older patients.

Plan
The practitioner should ascertain the degree of debilitation caused by the cataracts. If cataracts and signs of macular pathology are present, the practitioner should perform a potential acuity test (Potential Acuity Meter, interferometer, or super pinhole test) to estimate the postsurgical visual outcome. The patient with cataracts should be referred to a cataract surgeon if the patient can no longer perform desired tasks due to the opacity.

Advanced Open-Angle Glaucoma

Subjective
Patients with advanced glaucoma usually note peripheral vision loss and may complain of blurred vision once macular nerve fibers become involved.

Objective
Refraction or pinhole testing will not improve visual acuity if the loss is due to glaucomatous damage. Perimetry reveals significant defects in the visual field. Dilated fundus examination shows severe optic nerve cupping. Tonometry is used to measure intraocular pressure and to monitor effectiveness of or compliance with glaucoma therapy.

Plan
Patients with advanced glaucoma should be monitored closely to prevent central vision loss. Medical and surgical management should be carried out as indicated to prevent further vision loss.

Corneal Dystrophy

Subjective
Corneal dystrophies may occasionally elicit a complaint of reduced visual acuity. The complaints are often similar to cataract-related complaints.

Objective
Refraction or pinhole testing usually does not improve visual acuity. Biomicroscopy reveals corneal opacification. The depth, pattern, location, and extent of the opacification vary with the type of dystrophy.

Plan
The patient should be educated concerning the particular dystrophy that exists. In certain cases of advanced corneal dystrophy, a penetrating keratoplasty or therapeutic photokeratectomy may be of benefit.

Migraine Headache

Subjective
A positive family history of similar episodes is common among patients with migraine headaches. Patients with migraines often note a prodromal aura and may complain of transient episodes of blurred vision before an attack. The patient may describe the vision as shimmering or as having the appearance of looking through broken glass or water. A transient scotoma that changes in size or moves across the visual field may also be described. The episodes of visual disturbance typically last 15–60 minutes and are often followed by intense headache and nausea. Some patients can experience the ocular symptoms without the subsequent headache (acephalgic migraine).

Objective
Ocular examination is normal except that it may be possible to detect a visual field defect during the prodromal visual aura.

Plan
The vision examination is usually unremarkable in the migraine patient. Any refractive error should be corrected, because uncorrected refractive error is one factor

that can exacerbate migraine headaches. In rare cases, patients with migraines demonstrate signs of Horner's syndrome or persistent visual field defects. Patients with recurrent, prolonged, or debilitating migraines should be referred to their family physicians for further evaluation and treatment.

Binocular Optic Nerve Disease

Subjective
Binocular optic nerve disease can cause bilateral blurred vision.

Objective
Examination reveals optic nerve pallor or edema.

Plan
The patient with binocular optic nerve disease should be referred to a neurologist for MRI or CT.

SUGGESTED READING

Alexander LA. Primary Care of the Posterior Segment (2nd ed). Norwalk, CT: Appleton & Lange, 1995.

Bartlett JD, Jaanus SD. Clinical Ocular Pharmacology (3rd ed). Boston: Butterworth–Heinemann, 1995.

Fraunfelder FT, Roy FH. Current Ocular Therapy 4. Philadelphia: Saunders, 1995.

Cullom RD, Chang B. The Wills Eye Manual. Office and emergency diagnosis and treatment of eye disease (2nd ed). Philadelphia: Lippincott, 1994.

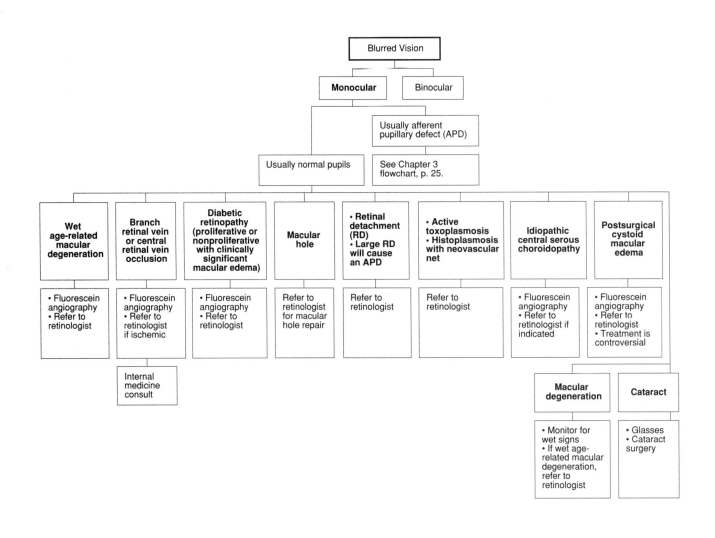

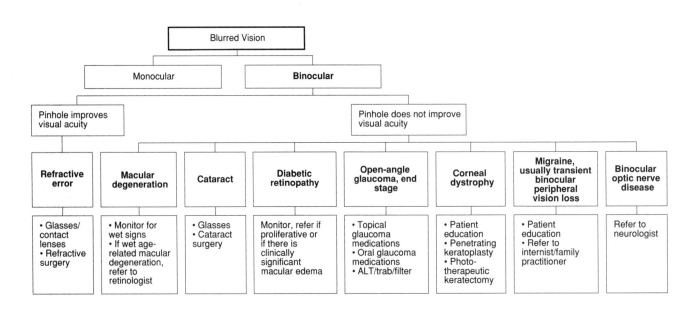

2

Sudden Vision Loss

CARL H. SPEAR

SUDDEN VISION LOSS AT A GLANCE

Amaurosis fugax
Ocular migraine
Vaso-occlusive disorders
    Central retinal vein occlusion
    Branch retinal vein occlusion
    Central retinal artery occlusion
    Branch retinal artery occlusion
    Ocular ischemic syndrome
Optic nerve disorders
    Inflammatory optic neuropathy
    Demyelinating optic neuropathy
    Compressive optic neuropathy
    Nonarteritic ischemic optic neuropathy
    Temporal arteritic ischemic optic neuropathy
Macular hole
Retinal detachment
Vitreous hemorrhage
Vertebrobasilar artery insufficiency
Others
    Syncope
    Postural hypotension
    Hysteria
    Papilledema
    Macular disorders
    Trauma
    Stroke

A patient who presents with sudden-onset vision loss presents the clinician with a diagnostic dilemma that must be rapidly resolved to prevent permanent vision loss and, in some cases, severe systemic sequelae or even death. A careful history to determine onset, duration, and extent of vision loss is essential. Objective findings cover a wide range of presentations, from the classic fundus picture of a central retinal vein occlusion to a completely normal fundus in retrobulbar optic neuritis. Often, management includes a systemic vascular evaluation to rule out an underlying systemic disease or consultation with a retinologist for therapy.

AMAUROSIS FUGAX

Subjective

Patients with amaurosis fugax report unilateral vision loss lasting from seconds to a few minutes. Vision returns to normal after the episode.

Objective

Ocular evaluation may be normal or retinal emboli may be visible on dilation. A carotid bruit may also be present.

Plan

A thorough medical examination is necessary and should include blood work (complete blood count, fasting blood sugar, and lipid profile). Carotid artery and cardiac evaluations are also indicated. The most common cause of amaurosis fugax is carotid artery disease. Other possible causes include ocular ischemic syndrome, cardiac disease, intravenous drug abuse, and hyperviscosity syndromes.

VERTEBROBASILAR ARTERY INSUFFICIENCY

Subjective

Patients with vertebrobasilar insufficiency present with bilateral blurred vision that lasts from seconds to a few minutes. Additional symptoms include hemiparesis, ataxia, and vertigo. Recurrent episodes are common.

Objective

Ocular findings are unremarkable.

Plan

Patients suspected of vertebrobasilar artery insufficiency should be referred for systemic evaluation.

OCULAR MIGRAINE

Subjective

Patients often report a visual aura lasting from minutes to 1 hour. Specific visual complaints include visual field defects, blurred vision, and flashing lights. It is important to differentiate ocular migraines from "true" migraines, which often have the same visual symptoms as a prodrome to the headache. Patients with migraines also may report nausea, vomiting, and photophobia.

Objective

The ocular examination will be normal. However, testing during an episode of an ocular migraine may reveal visual field loss or decreased vision that resolves when the episode subsides.

Plan

Treatment of patients with ocular migraines includes reassurance and education. Patients with true migraines should be referred to their primary care physicians for treatment.

CENTRAL RETINAL VEIN OCCLUSION

Subjective

Patients with a central retinal vein occlusion (CRVO) report a sudden, painless, unilateral vision loss. The systemic history typically includes hypertension, carotid artery disease, hyperlipidemia, or hyperviscosity syndrome, and the ocular history may include glaucoma.

Objective

Visual acuity is reduced by a variable amount depending on the extent of fundus changes. A positive afferent pupillary defect may be noted in some cases. The classic fundus appearance includes retinal hemorrhages and dilated, tortuous veins in all four quadrants. Cotton-wool spots, retinal edema, shunt vessels, and neovascularization may also be seen, depending on severity and duration.

Plan

Patients presenting with a CRVO should be referred for a complete systemic workup. Fluorescein angiography is indicated to determine the degree of retinal ischemia. If significant areas of retinal nonperfusion are detected, consultation with a retinologist is indicated to determine the possible benefit of panretinal photocoagulation. An electroretinogram may also be of some benefit in determining the degree of ischemia. All cases of CRVO should be closely monitored for the development of neovascular changes, specifically rubeosis iridis. Primary open-angle glaucoma should also be ruled out.

BRANCH RETINAL VEIN OCCLUSION

Subjective

Patients with a branch retinal vein occlusion (BRVO) may report a sudden, painless decrease in vision or may be asymptomatic. Careful history often reveals systemic hypertension or diabetes.

Objective

The classic fundus appearance of sectoral retinal hemorrhages may be accompanied by cotton-wool spots, retinal edema, and dilated retinal veins. Visual acuity may be dramatically reduced or unaffected.

Plan

Patients with a BRVO should be referred for a systemic evaluation. These patients should also be closely monitored for the development of retinal neovascularization. If neovascularization occurs, panretinal photocoagulation is the treatment of choice. Use of focal or grid laser therapy when macular edema is present is controversial.

CENTRAL RETINAL ARTERY OCCLUSION

Subjective

Patients with a central retinal artery occlusion (CRAO) present with a sudden, painless, total vision loss. Ocular history may include episodes of amaurosis fugax.

Objective

Visual acuity is reduced to finger counting or light perception. An afferent pupillary defect is present, and in early stages the fundus is characterized by a cherry red spot in the macula and whitening of the surrounding retina.

Plan

Digital massage and dramatic lowering of intraocular pressure with medications or paracentesis may be therapeutic if initiated within 24 hours of the onset of vision loss. Carbogen (95% O_2 and 5% CO_2) is advocated by some authorities. A systemic vascular workup and blood testing, including erythrocyte sedimentation rate (ESR), is indicated.

BRANCH RETINAL ARTERY OCCLUSION

Subjective

Patients with a branch retinal artery occlusion (BRAO) may present with sudden, painless, unilateral vision loss or may be asymptomatic. Ocular history may include episodes of amaurosis fugax.

Objective

A whitening of the retina adjacent to the occluded artery is observed. Retinal edema is also present. An embolus or narrowing of the artery is usually present proximal to the ischemic tissue. Cotton-wool spots may or may not be present.

Plan

Treatment is of questionable value, although digital massage may be attempted to dislodge the emboli. Carbogen is also recommended for BRAO by some authorities. More important, giant cell arteritis must be ruled out immediately, and a thorough systemic evaluation should be performed to eliminate the possibility of underlying systemic disorders.

INFLAMMATORY OPTIC NEUROPATHY

Subjective

Patients with inflammatory optic neuropathy present with sudden vision loss that may be unilateral or bilateral. The vision loss varies from moderate to severe and may be accompanied by orbital pain. These patients are typically under the age of 20. Pain on eye movements may also be reported by patients when the history is taken.

Objective

Color vision defects and an afferent pupillary defect are present. Optic disc edema with associated hemorrhages and a vitritis are apparent on dilation.

Plan

The etiology of the inflammatory optic neuropathy must be determined with a systemic evaluation. Possible causes include toxoplasmosis, herpes zoster, presumed ocular histoplasmosis syndrome, syphilis, and collagen vascular disorders, as well as many other systemic inflammatory conditions. Intravenous steroid therapy is advocated after consultation with a neurologist or neuro-ophthalmologist. Patients should be monitored at 1-month intervals.

DEMYELINATING OPTIC NEUROPATHY (RETROBULBAR OPTIC NEURITIS)

Subjective

Patients with demyelinating optic neuropathy report varying amounts of vision loss. The vision loss is often progressive over a 1-week period and tends to occur in patients from 20 to 45 years of age. Orbital pain and Uhthoff symptom (decreased vision when the body temperature rises) or Lhermitte's sign (electric-like shocks in the limbs or trunk when the head is flexed forward) may also be reported.

Objective

Visual acuity ranges from 20/20 to no light perception. Color vision defects, variable visual field defects, and a positive afferent pupillary defect are often present. Optic disc edema may sometimes be observed; however, the optic nerve is typically normal in appearance.

Plan

Patients suspected of having demyelinating optic neuropathy should be referred to a neurologist for magnetic resonance imaging (MRI) and a systemic workup.

COMPRESSIVE OPTIC NEUROPATHY

Subjective

Patients with compressive optic neuropathy report slowly progressive or acute vision loss.

Objective

Vision is reduced by a variable amount, and an afferent pupillary defect is observed. Patients may also have a central visual field defect. The optic nerve head may appear normal or may show varying degrees of pallor or edema.

Plan

A computed tomographic (CT) scan or MRI study is indicated for all patients with unexplainable loss of visual acuity, visual field defects, and an associated Marcus Gunn pupil. Patients suspected of compressive optic neuropathy should be referred to a neuro-ophthalmologist for diagnostic imaging and treatment.

NONARTERITIC ISCHEMIC OPTIC NEUROPATHY

Subjective

Patients with nonarteritic ischemic optic neuropathy (ION) present with sudden, painless, unilateral loss of vision. These patients are typically under the age of 50. Patients with ION often have systemic disorders such as hypertension, arteriosclerosis, or diabetes.

Objective

Vision loss varies from moderate to severe, and an afferent pupillary defect is usually present. Altitudinal visual field defect and color desaturation are also common findings in ION. Dilated fundus examination reveals optic disc edema with or without associated hemorrhages.

Plan

A systemic workup should be performed to determine underlying systemic etiology. These patients should be examined 1 month after the initial presentation.

ARTERITIC ISCHEMIC OPTIC NEUROPATHY

Subjective

Patients with arteritic ischemic optic neuropathy (AION) present with sudden, painless, unilateral loss of vision that may rapidly become bilateral. Patients are generally older than 50 years and may also report jaw claudication and scalp tenderness. Additional symptoms may include anorexia, weight loss, muscle and joint aches, and fever.

Objective

Visual acuity is often reduced to finger counting or worse with an associated afferent pupillary defect. The optic nerve is pale and swollen. ESR is markedly elevated.

Plan

Systemic steroid therapy should be initiated immediately. The patient should also be scheduled for a temporal artery biopsy if indicated to confirm the diagnosis.

MACULAR HOLE (IDIOPATHIC)

Subjective

Patients with macular holes present with sudden, painless, unilateral vision loss. Patients may complain of visual distortion. The typical patient is female and over the age of 60.

Objective

Visual acuity is usually in the 20/200 range for a full-thickness macular hole. Amsler grid findings reveal a large central scotoma surrounded by areas of metamorphopsia. A positive Watzke-Allen test is also noted with a full-thickness macular hole. Evaluation of the macula reveals a round, red, punched-out area approximately one-third to two-thirds of a disc diameter in size. Small yellow deposits are often seen at the base of the hole.

Plan

Patients with recent onset of idiopathic macular holes should be referred to a retinal specialist for consideration of macular hole repair.

RETINAL DETACHMENT (RHEGMATOGENOUS)

Subjective

Patients may report a significant decrease in vision or may be asymptomatic. The detachment is often described as a curtain or shadow moving over the field of vision. Flashes of light or floaters may also be reported.

Objective

Patients with a rhegmatogenous retinal detachment have varying degrees of vision loss depending on the extent of detachment. An afferent pupillary defect may also be present. The fundus evaluation reveals elevation of the retina, and a tear or flap is often visible. Scleral indentation may assist the clinician in appreciating the tear. A three-mirror lens may also be used to provide a more stable, magnified view. Cells in the anterior vitreous and a vitreous hemorrhage are also sometimes associated with a retinal detachment.

Plan

An immediate referral to a retinal surgeon is indicated in cases of acute rhegmatogenous retinal detachment.

VITREOUS HEMORRHAGE

Subjective

Patients with a vitreous hemorrhage report a sudden, painless, unilateral decrease in vision. They also may report spots or flashes of light, floaters, or erythropsia. It is important to determine if patients with vitreous hemorrhages are diabetic or have other systemic diseases.

Objective

Vision loss may be dramatically decreased or normal depending on the severity of the hemorrhage. Other findings such as an afferent pupillary defect are most often related to some underlying ocular disorder. Ophthal-moscopy may be of little benefit in cases of severe hemorrhage; however, in some cases it may allow the underlying cause to be determined. If no view of the retina is possible, B-scan ultrasonography is indicated to rule out a retinal detachment or intraocular tumor.

Plan

Consultation with a retinologist is indicated to determine the possible benefit of vitrectomy, particularly if the hemorrhage is long-standing.

SUGGESTED READING

Alexander LA. Primary Care of the Posterior Segment (2nd ed). Norwalk, CT: Appleton & Lange, 1994.

Bartlett JD, Jaanus SD. Clinical Ocular Pharmacology (3rd ed). Boston: Butterworth–Heinemann, 1995.

Fraunfelder FT, Roy FH. Current Ocular Therapy 4. Philadelphia: Saunders, 1995.

Kanski J. Clinical Ophthalmology (3rd ed). Oxford, UK: Butterworth–Heinemann, 1994.

Onofrey B. Clinical Optometric Pharmacology and Therapeutics. Philadelphia: Lippincott, 1994.

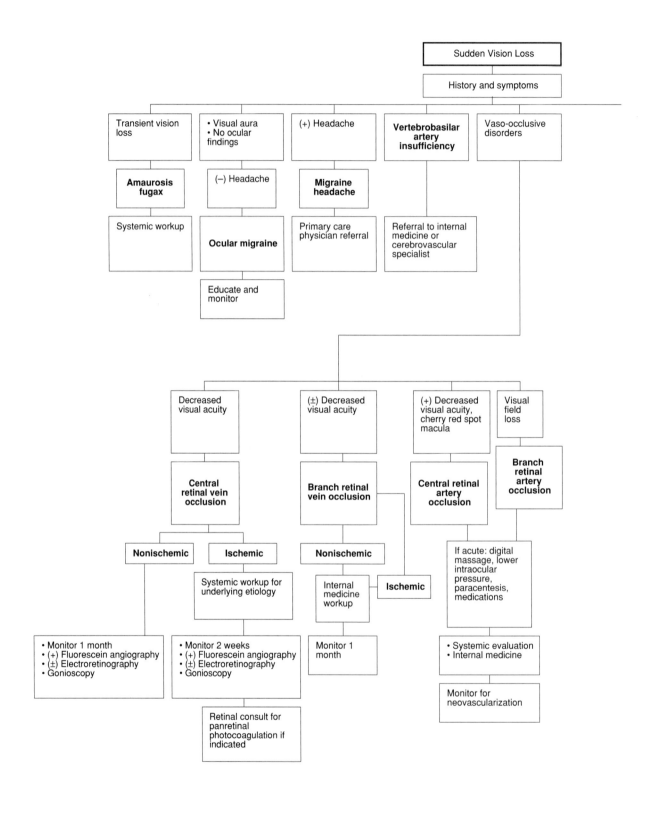

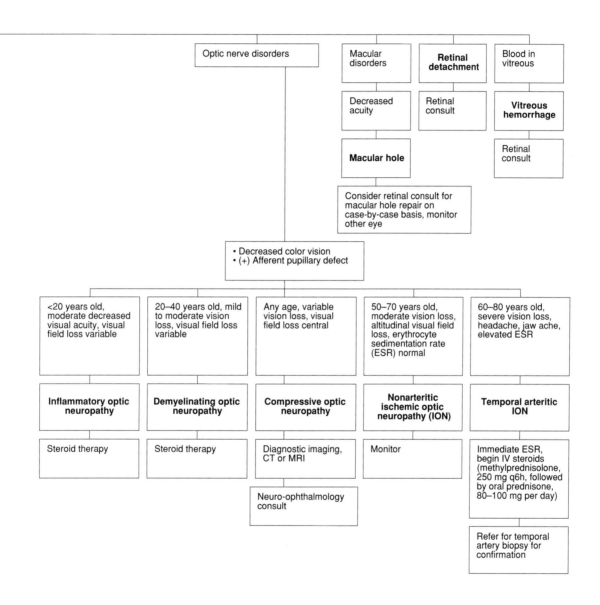

3

Visual Field Defects

FRANK P. LARUSSA

VISUAL FIELD DEFECTS AT A GLANCE

Monocular visual field defect with normal pupils
  Paracentral scotoma, arcuate scotoma, nasal step,
    enlarged blind spot
    Glaucoma
    Optic nerve head drusen
  Central defect
    Macular disease
Monocular field defect with an afferent pupillary defect
  Central defect
    Optic neuritis
    Optic atrophy
  Altitudinal defect
    Anterior ischemic optic neuropathy
Binocular visual field defect
  Homonymous hemianopsia, quadrantanopsia
    Cerebrovascular accident
    Tumor
    Aneurysm
    Trauma
  Bitemporal hemianopsia
    Chiasmal tumor
    Aneurysm
    Tilted discs
  Junctional scotoma
    Lesion at junction of optic nerve and chiasm
  Disjunctive scotomas
    Glaucoma
    Optic nerve head drusen
  Central scotomas
    Macular disease
  Enlarged blind spots
    Papilledema
    Glaucoma
    Optic nerve head drusen

Annular progressive midperipheral defects
    Retinitis pigmentosa
    Chorioretinal degenerations
Psychogenic field defects
    Malingering
    Hysteria

A patient with a visual field defect almost always has a significant ocular or systemic health problem. The practitioner must take a systematic approach to identify the underlying cause of the defect and select the appropriate treatment. The first step is to determine whether the condition is monocular or binocular. If it is monocular, pupillary testing will be useful. The flowchart at the end of the chapter and the accompanying text should help the practitioner to ascertain the cause of visual field loss.

MONOCULAR VISUAL FIELD DEFECT, USUALLY WITH NORMAL PUPILS

Paracentral Scotoma, Arcuate Scotoma, Nasal Step, Enlarged Blind Spot

Glaucoma
Subjective Although glaucoma is usually a bilateral disease, it is often asymmetric in its development and progression. Field loss may occur in one eye long before it becomes apparent in the other eye. Patients with early glaucoma are usually not symptomatic. They may complain of blurred vision or reduced visual fields in later stages of the disease.
Objective The patient with glaucoma usually has elevated intraocular pressures. The most common field defects are paracentral scotomas, arcuate scotomas, nasal step defects,

and enlarged blind spots. The optic nerve shows related cup changes. Severe monocular glaucoma or asymmetric bilateral glaucoma may restult in an afferent pupillary defect.

Plan Topical glaucoma agents (beta blockers, alpha-agonists, latanaprost, dipivefrin, dorzolamide, and pilocarpine) are the first line of defense against glaucoma. Oral carbonic anhydrase inhibitors, argon laser trabeculoplasty, trabeculectomy, and other surgical treatments may be used in nonresponsive cases.

Optic Nerve Head Drusen

Subjective Although most cases of optic nerve head drusen are bilateral, this condition is unilateral in approximately 30% of cases. Most patients with optic nerve drusen are asymptomatic, although a few may report noticeable field defects.

Objective Disc drusen cause an elevated optic nerve head or pseudopapilledema. Yellow, partially buried drusen may be visible. Occasionally drusen cause a flame hemorrhage at the disc margin. Field losses caused by disc drusen are quite variable and include enlarged blind spot and arcuate, sector, altitudinal, or nasal step defects. B-scan ultrasonography and autofluorescence studies are useful tests in the differential diagnosis of optic nerve head drusen.

Plan There is no specific treatment for optic nerve head drusen. Patients should be monitored annually to determine whether the field loss is progressing.

Monocular Central Field Defect

Macular Disease

Subjective A monocular central field loss can be caused by a number of macular conditions, including macular degeneration, macular hole, and toxoplasmosis. Patients with macular disease complain of decreased vision and distorted vision.

Objective Visual acuity is decreased when measured with standard testing techniques. Amsler grid or central automated visual field testing usually demonstrates a central defect. Ophthalmoscopy typically reveals pigmentary or other tissue changes in the macula, contingent on the specific condition. Color vision may be affected depending on the degree of retinal involvement.

Plan If the patient has dry macular degeneration, generally no treatment is indicated. Antioxidant vitamin therapy is currently controversial, but it is often recommended. The patient should be monitored carefully and educated about the symptoms of wet macular degeneration. If wet degeneration occurs, the patient should be referred to a retinologist as quickly as possible.

Patients with a macular hole, particularly if it is of recent onset, should be referred to a retinologist for possible treatment.

Inactive toxoplasmosis can be followed carefully. If the toxoplasmosis becomes active, the patient should be referred to a retinologist for treatment. In any case in which the primary care clinician is uncertain about the etiology of central vision loss, referral to a retinologist is indicated.

MONOCULAR FIELD DEFECT WITH AN AFFERENT PUPILLARY DEFECT

Central Field Defect

Optic Neuritis

Subjective The patient with optic neuritis usually complains of rapid reduction in vision in the involved eye. The patient may complain of pain on eye movements and may note a reduction in vision during exercise or after taking a hot bath (Uhthoff symptom). When the medical history is taken, the patient should be questioned about past systemic viral infections, inflammatory diseases, and multiple sclerosis.

Objective Optic neuritis is characterized by an afferent pupillary defect, decreased color vision, and a reduced perception of light intensity in the involved eye. Visual field testing usually reveals a central or cecocentral scotoma. The fundus examination may reveal a unilateral swollen disc with associated flame hemorrhages; however, it should be noted that, in retrobulbar cases, the disc often has a normal appearance. Later the disc may show pallor. Laboratory and radiologic testing—including erythrocyte sedimentation rate (ESR), complete blood count, fluorescent treponemal antibody absorption test, or magnetic resonance imaging (MRI)—may be used when an underlying systemic cause is suspected.

Plan Use of oral steroids is controversial and is no longer recommended as a primary treatment in optic neuritis cases. Observation is often recommended in cases when visual acuity is only mildly affected (acuity of 20/40 or better), and vision usually returns partially or fully with time. In more severe cases, intravenous steroids followed by oral steroids are often prescribed.

Optic Atrophy

Subjective Most cases of acquired optic atrophy occur in older patients. Optic atrophy also occurs in some congenital, inherited conditions such as Leber's and Behr's optic atrophy. Patients with acquired optic atrophy are usually aware of a nonprogressive field loss in one eye. It is often secondary to other ocular conditions such as ischemic optic neuropathy or central retinal artery occlusion. It also may be induced by certain drugs or by radiation.

Objective There is an afferent pupillary defect in the involved eye. Visual acuity is markedly reduced. The visual field reveals a central, cecocentral, or generalized defect. The optic nerve is pale.

Plan If the condition is long-standing, no treatment is indicated. If it is of recent onset, an MRI or computed tomographic (CT) scan should be performed to rule out a mass lesion.

Altitudinal Defect

Anterior Ischemic Optic Neuropathy
Subjective Patients with this condition are usually 40–60 years of age. They generally complain of a rapid, painless reduction of vision or visual field in one eye.

Objective Reduced acuity and a relative afferent pupillary defect are noted in the involved eye. The patient has a visual field defect in the affected eye only. The most common field defect is altitudinal. The patient may have reduced color perception in the involved eye. The optic nerve is swollen if the condition is acute and pale if it is long-standing.

Plan The patient should have an ESR test immediately to rule out giant cell arteritis. If the ESR is elevated, oral steroid therapy should be initiated. A temporal artery biopsy may be needed in equivocal cases. If ESR or temporal artery biopsy is normal and the vision loss is not progressive, the condition is assumed to be nonarteritic ischemic optic neuropathy, and no further treatment is indicated except to refer the patient to an internal medicine specialist for evaluation for underlying systemic disease.

BINOCULAR VISUAL FIELD DEFECT

Homonymous Hemianopsia, Homonymous Quadrantanopsia

Subjective
Patients with homonymous field loss may complain of poor side vision or may present with a history of bumping into objects on one side. They may complain of central vision difficulties if there is a macular splitting defect. Patients with homonymous field loss often have a history of a cerebral vascular accident or head trauma. Tumors and aneurysms are other causes for this type of field loss.

Objectives
Perimetry reveals similar visual field loss affecting the same hemispheres in each eye (left or right homonymous hemianopsia or quadrantanopsia).

Plan
Inferior homonymous quadrantanopsia ("pie on the floor") usually indicates a parietal lobe lesion. Superior homonymous quadrantanopsia ("pie in the sky") usually indicates a temporal lobe lesion. Complete homonymous hemianopsia usually indicates an occipital lobe or optic tract lesion. Generally speaking, the more congruent or symmetric the fields between the two eyes, the more posterior the lesion along the visual pathway. The more anterior the lesion in the visual pathway, the more likely it is secondary to a tumor. Other possible causes include aneurysm and trauma. The more posterior the lesion along the visual pathway, the more likely it is secondary to a vascular cause. Also, the older the patient, the more likely that the lesion is vascular in origin. Any patient who presents with a previously undetected homonymous visual field defect should undergo diagnostic imaging (CT or MRI) and should be referred to a neurologist for further evaluation.

Bitemporal Hemianopsia

Subjective
Patients with bitemporal hemianopsia are often asymptomatic. They may have vague complaints, peripheral vision loss, or other visual problems. Women with this condition may have associated changes in their menstrual cycles.

Objective
Perimetry reveals bitemporal visual field defects. Visual acuity may or may not be affected.

Plan
The primary cause of bitemporal visual field defects is chiasmal lesions. These lesions are due primarily to a pituitary adenoma, craniopharyngioma, or meningioma. An aneurysm may also cause a bitemporal field defect. The only benign cause of a bitemporal field defect is tilted discs. Diagnostic MRI should be performed for any patient with a bitemporal field defect, and the patient should be referred to a neurologist as soon as possible.

Junctional Scotoma

Subjective
Junctional scotomas are caused by lesions at the junction of the optic nerve and the chiasm. Patients with this condition usually complain of central vision loss in one eye. They may or may not note a superior temporal field defect in the opposite eye.

Objective
Perimetry reveals a central scotoma in one eye and a superior temporal field loss in the other eye.

Plan
The patient should be referred for diagnostic imaging and a neurologic evaluation.

Disjunctive Scotomas

Subjective
Disjunctive scotomas are bilateral scotomas that do not show the same pattern in each eye. Patients with these defects usually have no complaints unless the defects are quite extensive. The two primary causes of disjunctive scotomas are glaucoma and optic nerve head drusen.

Objective
Glaucoma patients usually have elevated intraocular pressures and notched, elongated, or enlarged optic nerve head cups. Patients with optic nerve head drusen display elevated discs that may have the appearance of rock candy. Paracentral, arcuate, and nasal step scotomas may be found in patients with both glaucoma and optic nerve head drusen.

Plan
Glaucoma patients should be treated initially with topical glaucoma medications such as beta blockers, dipivefrin, carbonic anhydrase inhibitors, prostaglandins, alpha-agonists, and pilocarpine. Oral carbonic anhydrase inhibitors, laser trabeculoplasty, and surgical trabeculectomy are reserved for cases that cannot be controlled with topical medications. There is currently no treatment for optic nerve head drusen.

Central Scotomas

Subjective
Bilateral central scotomas are usually caused by macular disease. Patients generally complain of reduced visual acuity or a blind spot right before their eyes. They often complain of not being able to read or recognize faces. Macular degeneration and macular holes are the most common causes. Additionally, a number of hereditary maculopathies can cause central vision loss, including Stargardt's disease, dominant drusen, and patterned dystrophies.

Objective
Patients with macular degeneration have RPE disruption/drusen in the macular region. An elevated grey/green region in the macular region is indicative of wet macular degeneration. Macular holes appear as a well-circumscribed red area in the macular region.

Plan
If the patient has dry macular degeneration, generally no treatment is indicated. Antioxidant vitamin therapy is controversial but often recommended. The patient should be monitored carefully and educated about the symptoms of wet macular degeneration. If wet degeneration occurs, the patient should be referred to a retinologist as quickly as possible. Patients with a macular hole, particularly if it is of recent onset, should be referred to a retinologist for possible treatment. Many patients with central field loss can be helped by the prescription of both optical and nonoptical low vision aids.

Enlarged Blind Spots

Subjective
The three most common causes of enlarged bilateral blind spots are papilledema (including that due to pseudotumor cerebri), glaucoma, and optic nerve drusen. These patients are often visually asymptomatic. Patients with papilledema may complain of transient episodes of vision loss or diplopia, headache, nausea, and vomiting.

Objective
Perimetry reveals bilateral enlarged blind spots. In the case of glaucoma or disc drusen, other field defects also may be present. Patients with papilledema have swollen optic nerve heads. They often have hemorrhages around the optic nerve and no spontaneous venous pulsation. Patients with glaucoma usually have elevated intraocular pressure and notched, elongated, or enlarged optic cups. Flame hemorrhages adjacent to the nerve head also may be present. Patients with optic nerve head drusen show elevated discs, often with partially buried drusen visible. Flame hemorrhages adjacent to the nerve head are occasionally noted. B-scan ultrasonography and autofluorescent techniques are helpful in the differential diagnosis of disc drusen.

Plan
Patients with papilledema should be referred for radiologic studies to rule out an intracranial mass. Glaucoma patients should be treated initially with one or more topical glaucoma medications. Oral glaucoma medications, laser trabeculoplasty, and surgical trabeculectomy are reserved for cases that cannot be controlled with topical medications. There is no treatment for optic nerve head drusen. The patient with this condition should have perimetry performed annually to determine whether the field loss is progressing.

Annular Progressive Midperipheral Field Defects

Subjective
The most common cause of annular progressive visual field defects is retinitis pigmentosa. Other chorioretinal

degenerations may also cause these types of defects. The patient with retinitis pigmentosa usually complains of reduced night vision and peripheral vision loss, and may have a family history of blindness.

Objective

In most cases of retinitis pigmentosa, the midperiphery of the retina displays pigment clumping. The field loss generally corresponds with the region of pigmentary change. Other signs include vessel attenuation and optic nerve head pallor. Posterior subcapsular cataracts are another common finding. An electroretinogram may be performed to confirm the diagnosis.

Plan

No established cure exists for retinitis pigmentosa; however, there is some evidence that vitamin A palmitate can slow the progression of the disease. Tinted spectacles and low vision devices can help patients use their existing vision.

PSYCHOGENIC VISUAL FIELD LOSS

Subjective

Psychogenic field loss is usually associated with malingering or hysteria. The patient may present with a variety of other visual or somatic complaints. The malingering patient usually hopes to achieve some personal gain, financial or otherwise, from proving disability. The hysterical patient, on the other hand, has an unconscious loss of function due to one or more stressful life events.

Objective

Psychogenic field defects include tunnel fields or concentrically contracting fields that do not change in size with a change in testing distance using the tangent screen. Spiraling isopters, crossing isopters, or monocular temporal hemianopsia also may occur. Other ocular findings are normal in psychogenic cases.

Plan

The management of hysterical psychogenic loss consists of providing reassurance and referring the patient for psychological counseling.

SUGGESTED READING

Alexander LA. Primary Care of the Posterior Segment (2nd ed). Norwalk, CT: Appleton & Lange, 1994.

Bajandas FJ, Kline LB. Neuro-Ophthalmology Review Manual (3rd ed). Thorofare, NJ: Slack, 1988.

Bartlett JD, Jaanus SD. Clinical Ocular Pharmacology (3rd ed). Boston: Butterworth–Heinemann, 1995.

Pau H. Differential Diagnoses of Eye Diseases. Philadelphia: Saunders, 1978.

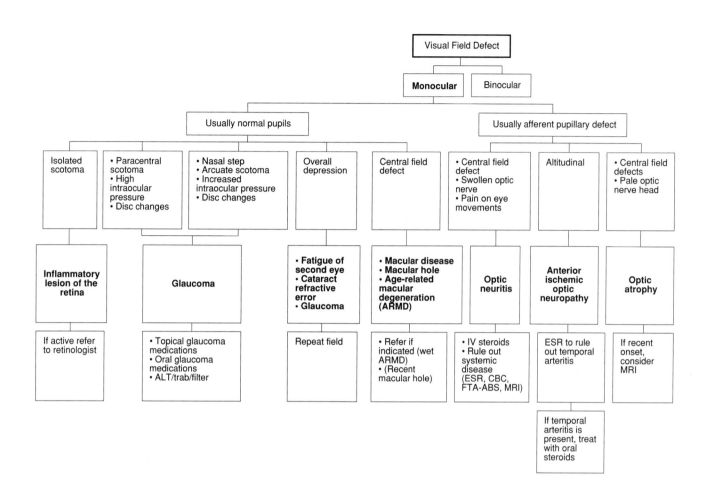

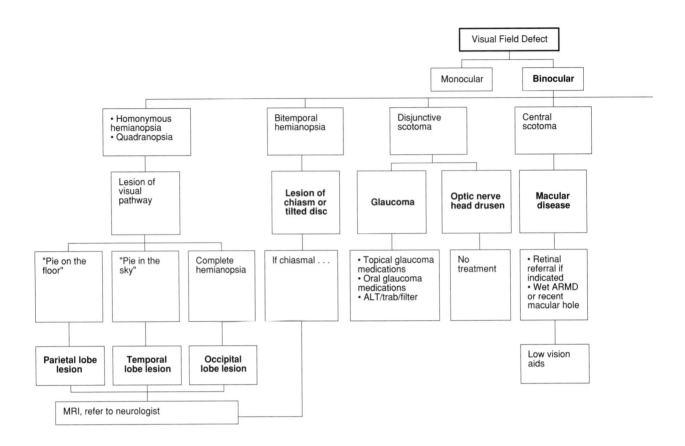

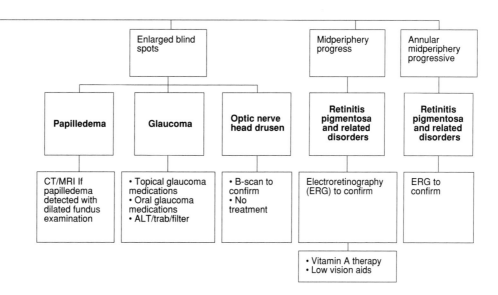

4

Nonphysiologic Vision Loss

CARL H. SPEAR AND TAMMY P. THAN

NONPHYSIOLOGIC VISION LOSS AT A GLANCE

Ocular hysteria
Malingering
Physiologic vision loss that may mimic nonphysiologic loss
    Retrobulbar optic neuritis
    Amblyopia
    Cortical blindness
    Toxic optic neuropathy

Essentially, only two causes of nonphysiologic vision loss exist: (1) ocular hysteria (conversion reaction) and (2) malingering. A complete examination reveals normal findings. Case history and careful observation of the patient are useful in arriving at either of the above diagnoses. Several physiologic conditions with which patients may present are also characterized by normal funduscopic findings and can mimic nonphysiologic vision loss.

OCULAR HYSTERIA (CONVERSION REACTION)

Subjective

The patient presents with variable nonspecific nonocular findings, a recent traumatic experience, and bilateral decreased vision. The patient is typically a young female who may have additional vague visual complaints or may have no other symptoms. Subjective responses from patients with ocular hysteria are often slow.

Objective

Objective findings will include decreased vision (distance vision is usually more reduced than near vision) and tubu-lar visual fields (determined by tangent screen testing). Thorough examination reveals a normal fundus, and all other ocular findings are also normal. Objective refractive error determination is inconsistent with visual acuity, and responses on subjective refraction vary widely.

Plan

The patient or parent needs to be reassured that the underlying cause of decreased vision is not pathologic. Inquiries should be made about potentially emotional experiences or recent traumatic events. The patient should be re-evaluated in 1 month. If no improvement has occurred, the practitioner should consider referral for counseling as indicated.

MALINGERING

Subjective

Patients may report vision loss that is either unilateral or bilateral. A careful history may reveal an underlying potential for financial gain or other benefit secondary to the recent onset of vision loss.

Objective

The decrease in visual acuity may be unilateral or bilateral, visual field loss varies, and other tests seem erratic and unreliable. The hallmark of malingering is a completely normal ocular health examination without any finding to account for the decrease in acuity. If at this point malingering is suspected, a variety of tests may be used to trick the patient into seeing better. The following tests may be used in an attempt to entrap the malingering patient and elicit a normal response:

- Mirror test
- Optokinetic test
- Fog test
- Menace reflex
- Intense light reflex
- 4Δ base-out prism test
- Schmidt-Rimpler test

If a definitive diagnosis of malingering cannot be made, diagnostic imaging should be considered to rule out a space-occupying lesion.

Plan

No treatment is indicated, but the patient often needs an opportunity to see better without confrontation. This objective can frequently be accomplished through dilation or other simple tests.

PHYSIOLOGIC VISION LOSS THAT MAY MIMIC NONPHYSIOLOGIC LOSS

Retrobulbar Optic Neuritis (Demyelinating Optic Neuropathy)

Subjective

Patients present with a unilateral vision loss that has progressed over the course of 1 week. The patient is typically between 20 and 40 years of age. Patients with retrobulbar optic neuritis also may report ocular tenderness and pain associated with eye movements.

Objective

Objective findings include decreased visual acuity, a positive afferent pupillary defect, color vision desaturation, and pain during extraocular muscle motilities. Various visual field defects can be present, but a central defect is the most common. The optic nerve usually appears normal. Associated cerebellar imbalance signs may be present.

Plan

Neuro-ophthalmologic consultation for magnetic resonance imaging (MRI) and institution of therapy is indicated in patients with retrobulbar optic neuritis. Use of corticosteroid therapy for these patients is controversial; the current belief is that intravenous steroid therapy followed by an oral steroid taper is the best treatment. However, some feel that no treatment is the best management for these patients.

Anisometropic or Strabismic Amblyopia

Subjective

Patients presenting with unilateral amblyopia have decreased vision in one eye that is greater than two lines of Snellen acuity compared with the other eye. History may include patching therapy or muscle surgery. Patients may also report that they have been told they have a "lazy eye."

Objective

Patients with anisometropic or strabismic amblyopia present with reduced visual acuity, but it is usually not below 20/200. Other findings include reduced stereopsis, possible anisometropia as determined with a cycloplegic refraction, possible strabismus, and a decreased amplitude and facility of accommodation. Visual acuity improves when a single letter is isolated for testing; the use of neutral density filters does not significantly reduce visual acuity. A complete baseline examination should be performed to rule out an organic cause for the vision loss because the anisometropia or strabismus may be due to an undetected ocular pathology.

Plan

If the amblyopia is due to anisometropia, treatment includes prescribing the full refractive error correction for both eyes and instituting patching therapy, which may be combined with additional vision therapy. If the amblyopia is strabismic in nature, the full refractive error correction should be prescribed along with patching and vision therapy. Surgical correction should be considered if the deviation is greater than 20Δ of esotropia or greater than 30Δ of exotropia.

Cortical Blindness

Subjective

Patients present with bilateral total vision loss. However, patients with cortical blindness may not think that they are blind (Anton's syndrome).

Objective

No light perception is present in either eye; however, it is possible to elicit a normal pupillary response in both eyes.

Plan

Referral to an internal medicine specialist for MRI is indicated. The most likely cause is bilateral occipital lobe infarct, but occasionally cortical blindness may be secondary to a neoplasm.

Toxic Optic Neuropathy

Subjective

Patients with toxic optic neuropathy present with bilateral painless, progressive vision loss. The patient may have a history of drug or alcohol abuse, or has taken medication known to be toxic.

Objective

The patient may appear to have signs of alcoholism or poor nutrition. Visual acuity is decreased but generally better than 20/200, and color vision is reduced. Visual field defects are present and typically central or cecocentral. The optic nerve may be normal or show varying degrees of atrophy and pallor.

Plan

Patients with toxic optic neuropathy should have complete laboratory testing, and the underlying cause should be treated. Once identified, the causative agent (i.e., alcohol or medication) should be eliminated. Because most of these patients are malnourished, vitamin therapy should be instituted.

SUGGESTED READING

Alexander LA. Primary Care of the Posterior Segment (2nd ed). Norwalk, CT: Appleton & Lange, 1994.

Amos JF. Diagnosis and Management in Vision Care. Stoneham, MA: Butterworth, 1987.

Fraunfelder FT, Roy FH. Current Ocular Therapy 4. Philadelphia: Saunders, 1995.

Kanski J. Clinical Ophthalmology (3rd ed). Oxford: Butterworth–Heinemann, 1994.

Rutstein RP. Problems in Optometry. Amblyopia. Philadelphia: Lippincott, June 1991;3.

Walsh TJ. Neuro-Ophthalmology: Clinical Signs and Symptoms (3rd ed). Philadelphia: Lea & Febiger, 1992.

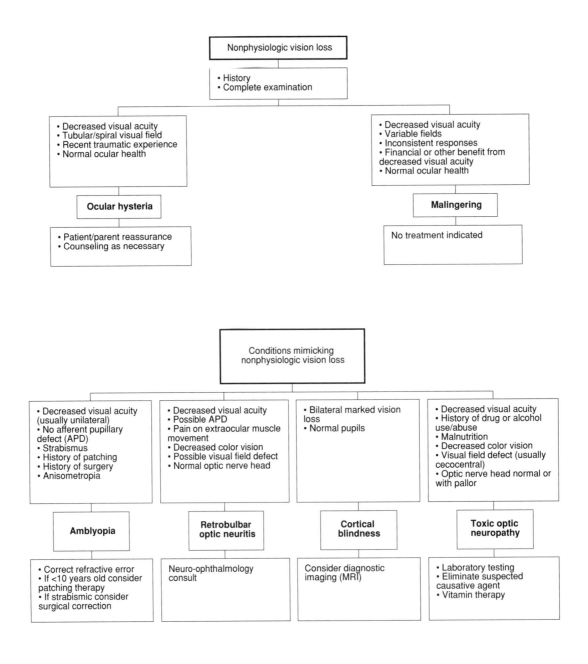

5

Color Vision Anomalies

David P. Sendrowski

COLOR VISION ANOMALIES AT A GLANCE

Inherited
  Down syndrome
  Guillain-Barré syndrome
  Dichromatopsia
  Monochromasy
  Trichromatopsia
  Albinism
  Retinitis pigmentosa
  Juvenile optic atrophy
Acquired
  Retinal dysfunction from drugs (blue/yellow)
  Optic nerve dysfunction from drugs (red/green)
  Anterior ischemic optic neuropathy
  Papillitis
  Diabetic retinitis
  Chorioretinitis
  Glaucoma
  Macular degeneration
  Optic atrophy
  Retinal detachment
  Central retinal arterial occlusion

Color vision testing can be a diagnostic tool in evaluating a patient with a disease process of the visual system. As with any diagnostic tool, it is up to the clinician to decide which test is most appropriate for each patient. The results of the testing should be considered in the context of the entire diagnostic profile.

In the use of color vision testing, the clinician should keep in mind that hereditary color defects are symmetric, and acquired deficiencies typically are different in the two eyes. It is important that color vision testing always be performed monocularly.

UNILATERAL OPTIC ATROPHY

Subjective

Acquired optic nerve disease is usually heralded by acute or subacute loss of visual acuity or visual field. Pain is not a complaint except with inflammatory diseases such as papillitis.

Patients with acquired optic atrophy normally complain of a change in color perception, a change in light perception, or vision loss. Each of these complaints varies depending on the degree of nerve involvement.

The medical history should be thoroughly evaluated for hypertension, diabetes, acquired immunodeficiency syndrome, headaches, trauma, and congenital diseases that may affect the optic nerve. The clinician should always look for a systemic cause for acquired optic atrophy.

Objective

Visual acuity varies depending on the degree of nerve head involvement. The pupil examination may demonstrate a decreased response to direct light stimulation and a positive afferent pupillary defect. If present, this finding strongly suggests a unilateral optic atrophy. Amsler grid testing may reveal scotomatous loss without metamorphopsia. A color vision test should be performed to look for unilateral loss of saturation. Such loss is particularly evident with a red stimulus. The intraocular pressure should be measured to rule out glaucoma. The examination should concentrate on the visual field and optic nerve head appearance. A dilated fundus examination should be performed with high plus lenses to evaluate the optic nerve head. The nerve head usually shows some degree of pallor and corresponding retinal nerve fiber layer loss.

The disc margins are clear and distinct. The macula should be evaluated to rule out leakage. Threshold visual field testing is very diagnostic in determining the areas of optic nerve or visual pathway involvement.

Additional testing may include electrodiagnostic evaluation such as measurement of visual evoked potentials (VEPs). VEP testing shows diminished wave amplitudes. Blood pressure evaluation can help to rule out undiagnosed hypertension.

Plan

If the optometric examination fails to reveal a cause for the unilateral optic atrophy, such as glaucoma or old injury, the patient should be referred to an internist for further testing. If a neoplastic lesion is suspected to be the cause, then a magnetic resonance imaging (MRI) scan or computed axial tomographic (CAT) scan should be performed.

NUCLEAR SCLEROTIC CATARACTS

Subjective

Patients with nuclear sclerotic cataracts (NSCs) are usually older and complain of a gradual loss of visual acuity. The loss of acuity is generally greater for distance vision than for near vision. The patient may complain of losing an appreciation for color, especially blue and yellow. Glare may be a distinctive problem when the patient drives at night. Occasionally, the patient may note noncolored halos around lights due to nuclear sclerotic cataracts.

Objective

The refractive error usually shows a myopic shift. Visual acuities may be diminished, but ocular motilities and pupil responses are normal. A biomicroscopic examination of the dilated eye shows the nucleus of the lens to be yellowed and differentiated from the rest of the lens. Use of a cobalt filter may show blue light to be absorbed and transmitted through the lens to a lesser degree than normal. Visual field testing may show a generalized depression. The optic nerve head and macula appear normal.

Additional testing can include use of a potential acuity meter or interferometer to evaluate the macular potential. Ultrasonography can be used for retinal disease assessment or presurgical determination of the intraocular lens power.

Plan

Refractive correction may be all that is required in the early stages of cataract development. If changes in spectacle correction do not satisfactorily increase visual acuity, referral to an ophthalmic surgeon should be considered. Patients should be educated about the need for prescription spectacles to include UV protection after cataract surgery, especially if they are in the sunlight for extended periods.

Before surgery, examinations should be performed annually or more frequently, depending on the severity of the cataract formation.

AGE-RELATED MACULAR DEGENERATION

Subjective

Older patients with age-related macular degeneration (ARMD) present with a gradual loss of central vision. Patients may complain of difficulty in seeing signs, faces, and printed material. Patients usually complain that they are unable to appreciate colors as well as they used to. Many patients with ARMD are white and have light skin pigmentation. A family history of the disorder may be present. The clinician should also inquire about the patient's history of tobacco smoking.

Objective

External and entrance examination are usually normal. Amsler grid and photostress testing are helpful in diagnosing macular changes. Fluorescein angiography can be performed to determine whether leakage is present in the macular area. Because ARMD occurs in the older population, some lens changes may also be associated. These lens changes do not correlate with the amount of visual acuity loss. Potential acuity meter readings may be very helpful in assessing macular potential through a media opacity.

Examination with high plus lenses through a dilated pupil is extremely helpful in evaluating the macula for changes in pigmentation and development of drusen. Depigmented areas of atrophy may progressively appear throughout the macula as well.

Plan

The patient should be given an Amsler grid to be used regularly at home to monitor for the development of subretinal neovascular nets. The patient should be re-examined every 6 months. Although no proven cures for ARMD currently exist, a number of therapies have been proposed, including the use of UV-protective sunglasses while outside and the use of vitamin tablets (e.g., Ocuvite) or consumption of green leafy vegetables (e.g., spinach). If the patient is a smoker, cessation or reduction of smoking may be an excellent behavioral modification.

If the fluorescein angiogram shows leakage from a subretinal neovascular net, the patient should be referred immediately to a retinologist to determine whether the patient is a candidate for argon laser photocoagulation to repair the retinal leakage.

PAPILLITIS

Subjective

Papillitis commonly occurs in patients between the ages of 18 and 45 years and is unilateral. The patient with papillitis may complain of a loss of vision developing over several hours or days. The vision loss can range from very slight to profound. The patient may complain of orbital pain, especially on eye movement. There may also be a noticeable loss of color vision and light intensity in the affected eye.

The clinician should ask about visual deficit with increase in body temperature or after exercise (Uhthoff symptom). The patient should be questioned regarding other neurologic symptoms, upper respiratory infections, and urinary tract or gastrointestinal problems as well.

Objective

The entrance tests should include pupillary testing to evaluate for a relative afferent pupillary defect and color testing to reveal a loss in color perception. An Amsler grid or threshold visual field testing may reveal a central or paracentral scotoma. Other types of visual field defects are possible as well. Visual acuity varies.

The dilated examination should include evaluation of the macula, which should be normal. Central serous choroidopathy occurs in roughly the same age group. High plus lenses are helpful in revealing a swollen disc with or without peripapillary flame hemorrhages. A diagnostic finding is the presence of white blood cells in front of the nerve head. It may take several attempts to visualize them. It should be noted that, in retrobulbar optic neuritis, the ophthalmoscopic appearance of the disc is essentially normal.

Additional testing to confirm the diagnosis or rule out other conditions may include blood pressure assessment, blood tests (e.g., complete blood count [CBC], rapid plasma reagin, fluorescent treponemal antibody absorption), chest radiography, lumbar puncture, and MRI or CAT scan of the orbits and brain.

Plan

The treatment is somewhat controversial. The initial use of orally administered low-dose steroids should be avoided, because they may precipitate more frequent attacks of papillitis. Intravenous administration of methylprednisolone has been shown to reduce the symptoms and delay the next attack, but not to affect the final visual outcome for the patient.

The patient should be followed up every 3–5 days to evaluate the recovery of visual function. An MRI scan to detect periventricular white lesions (plaques) and lumbar puncture can be helpful in determining whether multiple sclerosis is the cause of the optic neuritis. Referral to a neurologist for further evaluation and management is indicated.

ARTERITIC ANTERIOR ISCHEMIC OPTIC NEUROPATHY

Subjective

The patient with arteritic anterior ischemic optic neuropathy (AION) is usually 65 years or older. The complaints include a sudden, painless, initially unilateral vision loss. Headache, jaw claudication, scalp tenderness, joint ache, weight loss, fever, and depression may occur before or coincident with the vision loss.

Medical history should include questioning about present illnesses such as arthritis, polyarteritis, scleroderma, and other rheumatoid disorders.

Objective

The entrance testing should evaluate pupillary response and look for a relative afferent pupillary defect, loss of color vision, palpable tender and nonpulsable artery, and ocular motility. A quick confrontation field screening may reveal an altitudinal loss, which is an important diagnostic finding in arteritic AION.

The dilated examination may reveal a pale, swollen disc, sometimes with flame hemorrhages. The macula appears normal. There is no evidence of white blood cells in front of the optic nerve head.

Additional testing should include blood pressure assessment, an immediate CBC, and Westergren method erythrocyte sedimentation rate (ESR). Temporal artery biopsy should be performed if the ESR is equivocal or to confirm the diagnosis.

Plan

Arteritic AION is a true ocular emergency. Systemic steroids (e.g., prednisone) should be given immediately once the diagnosis of arteritic AION is strongly suspected. Administration of steroids should begin before obtaining biopsy results. The initial steroid dose should be maintained for 2–4 weeks until symptoms reverse and the Westergren rates normalize. Treatment dosage should be adjusted up or down according to the Westergren rates. The treatment may last from 3 months to 1 year. The patient should be followed up every 2–4 weeks during treatment, and intraocular pressure and lenticular clarity should be assessed.

NONARTERITIC ANTERIOR ISCHEMIC OPTIC NEUROPATHY

Subjective

The ocular symptoms for nonarteritic AION may be the same as for arteritic AION except that the patient is usually younger, between the ages of 40 and 60. In most cases, the vision loss is less dramatic in the nonarteritic form. The clinician should look for hypertension and diabetes as the underlying cause, but many cases are idiopathic.

Objective

The changes seen in nonarteritic AION are very similar to those seen in arteritic AION. Part or all of the optic disc may be involved. Optic atrophy develops approximately 3 months after the acute phase of the disease.

Plan

The patient should be treated as for arteritic AION until the laboratory testing shows no elevation in Westergren ESR. At the same time, the patient should be evaluated for cardiovascular disease, diabetes, and hypertension. If no evidence of any of these disorders is found, the patient is considered to have an idiopathic type of nonarteritic AION.

The patient should be educated concerning the potential for a similar event to occur in the other eye. The patient

should be followed up every month to evaluate any progression of the visual field changes and assess resolution of the disc edema. Currently, no proven treatment for nonarteritic AION exists.

INHERITED COLOR VISION DEFECT

Subjective

It is very unusual for patients to have complaints about an inherited loss of color vision. Protanomalies and deuteranomalies are red-green deficiencies and are found in approximately 8% of all males. These deficiencies are much less common in females. Commonly, the deficiencies are discovered during a routine vision examination, in the classroom, or when the individual has applied for a job for which a color vision test is required.

Objective

Color vision testing should be performed to confirm the type of color vision deficiency. The results of all other tests should be normal or unrelated to the color defect. Special attention should be given to pupils, lens, macula, and optic nerve head to make sure that all are normal.

Plan

No treatment for inherited color deficiencies exists. The patient should be made aware of the defect and the potential visual problems that may be encountered with certain tasks or careers. The patient should be examined routinely.

DRUG-INDUCED OPTIC ATROPHY/RETINAL DISEASE

Subjective

The patient usually complains of a bilateral loss of vision that is painless and progressive. The history should assess possible tobacco or alcohol abuse. This condition can also be caused by vitamin B_1 deficiency and pernicious anemia. Certain drugs and other agents can cause toxic neuropathy as well; these include chloramphenicol, ethambutol, isoniazid, digitalis, chloroquine, streptomycin, amphetamines, aspirin, acetaminophen, ibuprofen, erythromycin, nalidixic acid, sulfonamides, tetracycline, phenytoin, quinine, phenothiazines, diuretics, quinidines, vitamin A, chlorpropamide, disulfiram, and lead. The use of medications and recreational drugs should be thoroughly investigated.

Objective

The entrance tests should include pupil testing, color vision evaluation, and motility testing. Pupil testing may not reveal an afferent pupillary defect, but the direct response should be diminished. Threshold visual field testing should be performed with specific concern for the papillomacular bundle. Visual field loss can include cecocentral and central visual field loss. A dilated examination should be performed with high-plus-lens examination of the optic nerve head and macular region.

Additional tests that may be of benefit include a CBC, serum B_{12} level, and heavy-metal screen.

Plan

Whenever possible, the offending agent or drug should be eliminated. The patient should be referred to an internist for a workup. Once the agent is found and eliminated, the patient should be re-examined every month until the field defects stabilize or resolve. The patient can then be followed up every 6–12 months.

SUGGESTED READING

Fraunfelder FT. Drug Induced Ocular Side Effects and Drug Interactions. Philadelphia: Lea & Febiger, 1989.

Glaser JS (ed). Neuro-Ophthalmology, Vol 2 (2nd ed). Philadelphia: Lippincott, 1990;1–23.

Pease PL, Allen J. A new test for screening color vision: concurrent validity and utility. Am J Optom Physiol 1988;65: 729–738.

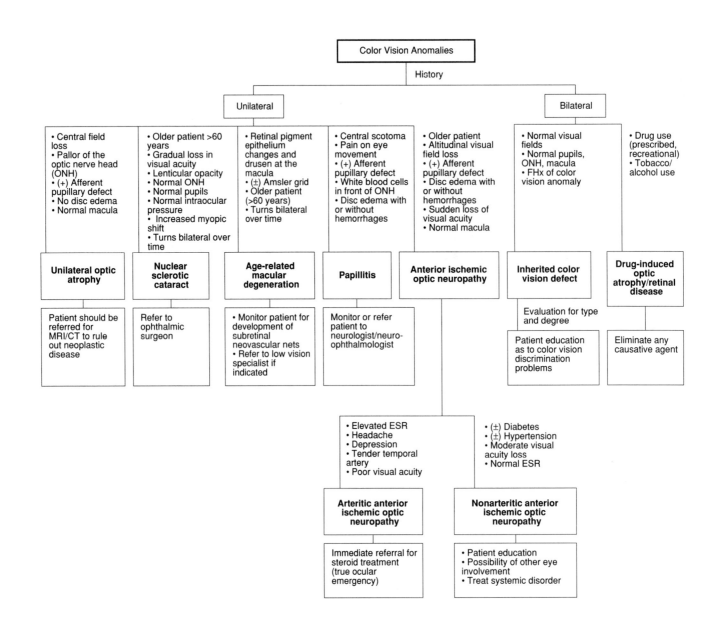

6

Poor Night Vision (Nyctalopia)

Debra J. Bezan

POOR NIGHT VISION (NYCTALOPIA) AT A GLANCE

Uncorrected refractive error
Media opacity
Pupillary miosis
  Age-related
  Drug-induced
Post–refractive surgery
Post–panretinal photocoagulation
Retinal detachment
Advanced glaucoma
Retinitis pigmentosa
Cone-rod degeneration
Choroideremia
Gyrate atrophy
Refsum's syndrome
Bassen-Kornzweig syndrome
Laurence-Moon-Bardet-Biedl syndrome
Mucopolysaccharidoses
Achromatopsia
Congenital stationary night blindness
Oguchi's disease
Fundus albipunctatus
Retinitis punctata albescens
Vitamin A deficiency
Siderosis
Chalcosis
Drug toxicity

The initial evaluation of a patient who complains of having difficulty seeing at night should consist of taking a good history and conducting a comprehensive eye examination. Some pertinent areas to be explored in the history include onset and progression of the reduced night vision, history of a similar condition in blood relatives, history of ocular disease or surgery, and associated symptoms such as reduced central or peripheral vision. Specialized tests that can be useful in the differential diagnosis of nyctalopia include dark adaptometry, electroretinography (ERG), and color vision assessment.

UNCORRECTED REFRACTIVE ERROR

Subjective

Patients with uncorrected refractive error typically complain of blurred vision that may be more noticeable at night. This complaint is seen especially with myopia. This condition is different from "night myopia," which is a state of intermediate accommodation that occurs under minimal lighting conditions.

Objective

Uncorrected refractive error and anomalous accommodative states are generally detected in the course of routine refraction and phorometric examination.

Plan

Correcting the refractive error is the primary means of managing this problem.

POST–REFRACTIVE SURGERY

Subjective

Patients who have had refractive surgery, particularly radial keratotomy, frequently complain of problems with their night vision. When the problem is evaluated further, it is usually found to stem from excessive glare that occurs when the dilated pupil is larger than the surgical optical zone.

Objective

Gross observation and slit-lamp evaluation of the pupil size in relation to the surgical zone under different lighting conditions are usually all that is needed to identify the cause of the problem. Glare testing can be useful to confirm the problem and demonstrate it to the patient in an office setting.

Plan

Patient education and reassurance are usually all that can be done to manage these cases.

MEDIA OPACITY

Subjective

Patients with media opacities, particularly cataracts or opacified posterior capsules, often complain of reduced night vision with a gradual onset. Driving at night is often the first activity that is significantly impaired in patients with age-related progressive cataracts. Reduction in the amount of light reaching the retina and increased glare from the light-scattering effect of the opacity contribute to the problem. These patients often complain of reduced vision under normal lighting conditions as well.

Objective

The location and extent of the media opacity can be evaluated with a slit-lamp biomicroscope through both an undilated and dilated pupil. Glare testing can be useful in determining the degree of impairment under different lighting conditions.

Plan

If the patient feels that his or her daily functioning is significantly impaired by the media opacity, an evaluation for cataract surgery is indicated. Patients who have already had cataract surgery should be evaluated for capsule opacification. Laser capsulotomy should be performed if indicated.

PUPILLARY MIOSIS

Subjective

Relative pupillary miosis due to the inability of the pupil to dilate well contributes to poor night vision. This complaint is common among the elderly. The problem is compounded by age-related media opacification and a reduced level of dark adaptation. Pupillary miosis can also be caused by a number of drugs, including narcotic agents for pain control and miotic agents for glaucoma management.

Objective

A careful history should be taken to determine whether the patient is taking any drugs—prescription, over-the-counter, or recreational—that could cause pupillary miosis. Routine pupil assessment is also used to determine pupil size and reactivity.

Plan

Modification of drug usage, when appropriate, can be helpful in eliminating drug-induced miosis. Education and reassurance are used to manage the patient with age-related miosis.

RETINAL DETACHMENT

Subjective

Sudden onset of reduced night vision can be caused by retinal detachment. Patients with detachments may also note flashes or floaters, or report feeling as if there were a curtain over a portion of their vision.

Objective

A dilated fundus examination is indicated to evaluate a retinal detachment. A three-mirror contact fundus lens or scleral indentation may be needed to examine the peripheral extent of the lesion. When a serous or exudative detachment is noted, the clinician should rule out the possibility of an underlying tumor.

Plan

Most patients with retinal detachments should be referred to a retinal specialist for surgical reattachment.

POST–PANRETINAL PHOTOCOAGULATION

Subjective

A significant number of patients who have undergone panretinal photocoagulation for proliferative retinopathy complain of nyctalopia. The destruction of peripheral retinal tissue appears to cause a further reduction in dark adaptation in eyes that already have reduced scotopic vision secondary to proliferative retinopathy.

Objective

A dilated fundus examination can help the clinician determine the location and extent of the photocoagulation. Dark adaptometry is a helpful adjunct test to demonstrate changes in the rod-cone curve.

Plan

Management of this condition consists of education and reassurance. Frequent examinations to evaluate the retinopathy are also indicated.

CONGENITAL STATIONARY NIGHT BLINDNESS

Subjective

Congenital stationary night blindness (CSNB) is a condition with various modes of inheritance, including autosomal dominant, recessive, and X-linked. As the name implies, the primary symptom is a nonprogressive impairment in night vision. Mildly reduced central vision (acuity ≥ 20/40) is often associated with this condition.

Objective

Patients with CSNB are often myopic. Their retinas generally appear normal except for loss of foveal reflex. Tilted optic nerve heads are present in some cases. Dark adaptometry levels are reduced, and ERG findings are abnormal but variable. Color vision is normal.

Plan

Due to the stable nature of the condition, no specific management is indicated other than regular examinations and vision rehabilitation when needed. Genetic counseling is also recommended.

OGUCHI'S DISEASE

Subjective

Oguchi's disease is thought by some to be a variant of CSNB. It has an autosomal recessive mode of inheritance. The symptoms of Oguchi's disease are very similar to those of CSNB.

Objective

The hallmark of Oguchi's disease is Mizuo's sign, an unusual grayish-yellow discoloration of the retina that reverts to a normal color after 2–3 hours of dark adaptation.

Plan

The management of Oguchi's disease consists of routine monitoring and genetic counseling.

FUNDUS ALBIPUNCTATUS

Subjective

Fundus albipunctatus is an inherited condition with an autosomal recessive mode of inheritance. The main symptom associated with this condition is nonprogressive nyctalopia.

Objective

The name of this condition is derived from its clinical appearance: that of discrete dull white dots scattered throughout the central and midperipheral retina. There are no associated color vision changes, reduction in acuity, retinal pigment epithelial (RPE) degeneration, or field loss. Lack of such changes differentiates fundus albipunctatus from retinitis punctata albescens. However, ERG findings are abnormal and dark adaptation is delayed in both conditions.

Plan

Fundus albipunctatus is managed by conducting routine monitoring and reassuring the patient about its nonprogressive nature. Genetic counseling is also recommended.

MUCOPOLYSACCHARIDOSES (MUCOPOLYSACCHARIDE DISORDERS)

Subjective

The mucopolysaccharidoses are a group of mucopolysaccharide (MPS) storage disorders. They all have an autosomal recessive mode of inheritance except MPS II-A (Hunter's syndrome), which is X-linked recessive. The most common ocular symptoms associated with the MPS disorders are night blindness and reduced acuity.

Objective

The posterior segment signs of the MPS disorders resemble those of retinitis pigmentosa. Many of the MPS subtypes also exhibit corneal clouding. The systemic manifestations of the MPS disorders are quite varied. They include skeletal and facial anomalies, cardiac disease, deafness, and mental retardation. Laboratory tests are available to help differentiate between the MPS subtypes.

Plan

Patients with MPS disorders should be routinely monitored. Some may benefit from keratoplasty. These patients should also be referred for management of their systemic conditions when appropriate.

CHOROIDEREMIA

Subjective

Choroideremia is a degenerative condition of the choriocapillaris and overlying RPE that has an X-linked mode of inheritance. The initial symptom of this disorder is nyctalopia, which becomes apparent in childhood. Loss of peripheral vision also begins in childhood and progresses to loss of central vision later in life.

Objective

The clinical evidence of RPE degeneration begins as a pigment stippling in the midperiphery (the midperiphery of the female carrier exhibits a similar appearance). The degenerative changes spread both centrally and peripherally, and the end stage of the disease shows generalized loss of RPE pigmentation. Associated signs include posterior subcapsular cataracts, vitreous degeneration, and temporal pallor or abnormal vessels at the optic nerve head. Findings of dark adaptometry, ERG, and visual field testing are all abnormal. Fluorescein angiography is useful in demonstrating RPE changes.

Plan

Choroideremia is managed by monitoring its progression and prescribing low vision aids or other means of vision rehabilitation. Genetic counseling is also indicated to help prevent this visually devastating condition.

GYRATE DYSTROPHY OF THE RETINA AND CHOROID (GYRATE ATROPHY)

Subjective

Gyrate dystrophy is a progressive condition with an autosomal recessive mode of inheritance. It is associated with a deficiency in the enzyme ornithine ketoacid aminotransferase. The symptoms usually appear during the teenage to young adult years and include peripheral field loss and night blindness. Loss of central and color vision appear later in the disease course, and legal blindness usually occurs by middle age.

Objective

The midperipheral choroid and RPE begin to atrophy in the early stages of this disease. As these areas coalesce, they appear as large yellow patches with scalloped, pigmented borders. The lesions spread both peripherally and centrally until the entire retina is involved. Other associated ocular manifestations include myopia, macular edema, and early-onset posterior subcapsular cataracts.

Elevated plasma ornithine and reduced serum lysine levels help to confirm the diagnosis of this disease. Abnormal ERG, electro-oculography (EOG), and dark adaptometry findings, as well as peripheral field defect, are useful in diagnosing gyrate dystrophy. ERG, EOG, dark adaptometry, and field testing can be used to monitor the progression of the disease.

Plan

In some cases, dietary modification through supplementation with vitamin B_6 or proline, or reduction of protein intake has been effective in slowing the progression of gyrate dystrophy. Vision rehabilitation may be very helpful for those patients who have already experienced significant vision loss. Genetic counseling is also indicated, because this is an inherited disease.

RETINITIS PIGMENTOSA

Subjective

Retinitis pigmentosa is cone-rod dystrophy that has autosomal dominant, recessive, X-linked, and sporadic modes of inheritance. It is characterized by night blindness and progressive peripheral field loss. Central vision generally remains intact until late in the disease; however, it can be reduced due to cataracts or macular edema.

Objective

Signs of retinitis pigmentosa include peripheral "bone spicule" pigment clumping, waxy pallor of the optic nerve, vessel attenuation, and occasionally macular edema and posterior subcapsular cataracts. ERG, perimetry, and dark adaptometry are all useful in diagnosing and monitoring the progression of retinitis pigmentosa. A diminished ERG pattern may be noted before other signs are clinically apparent.

Plan

Patients with retinitis pigmentosa should be monitored routinely. Patients with vision loss often benefit from low vision aids. Vitamin A palmitate therapy may have some benefit in slowing the progression of this disease. Genetic counseling is also indicated when the mode of inheritance can be determined.

REFSUM'S SYNDROME

Subjective

Refsum's syndrome is an inherited condition caused by an error in fatty acid metabolism, which results in elevated plasma levels of phytanic acid. This condition has an autosomal recessive mode of inheritance. Its primary symptoms are nyctalopia and peripheral vision loss. Central vision can also be affected due to cataract formation or corneal clouding.

Objective

Refsum's syndrome exhibits a bone spicule–like pigmentary retinopathy similar to that of retinitis pigmentosa. Associated ocular findings are posterior subcapsular cataracts and corneal clouding. Systemic signs and symptoms include ataxic gait, peripheral neuropathy, scaly skin (ichthyosis), and deafness. Assessment of plasma phytanic acid levels is needed to confirm the diagnosis.

Plan

Refsum's disease may be slowed or reversed by placing the patient on a restrictive diet that decreases phytanic acid in the plasma. Genetic counseling is also recommended.

VITAMIN A DEFICIENCY

Subjective

Vitamin A deficiency due to improper diet is uncommon in the United States and other developed countries; however, the deficiency can occur secondary to lipid disorders or malabsorption syndromes. The primary ocular symptoms associated with avitaminosis A are poor night vision and discomfort secondary to dry eye. Loss of peripheral vision occasionally occurs.

Objective

External ocular signs of vitamin A deficiency include marked desiccation of the cornea and conjunctiva with formation of Bitot's spots. The effects can progress to corneal opacification, keratomalacia, ulceration, and per-

foration. Internal signs include retinal pigment migration and degeneration. The findings of dark adaptometry are helpful in the diagnosis of this condition and may be even more reliable than serum vitamin A levels.

Plan

The management of vitamin A deficiency consists of supplementation with oral or intramuscular doses of vitamin A. Topically applied tretinoin can be beneficial in treating dry eye and promoting corneal healing. In addition to managing the ocular manifestations, the clinician should refer patients with avitaminosis A to an internist, who can rule out underlying systemic diseases such as gastroenteritis, liver disease, cystic fibrosis, or abetalipoproteinemia.

ADVANCED GLAUCOMA

Subjective

Although glaucoma can occur at any age, its incidence increases with age. In its early stages, primary open-angle glaucoma is an asymptomatic disease; however, as it progresses, the patient loses peripheral vision and ultimately central vision. Reduced night vision and changes in color perception are less common complaints.

Objective

Signs of primary open-angle glaucoma include elevated intraocular pressure, optic nerve cupping, nerve fiber layer defects, and scotomas.

Plan

The primary therapeutic goal for the glaucoma patient is to maintain intraocular pressure at a level at which no further nerve damage occurs. This objective is attempted through the use of topical agents such as beta blockers, adrenergic agonists, prostaglandins, carbonic anhydrase inhibitors, and miotics; through oral administration of carbonic anhydrase inhibitors; and through laser or other surgical procedures.

DRUG TOXICITY

Subjective

The toxic effects of numerous drugs can cause problems in night vision. Drugs with these effects include quinidine, chloroquine, phenothiazine, and ethyl alcohol. Retained iron or copper intraocular foreign bodies can also cause toxic nyctalopia.

Objective

The signs of drug toxicity vary depending on the offending agent but often include pigmentary retinopathy.

Plan

Management consists of discontinuing the use of the toxic substance whenever possible. In many cases, the damage that has already occurred is irreversible.

SUGGESTED READING

Alexander LA. Primary Care of the Posterior Segment (2nd ed). Norwalk, CT: Appleton & Lange, 1994.

Bartlett JD, Jaanus SD. Clinical Ocular Pharmacology (3rd ed). Boston: Butterworth–Heinemann, 1995.

Carr RE, Seigel IM. Electrodiagnostic Testing of the Visual System: A Clinical Guide. Philadelphia: Davis, 1990.

Fraunfelder FT, Roy FH. Current Ocular Therapy 4. Philadelphia: Saunders, 1995.

Gilbert ML, McDonald M. RK and PRK: a future of choices. Eyecare Technol 1995;5:31–33.

Goss DA. Ocular Accommodation, Convergence, and Fixation Disparity (2nd ed). Boston: Butterworth–Heinemann, 1995.

Rosenbloom AA, Morgan MW. Vision and Aging (2nd ed). Boston: Butterworth–Heinemann, 1993.

Roy FH. Ocular Differential Diagnosis (5th ed). Philadelphia: Lea & Febiger, 1993.

van Heuven WAJ, Zwaan JT. Decision Making in Ophthalmology. St. Louis: Mosby–Year Book, 1992.

Weingeist TA, Sneed SR. Laser Surgery in Ophthalmology: Practical Applications. Norwalk, CT: Appleton & Lange, 1992.

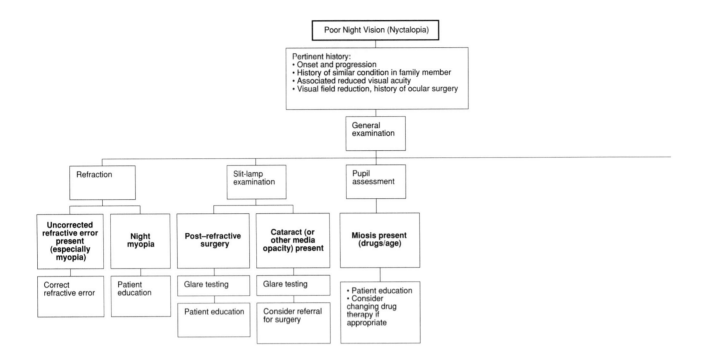

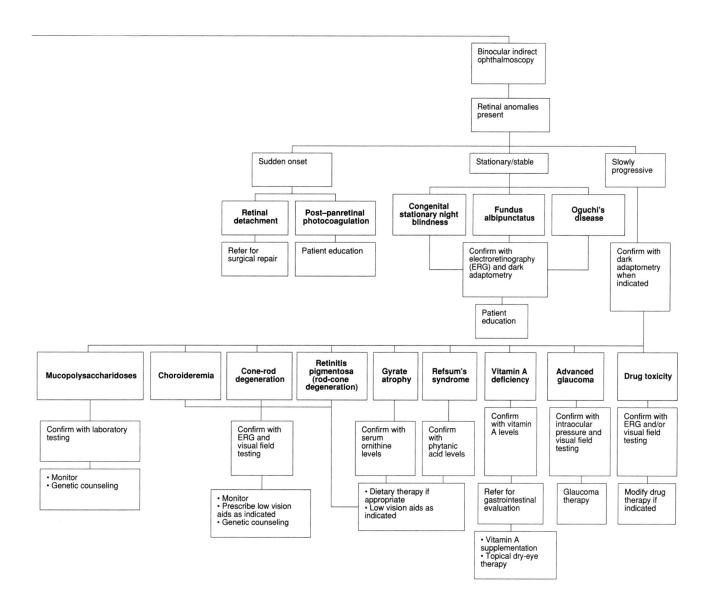

7

Flashes and Floaters

DEBRA J. BEZAN

FLASHES AT A GLANCE

Posterior vitreous detachment
Retinal break
Retinal detachment
Retinal traction
Migraine
Pressure phosphenes
Pseudoflashes
Glare
Photophobia

FLOATERS AT A GLANCE

Posterior vitreous detachment
Vitreous condensation
"Galloping gadgets"
Vitreous hemorrhage
Asteroid hyalosis
Synchysis scintillans
Retinal break
Retinal detachment
Intermediate or posterior uveitis
Neoplasm (masquerade syndrome)

Flashes and floaters are relatively common visual complaints. The conditions associated with these symptoms, although often benign, may be vision threatening. Therefore, these symptoms should not be taken lightly. When a patient presents with a complaint of flashes or floaters, a thorough history of the symptoms should be taken, including onset and time course. Other pertinent aspects of the initial history include information regarding the patient's age, prior trauma, ocular surgery, systemic diseases such as diabetes mellitus, prior ocular infection or

inflammation, and headaches or reduced vision associated with the flashes or floaters.

POSTERIOR VITREOUS DETACHMENT

Subjective

Posterior vitreous detachment (PVD) is one of the most common causes of flashes and floaters. It is associated with degenerative changes in the aging vitreous and thus is found primarily in patients over the age of 45. However, certain conditions—including trauma, inflammation, diabetic retinopathy, degenerative myopia, and other vitreoretinal degenerations—can cause an earlier onset of PVD.

The floaters noted by patients with PVD typically have a sudden onset and appear as a well-defined shape that shifts with fixation. The flashes occur when movements of the vitreous cause traction on the retina at areas of firm vitreoretinal attachment, such as the vitreous base. Cessation of the flashes usually indicates progression of the PVD and release of traction on the retina.

Objective

Centrally located PVDs can often be observed with a direct ophthalmoscope. Fundus biomicroscopy and binocular indirect ophthalmoscopy are two other techniques for viewing a PVD through a dilated pupil. A PVD often appears as a ring- or crescent-shaped opacity just anterior to the optic nerve head (Weis' ring). Large PVDs may present as a wispy or corrugated veil suspended in the vitreous cortex.

Plan

Patients presenting with a recent onset of PVD should have their peripheral retinas carefully evaluated for the presence of breaks with scleral indentation or a three-mirror contact fundus lens. Breaks occur in 15–30% of cases of symptomatic PVD. Patients with PVD should be educated about the condition and informed about the symptoms of retinal detachment. They should be monitored closely for the first 1–2 months after the onset of symptoms and then annually thereafter.

RETINAL TEARS OR DETACHMENTS

Subjective

Breaks in the retina, either round holes or linear tears, provide a route for liquefied vitreous to flow underneath the sensory retina, and thus pose a risk for retinal detachment. Such breaks may be idiopathic or secondary to another condition such as ocular trauma. In addition to the presence of retinal degenerations or breaks, other risk factors for retinal detachment include high myopia, aphakia or pseudophakia, proliferative retinopathy, a history of detachment in the opposite eye, and symptoms of flashes and floaters. The lightning streak–like flashes are caused by vitreoretinal traction and are similar to those experienced in PVD. The floaters associated with a retinal break, however, are often multiple and resemble a swarm of insects. The symptom of feeling as if a curtain or veil were dropping over a portion of the visual field may indicate a retinal detachment.

Objective

Retinal holes are small, round, red lesions usually located near the ora. There may be a free-floating operculum in the vicinity. Retinal tears are linear or horseshoe shaped. There may be an adjacent vitreoretinal adhesion forming a flap tear. A white cuff surrounding a retinal break indicates the accumulation of fluid under the sensory retina forming a retinal detachment.

Larger retinal detachments have a milky appearance that obscures underlying details and often have an elevated, corrugated surface. Small, pigmented, tobacco dust–like particles in the anterior vitreous (Shafer's sign) indicate that the clinician should evaluate the peripheral retina carefully for a break or detachment. Ultrasonography is indicated to evaluate suspected retinal detachments if a direct view is obscured by media opacification.

Plan

Symptomatic retinal breaks should be monitored carefully. When other risk factors are present, including a significant zone of surrounding subretinal fluid or a patient

history of high myopia, aphakia or pseudophakia, or detachment in the opposite eye, the retinal break may be treated prophylactically with a laser to prevent detachment. If detachment has already occurred, retinal reattachment should be attempted through the use of pneumatic retinopexy, scleral buckling, and laser photocoagulation or cryotherapy procedures.

PSEUDOFLASHES

Subjective

A number of conditions can cause chronic or intermittent symptoms that a patient may describe as flashes. These may more accurately be characterized as visual hallucinations associated with certain drugs, glare associated with media opacities, halos around lights associated with corneal edema, or photophobia.

Objective

Evaluation of the patient who complains of nonspecific chronic or recurrent flashes should include a thorough dilated fundus examination to rule out PVD and other types of retinal traction. The clinician should also investigate the use of any prescription, over-the-counter, or recreational drugs that may be causing visual hallucinations. Gonioscopy and tonometry are helpful in ruling out narrow-angle or angle-closure glaucoma, which may cause the symptom of halos around lights. Slit-lamp evaluation should also be performed to rule out other causes of corneal edema and to look for media opacities or evidence of anterior uveitis.

Plan

When indicated, modification of drug therapy, cataract extraction, peripheral iridotomy for angle closure, or topical therapy for corneal edema or anterior uveitis should be instituted. Reassurance is often helpful to the patient with nonspecific flashes after pathologic causes have been ruled out. Prescribing tinted spectacle lenses may also be helpful in some cases.

MIGRAINE

Subjective

Migraines most commonly occur in females with a family history of this condition although they occur commonly in males as well. Migraines are sometimes associated with visual auras or scintillating scotomas that the patient may describe as flashes. These often appear as bright or multicolored zigzag lines that migrate slowly across the visual field. They usually last 15–60 minutes and often precede a unilateral headache in classic migraine. They may occur without an associated headache in acephalic migraine. Other associated symptoms include nausea, fatigue, mood changes, and photophobia.

Objective

Few objective signs are associated with migraines; however, patients can experience a permanent visual field defect in rare cases.

Plan

The visual disturbances associated with migraines can be quite alarming, and often reassurance is very helpful to the patient. Referral for evaluation and systemic treatment of migraine is indicated in many cases. The clinician should also consider referring the patient for a cerebrovascular evaluation if the migraine-like symptoms are first experienced in middle age or later.

PRESSURE PHOSPHENES

Subjective

Pressure phosphenes are light flashes that are perceived when pressure is applied to the globe, such as during eye rubbing.

Objective

There are no objective signs associated with pressure phosphenes.

Plan

Education and reassurance are indicated if the patient is concerned about pressure phosphenes.

VITREOUS CONDENSATION

Subjective

Focal condensation of vitreous protein and collagen is the most common type of benign degenerative vitreous floater. Remnants of the fetal vascular system suspended in the vitreous can also cause the patient to experience floaters. Both of these types of floater are chronic. The floaters are relatively stable in size and shape and tend to shift with changes in fixation.

Objective

Focal vitreous condensations can sometimes be visualized with the slit-lamp biomicroscope.

Plan

No treatment beyond reassurance and routine monitoring is indicated for cases of vitreous condensation.

ASTEROID HYALOSIS

Subjective

Asteroid hyalosis is a vitreous condition most often seen in patients over the age of 60. It is usually unilateral and may be found in association with certain systemic vascular diseases, particularly diabetes mellitus. Although most patients with asteroid hyalosis are asymptomatic, some report floaters or blurred vision.

Objective

Asteroid hyalosis appears as multiple small, white spheres composed of calcium soaps that are suspended in the vitreous. They are visible with ophthalmoscopy or slit-lamp biomicroscopy. The spheres suspended in the vitreous gel shift slightly after eye movements then return to their original position. In contrast, the particles seen in synchysis scintillans sink to the bottom of the liquefied portion of the vitreous after eye movements.

Plan

In most cases, asteroid bodies are benign and require only routine observation. Patients with this condition should be evaluated for diabetes mellitus and hypertension if these conditions have not been diagnosed previously. If vision is significantly affected by asteroid bodies or if they prevent adequate visualization of the retina needed to monitor diabetic retinopathy, vitrectomy may be indicated.

GALLOPING GADGETS

Subjective

"Galloping gadgets" are floaters caused by the shadows cast by the corpuscles in the retinal blood vessels. They are often noted by the patient when gazing up at the sky or at a bright blank wall and appear as rapidly moving small particles. They can also be visualized by the patient while looking in a blue-field entoptoscope and can be used to assess macular function.

Objective

There are no objective signs of galloping gadgets.

Plan

Education and reassurance are indicated for patients who are concerned about this type of floater.

VITREOUS HEMORRHAGE

Subjective

Vitreous hemorrhages are associated with a number of ocular conditions, including PVD, proliferative retinopathies, ocular trauma, retinal breaks, and intraocular tumors. The patient with a vitreous hemorrhage often experiences a sudden onset of cobweb-like floaters or hazy vision that may have a reddish hue.

Objective

There are two forms of vitreous hemorrhage, with differing clinical presentations. Retrovitreous (preretinal) hemorrhages are initially bright red and well-defined, and usually settle into a boat shape due to gravity. Intravitreous hemorrhages are more diffuse and are initially dark red or reddish gray in color.

Plan

Vitreous hemorrhages usually resolve over time. Patients who present with vitreous hemorrhages should be evaluated for underlying systemic conditions such as diabetes mellitus or sickle-cell disease if these have not been diagnosed previously. Patients with proliferative retinopathies often benefit from laser photocoagulation to prevent further vitreous hemorrhaging. Vitrectomy may be indicated in patients with unresolving vitreous hemorrhage that affects vision.

INTERMEDIATE OR POSTERIOR UVEITIS

Subjective

A number of conditions causing intermediate or posterior uveitis can lead to the release of inflammatory debris into the vitreous. Pars planitis, sarcoidosis, toxoplasmosis, toxocariasis, syphilis, Behçet's disease, Vogt-Koyanagi-Harada's disease, acute retinal necrosis, and endophthalmitis are some of the conditions that can cause significant vitritis. Debris in the vitreous can cause the patient to complain of blurred vision or floaters.

Objective

In addition to haze and clumps of debris in the vitreous, other ocular signs often present in intermediate and posterior uveitis can aid in differential diagnosis. These include anterior chamber reaction, chorioretinal scars, perivasculitis, and cystoid macular edema. Laboratory and radiologic testing can help confirm the diagnosis of many types of posterior uveitis. (For more detail, see Chapter 42.) Occasionally, analysis of a vitreous aspirate is needed to rule out a masquerade syndrome or to arrive at a definitive diagnosis of an infectious condition.

Plan

Infectious forms of posterior uveitis are managed by using anti-infective agents to treat the underlying infection as well as anti-inflammatory agents to manage the inflammatory component. The management of noninfectious forms consists primarily of controlling symptoms with steroidal and nonsteroidal anti-inflammatory agents. Antimetabolites and other immunosuppressive agents are needed in some cases of severe inflammation.

SUGGESTED READING

Alexander LA. Primary Care of the Posterior Segment (2nd ed). Norwalk, CT: Appleton & Lange, 1994.

Margo CE, Hamed LM, Mames RN. Diagnostic Problems in Clinical Ophthalmology. Philadelphia: Saunders, 1994.

Roy FH. Ocular Differential Diagnosis (5th ed). Philadelphia: Lea & Febiger, 1993.

Smith RE, Nozik RA. Uveitis: A Clinical Approach to Diagnosis and Management (2nd ed). Baltimore: Williams & Wilkins, 1989.

van Heuven WAJ, Zwaan JT. Decision Making in Ophthalmology. St. Louis: Mosby–Year Book, 1992.

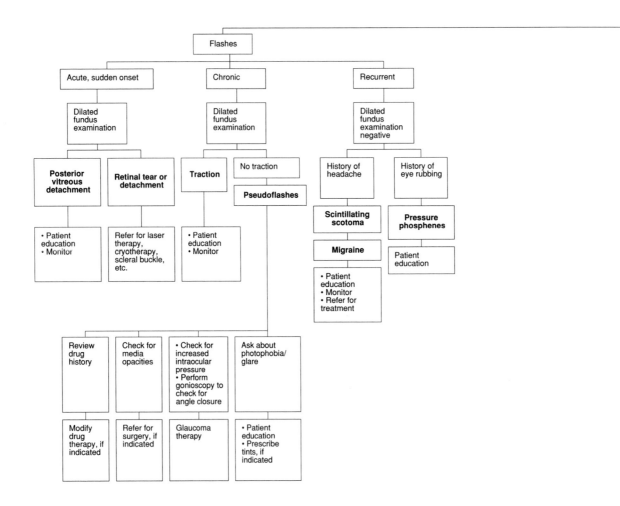

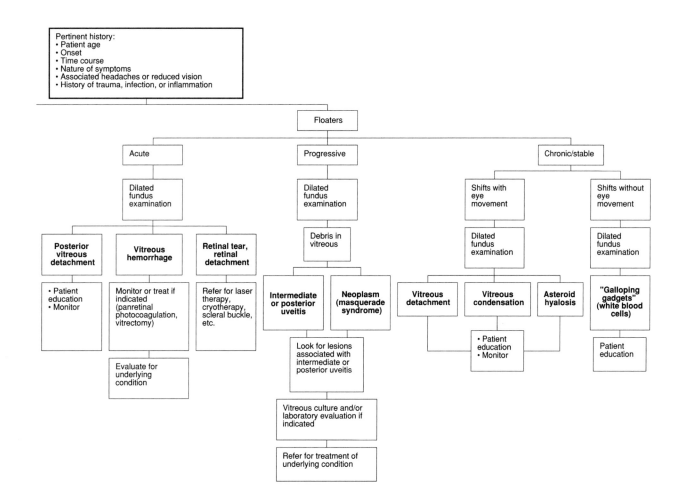

8

Diplopia

David P. Sendrowski

DIPLOPIA AT A GLANCE

Monocular
  Astigmatism
  Cataract
  Keratoconus
  Polycoria
  Intraocular tumor
  Macular disease
  Retinal detachment
  Ectopia lentis
  Intraocular lens dislocation
  Postiridectomy
  Post–radial keratotomy
Binocular
  Uncompensated phoria
  Convergence insufficiency
  Orbital disease
  Trauma
  Diabetes
  Hypertension
  Atherosclerosis
  Stroke
  Aneurysm
  Tumor
  Increased intracranial pressure
  Post–strabismus surgery
  Anomalous retinal correspondence
  Physiologic diplopia

True diplopia is the awareness of seeing the same object in two different places in visual space. It implies misalignment of the eyes. Patients frequently describe refractive blur of an object as object doubling. The astute clinician should determine whether the patient is describing refractive blur or true diplopia before embarking on further diagnostic testing.

It is important to determine whether the diplopia is monocular or binocular at the beginning of the examination. Monocular diplopia reflects optical aberrations within the refracting media of the eye. Binocular diplopia is much more serious and may be an early sign of neurologic, orbital, neoplastic, or vascular disease.

REFRACTIVE DIPLOPIA

Subjective

The patient with a refractive problem may sometimes complain of diplopia. The approach in taking the history is first to delineate whether the complaint is monocular or binocular. The astute clinician asks the patient whether the images are together or separated. In refractive "diplopia," the images are blurred and together, rather than separated; there is no history of recent trauma; and the diplopia is usually of a gradual rather than sudden onset.

Common refractive problems such as uncorrected astigmatism, especially oblique astigmatism, may cause blur or doubling. Other conditions that may cause a monocular diplopia are keratoconus and cataract.

Objective

The examination should start by ruling out the less threatening causes of the double vision. The use of a pinhole during visual acuity assessment is an excellent means of telling very quickly that the diplopia may be refractive in nature. Keratometry and retinoscopy should help determine astigmatic and keratoconic causes of the diplopia. Additional tests should include Amsler grid or photostress testing to rule out macular disease.

A dilated fundus examination is warranted to evaluate the lens for dislocation and to allow a complete exploration of the retina to rule out a retinal detachment. Threshold visual field testing is usually not helpful in the diagnosis, and a confrontation screening field gives the needed information.

Plan

Uncorrected astigmatism can easily be corrected with a change in the refractive prescription. The patient with keratoconus may benefit from correction with rigid gas-permeable contact lenses. In the case of cataract, if the spectacle correction cannot alleviate the complaint of diplopia, the patient should be referred for surgical evaluation. All of these cases are nonemergent and can be followed at the doctor's discretion.

NONREFRACTIVE DIPLOPIA

Subjective

In contrast to patients with refractive diplopia, patients with nonrefractive diplopia complain that the images are distinct and separated. A history of recent trauma may be helpful in the diagnosis of polycoria or retinal detachment. History of a recent cataract surgery may assist in isolating the cause of the diplopia as a dislocated intraocular lens.

Objective

The patient should be evaluated with pinhole testing, keratometry, and phorometry to rule out any refractive cause. Additional testing with an Amsler grid and photostress test may be helpful in isolating an exudative (wet) type of maculopathy.

A dilated fundus examination should be performed to rule out a retinal detachment and to allow the use of high plus lenses for macular evaluation. Where there is a subtle form of macular disease or tumor formation in the posterior pole, threshold visual field testing of the macular or posterior pole area may be very helpful for the diagnosis. Otherwise, a confrontation method of visual field examination is sufficient.

In the case of macular disease, a retinal fluorescein angiogram may be of aid in the diagnosis. Ultrasonography and a magnetic resonance imaging (MRI) or computed tomographic (CT) scan may also aid in the diagnosis of intraocular tumor.

Plan

The management plan varies in accordance with the initial diagnosis. In the case of traumatic polycoria, intraocular tumor, retinal detachment, or dislocated intraocular lens, the patient will benefit from referral to an ophthalmic surgeon for evaluation and management.

COMITANT DEVIATION, DUE TO UNCOMPENSATED PHORIA OR CONVERGENCE INSUFFICIENCY

Subjective

Comitant deviations due to uncompensated phorias or convergence insufficiency can cause the patient to experience diplopia. The patient with comitant deviation may complain of a binocular diplopia that occurs more commonly while reading or performing other near work. There may also be associated findings of sleepiness after near work, headaches, and ocular asthenopia. The condition tends to occur more frequently in young adults and teenagers but can also occur in the presbyopic population. The key point in the history is that the diplopia is not constant and is initiated by performing some near task. The diplopia almost never occurs in distance vision. It should be noted that symptoms of diplopia are uncommon in the patient with comitant esotropia or exotropia due to the age of onset or duration of the condition. In these patients, suppression is more common.

Objective

The entrance testing should include a cover test. There is commonly an exophoria that is greater at near than at distance. There may also be a decrease in the near point of convergence. The key to the diagnosis is the results of the phorometry testing. The amplitude of accommodation may be low, and the compensating convergence is reduced. In younger patients, a cycloplegic refraction may be indicated.

Plan

The best possible spectacle correction should be prescribed for the patient. A regimen of vision therapy exercises should be prescribed to improve the accommodative and binocular status. These procedures can be done in office, or the patient may be referred to a specialist in vision training for evaluation and treatment. The results are usually very beneficial for the patient.

NONCOMITANT DEVIATION

Orbital Disease

Subjective

The patient with orbital disease may present with a variety of complaints, but one of the more common complaints is diplopia. The diplopia is binocular and goes away when one eye is covered. The patient may also complain of eyelid swelling, proptosis (bulging of the eye), pain, and loss of visual acuity.

The history should include questions about the onset of the diplopia to determine if it was rapid or gradual. The patient should be questioned about any recent fever or other systemic symptoms such as heat intolerance or irritability. The clinician should also determine whether the past medical history includes thyroid disease, cancer, diabetes, pulmonary disease, renal disease, dermatologic conditions, or recent trauma. Medications should be evaluated for their potential ocular side effects.

Objective

The external examination should include an evaluation for periorbital changes, pulsatile motion of the globe, resistance to retropulsion of the eyes, and, most importantly, displacement of the globe. The pupils, ocular motility, intraocular pressure, and visual fields should all be tested. Exophthalmometry should be considered to rule out exophthalmus from orbital disease. Pupil dilation allows the clinician to examine the retina for choroidal folds and to assess the integrity of the optic nerve head and the peripheral retina.

Additional tests that should be considered based on the clinical picture include laboratory studies such as a complete blood count (CBC), free levorotatory thyroxine and thyrotropin levels, erythrocyte sedimentation rate (ESR), antinuclear antibody level, fasting blood glucose level, and blood cultures. An orbital CT or MRI scan helps to localize inflammations or neoplastic growths. Ultrasonography can also be helpful in the diagnosis.

Plan

Treatment and management vary depending on the cause of the orbital disease. The patient can benefit from a referral to an internist or endocrinologist for evaluation of any suspected disease states and to an ophthalmic surgeon for evaluation of ocular inflammatory or neoplastic conditions.

Third Nerve Palsy

Subjective

The patient with a third nerve palsy almost always complains of double vision. The diplopia disappears when one eye is closed. Because the third nerve controls the levator muscle of the upper lid, the patient has an associated ptosis as well. The ptosis is usually greater than 3 mm. There may or may not be a complaint of pain with the onset of the diplopia. When present, the pain is usually severe and may be described as a sharp, boring type of pain.

It is important to the medical history to establish whether the patient has diabetes or any other type of microvascular disease.

Objective

It is important for the clinician to establish the motility status. If the patient has limitation of motion in all fields of gaze, then the patient may have a complete palsy. If the patient has partial limitation, then the patient has a partial palsy. Ptosis and the inability to look upward may suggest a superior division palsy; inability to look nasally or downward may indicate an inferior division palsy.

The pupillary response is very important. If the pupil is fixed and not responsive to light and constricts to 0.5% pilocarpine, then an aneurysm at the posterior communicating artery is a possible cause. If the pupil does not constrict to 0.5% or 1% pilocarpine, a pharmacologic block may be present. If the pupil is reactive, the cause could be a microvascular disease such as diabetes.

Additional entrance tests should include testing of the confrontation fields, evaluation for proptosis, test for orbital retropulsion, a complete cranial nerve evaluation, and blood pressure assessment. A cover test may reveal excyclorotation produced by an intact fourth nerve. Such a finding would suggest that the condition is an isolated third nerve and not a cavernous sinus disorder.

Other testing that should be considered includes CBC with blood glucose assessment and ESR, and MRI or CT scanning, especially for patients with pupil involvement. There is less immediate need for an imaging series for patients with a pupil-sparing third nerve disease.

Plan

If the pupil is involved, the patient should be referred to the hospital for evaluation immediately. A neurologic consultation should be sought for the patient as soon as possible. If the pupil is spared, the patient should be referred to an internist for evaluation for microvascular disease. The referral appointment should be the same or next day.

In the case of microvascular disease, the diplopia can be treated by patching the involved eye. As the third nerve begins to recover, the diplopia should also resolve. The patient should be considered for visual training to regain full motor control of the involved eye.

The patient should be comanaged by the internist and the eye care practitioner.

Sixth Nerve Palsy

Subjective

The patient with a sixth nerve palsy usually complains of a binocular horizontal diplopia. The diplopia may be worse at distance than near. It may also be more pronounced in the direction of the lateral muscle that is involved. The patient should be asked if the diplopic symptoms fluctuate during the day. If a bilateral palsy is suspected, the patient should be asked about headaches. An increase in intracranial pressure may produce a bilateral sixth nerve involvement.

Additional history questions should inquire about any past history of cancer, thyroid eye disease, diabetes, multiple sclerosis, sarcoidosis, or stroke. The patient should also be asked about any recent neurologic testing such as lumbar puncture, which can also cause an isolated sixth nerve palsy. Other disease entities that may effect the sixth nerve are Möbius' syndrome, Duane's syndrome (type 1), orbital pseudotumor, myasthenia gravis, and Gradenigo's syndrome. If Gradenigo's syndrome is suspected, the patient should be asked about pain in the division of the fifth nerve around the face.

Objective

The entrance testing should include motility testing, confrontation visual field testing, pupillary evaluation, blood pressure measurement, and a complete cranial nerve evaluation. During the cranial nerve evaluation, the clinician should pay close attention to the fifth cranial nerve because of its close association with the sixth nerve. A forced duction test may be helpful to rule out a restrictive myopathy. The dilated fundus examination should include a high plus lens evaluation of the optic nerve heads to rule out papilledema.

Additional testing that should be considered includes CBC and evaluation for blood glucose level and ESR. MRI scans are warranted if there is any suspicion of underlying neurologic causes of the sixth nerve involvement. There may be such a neurologic cause in young children, who may have a sixth nerve involvement from a pontine glioma.

Plan

Patients with sixth nerve palsy, especially young children, should be sent for neurologic evaluation immediately. If the patient is older and there are no signs of elevated intracranial pressure, the patient should be referred to an internist, who can rule out an underlying vasculopathy.

Patching should be considered for the paretic eye until the condition resolves. This step should be approached with caution in young children, who may develop amblyopia as a result of the patching. Fresnel prisms may be used in milder cases of diplopia.

The patient should be followed every 2–3 weeks to check for the resolution of the diplopia.

Fourth Nerve Palsy

Subjective

The patient with a fourth nerve palsy usually complains of vertical diplopia. The diplopia is worse when the patient attempts near tasks such as reading. It is possible for the patient to be asymptomatic and the palsy to be found during a routine eye examination.

The history should include questions regarding head trauma. The fourth nerve is most vulnerable to the effects of trauma. The patient should also be asked about diabetes, hypertension, multiple sclerosis, thyroid eye disease, myasthenia gravis, and orbital pseudotumor.

The patient may have assumed a head tilt as a result of the palsy. The patient can be asked for any pictures of the patient as a child; these may reveal that the head tilt was present at an early age.

Objective

The entrance testing should include pupillary evaluation, confrontation visual field testing, and motility testing. Orbital examination for proptosis and retropulsion may be useful to help rule out orbital disease. A Park's three-step test or a cover test with a Maddox rod over the affected eye is an excellent test to isolate the affected muscle. Measurement of the vertical fusional amplitudes may be used to distinguish between an acquired and a congenital fourth nerve palsy. The fusional amplitude is often much greater (usually $>3\Delta$) with congenital fourth nerve palsy than with acquired fourth nerve palsy, which shows an amplitude in the normal range (usually $1–3\Delta$).

A dilated examination should be performed to rule out any involvement of the optic nerve head. Evaluation of the retina is also strongly recommended.

Additional tests that should be considered are measurement of blood glucose levels and ESR. An MRI scan is recommended for children with additional evidence of a neurologic cause or a recently acquired fourth nerve palsy. It can also be helpful in adults if all other blood work is negative.

Plan
Children with recently acquired fourth nerve palsy without a history of trauma should be sent for a neurologic evaluation. Adult patients without a history of trauma should be sent to an internist for evaluation for an underlying vascular event.

Once the underlying cause is treated, the eye with the palsy should be patched. Patching should be approached cautiously in the younger child so as not to cause amblyopia. When the deviation is small, patching may not be necessary, because prism correction can be helpful in alleviating the diplopia.

When patching or prism correction is not effective for relief of the diplopia or cosmetic correction of the head tilt, surgical intervention is recommended. The surgery should not be considered for at least 6 months to allow for spontaneous resolution.

SUGGESTED READING

Glaser JS. Topical Diagnosis: Prechiasmal Visual Pathways. In: Neuro-Ophthalmology, Vol 2 (2nd ed). Philadelphia: Lippincott, 1990;1–85.

Miller NE (ed). Walsh and Hoyt's Clinical Neuro-Ophthalmology (5th ed). Baltimore: Williams & Wilkins, 1998.

Nelson B, Calhoun JH, Harley RD. Pediatric Ophthalmology (4th ed). Philadelphia: Saunders, 1998.

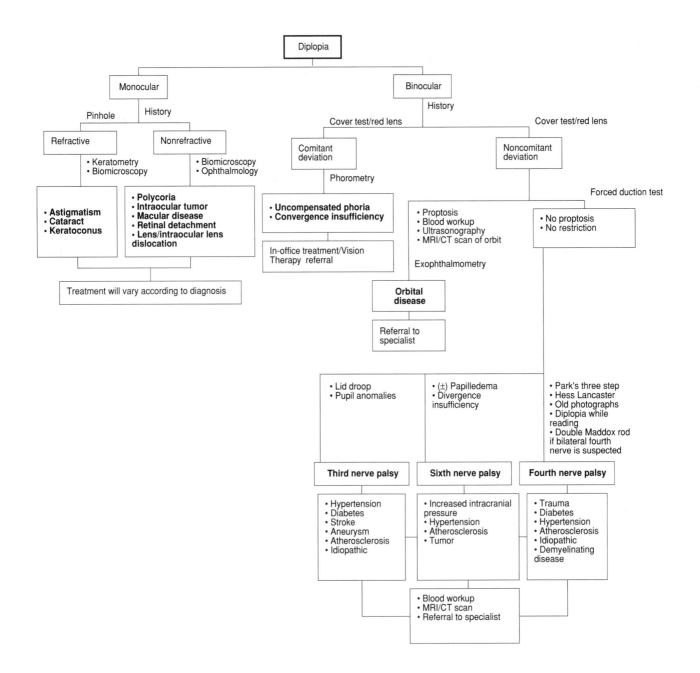

9

Lid Twitch

Debra J. Bezan

LID TWITCH AT A GLANCE

Blepharospasm associated with corneal irritation
  Dry eye
  Abrasion
  Foreign body
Benign tic
Benign essential blepharospasm
Blepharospasm or myokymia associated with neurologic
    disorders
  Multiple sclerosis
  Parkinson's disease
  Myasthenia gravis
  Trigeminal neuralgia
  Meige's syndrome
  Brueghel's syndrome
  Craniocervical dystonia
  Nuchal dystonia
  Huntington's disease
  Brain stem lesions
  Guillain-Barré syndrome
  Tourette's disease
  Wilson's disease
Simple myokymia (not associated with neurologic dis-
    orders)

The diagnostic evaluation of a patient complaining of
lid twitch begins with taking a good history. Questions
should be asked concerning the onset, duration, and recurrence of the twitching. Associated symptoms such as foreign body sensation, fatigue, muscle weakness, and
tremors should be investigated. A social history—including questions about stress, anxiety, and the use of tobacco,
alcohol, or other drugs—can be useful in the evaluation

of lid twitch. After taking the history, the clinician should
perform a gross evaluation to determine the nature of the
lid twitch (tremor vs. forced closure) and should follow
with a slit-lamp evaluation of the external eye.

REFLEX BLEPHAROSPASM ASSOCIATED WITH OCULAR IRRITATION

Subjective

In blepharospasm associated with ocular irritation, the chief
complaint is often a dry, scratchy, painful, or photophobic eye. Symptoms are relieved somewhat with lid closure.
The history may reveal other associated factors such as
recent ocular trauma, infection, or chronic dry eye.

Objective

Slit-lamp evaluation alone and with the aid of sodium
fluorescein staining is used to detect anterior chamber
reaction, foreign bodies, areas of epithelial disruption,
and rapid tear break-up time.

Plan

The initial treatment of dry eye typically involves application of topical lubricants in drop or ointment form. If
this treatment is unsuccessful, punctal occlusion, moisture shields, or bandage contact lenses may provide relief.
    When there is a superficial corneal or conjunctival for-
eign body or abrasion, management involves removal
of any foreign material and evaluation for secondary
uveitis. This step is followed by topical instillation of a

prophylactic broad-spectrum antibiotic and a cycloplegic agent. The eye is usually pressure patched unless the patient wears contact lenses. Bandage contact lenses may be used as an alternative to pressure patching in many cases.

BENIGN TIC

Subjective

In benign tic, lid twitch is not specifically associated with neurologic disorders; however, it may be exacerbated by stress or fatigue.

Objective

The condition is characterized by a unilateral intermittent lid twitch.

Plan

Treatment consists of reassurance and counseling about lifestyle factors.

BENIGN ESSENTIAL BLEPHAROSPASM

Subjective

Benign essential blepharospasm is a chronic, bilateral, usually progressive condition that primarily affects older persons. It is more common among women than men. It may be exacerbated by fatigue, stress, bright lights, television viewing, or driving, and can be quite debilitating.

Objective

Benign essential blepharospasm is characterized by constant or intermittent involuntary forced closure of the eyelids. It may be found in isolation or in association with spasms of the lower face, oropharynx, or cervical muscles (Meige's syndrome, Brueghel's syndrome, orofacial dystonia).

Plan

Management of benign essential blepharospasm consists of an initial trial with oral pharmaceutical agents, including anticholinergics, benzodiazepines, dopamine agonists, or antidepressants. If none of the oral agents works, injection of botulinum toxin may provide

extended relief. If this therapy is ineffective, surgical management may be indicated.

MYOKYMIA ASSOCIATED WITH NEUROLOGIC DISORDERS

Subjective

Myokymia may be a manifestation of underlying neurologic disease. Associated symptoms can provide useful clues. For example, complaints of muscle weakness may suggest myasthenia gravis or multiple sclerosis. In addition, the multiple sclerosis patient may complain of episodes of decreased vision. Intense facial pain is associated with trigeminal neuralgia. Muscle rigidity, resting tremor, and postural instability are associated with Parkinson's disease.

Objective

Myokymia is characterized by a spontaneous fascicular contraction of the eyelid muscle.

Plan

Patients with myokymia that is suspected to be a manifestation of neurologic disease should be referred to a neurologist for further evaluation and management.

MYOKYMIA NOT ASSOCIATED WITH NEUROLOGIC DISORDERS (SIMPLE MYOKYMIA)

Subjective

Simple myokymia is not associated with organic disease; however, it may be exacerbated by fatigue, stress, overexertion, or excessive intake of tobacco, alcohol, or caffeine.

Objective

Simple myokymia is characterized by a fine contraction of the eyelid muscle that is not associated with weakness or other neurologic disorders.

Plan

Treatment of simple myokymia initially involves patient reassurance and counseling about lifestyle factors, including stress, sleep habits, smoking, and ingestion of caffeine or alcohol. More severe cases may be managed with topical or oral antihistamines or oral quinine therapy.

SUGGESTED READING

Bartlett JD, Jaanus SD. Clinical Ocular Pharmacology (3rd ed). Boston: Butterworth–Heinemann, 1995.

Berkow R, Fletcher AJ. The Merck Manual of Diagnosis and Therapy (16th ed). Rahway, NJ: Merck, 1992.

Fraunfelder FT, Roy FH. Current Ocular Therapy 4. Philadelphia: Saunders, 1995.

Margo CE, Hamed LN, Mames RN. Diagnostic Problems in Clinical Ophthalmology. Philadelphia: Saunders, 1994.

Roy FH. Ocular Differential Diagnosis (5th ed). Philadelphia: Lea & Febiger, 1993.

van Heuven WAJ, Zwaan JT. Decision Making in Ophthalmology. St. Louis: Mosby–Year Book, 1992.

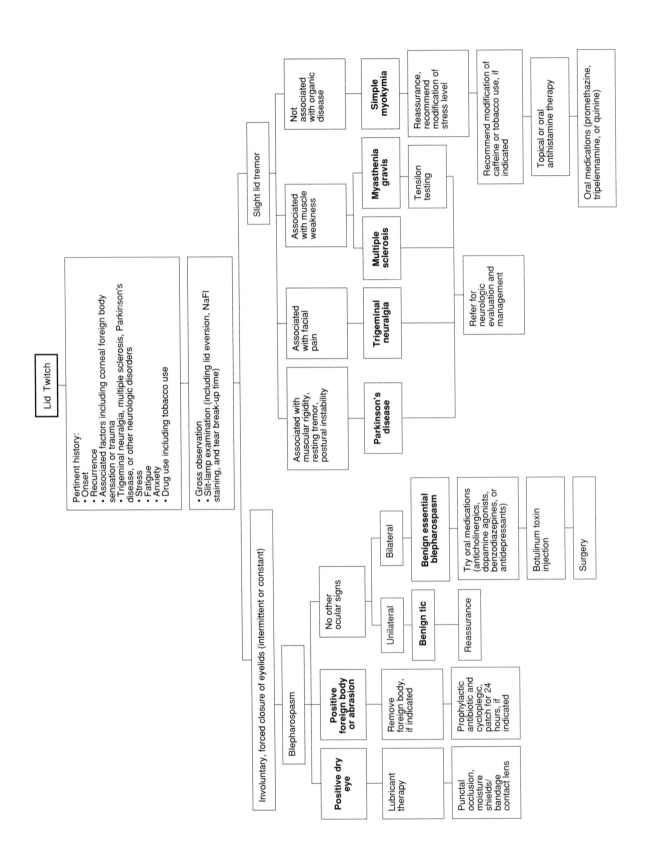

10

Eye Itch

Debra J. Bezan

EYE ITCH AT A GLANCE

Allergic reactions
 Type I
 Type IV
 Mixed
Poorly fitting contact lens
Exposed suture barb
Parasitic infestation
 Demodicosis
 Pediculosis

When a patient presents complaining of itching eyes, the case history is vital to making the differential diagnosis. Pertinent questions to ask include the following: When did the itching start? How long has it persisted? Have you been exposed to any new drugs or chemicals recently (including soaps, shampoos, cosmetics)? Have you been exposed to anything you might be allergic to lately (including pets, pollen, mold)? Do you or members of your family have asthma, hay fever, eczema, or other allergic reactions? Do you wear contact lenses? Have you had cataract surgery? A thorough slit-lamp examination also adds clinical data valuable in the differential diagnosis of an itching eye.

TYPE I HYPERSENSITIVITY REACTIONS TO DRUGS OR CHEMICALS

Subjective

Type I (anaphylactoid, IgE-mediated) hypersensitivity reactions can occur in response to topical or systemic administration of a number of drugs. Symptoms of itching or burning and signs develop rapidly after exposure to the offending agent.

Objective

Ocular signs of type I hypersensitivity reactions to medications include lid edema, conjunctival injection, and chemosis.

Plan

Application of cool compresses and topical vasoconstrictors and antihistamines, as well as use of oral antihistamines, can be helpful in providing symptomatic relief. Although full-blown systemic anaphylactic reactions are rare, they should be considered when dealing with type I reactions. As with other allergies, the definitive treatment is to avoid contact with the allergen.

TYPE IV HYPERSENSITIVITY REACTIONS TO DRUGS OR CHEMICALS

Subjective

Contact dermatitis is one manifestation of type IV (cell-mediated) hypersensitivity. After the initial exposure to an allergen, subsequent exposures result in symptoms (intense itching) and signs that occur after a delay of 24–72 hours. Common offending allergens include certain topical ophthalmic preparations, cosmetics, soaps, and perfumes.

Objective

Signs of contact dermatitis include lid edema, erythema, and a scaly eczema.

Plan

Application of cool compresses and topical corticosteroids is helpful in providing symptomatic relief in contact dermatitis. When possible, the allergen should be avoided to prevent recurrence.

HAY FEVER CONJUNCTIVITIS

Subjective

Hay fever conjunctivitis is a type I hypersensitivity reaction to an environmental allergen such as pollen, dust, mold, or animal dander. The symptoms of itch and signs of this condition can be seasonal or chronic depending on the duration of exposure to the allergen.

Objective

Ocular signs of hay fever conjunctivitis include conjunctival injection, chemosis, and tearing. Associated signs include allergic rhinitis, mild asthmatic reaction, and sinusitis.

Plan

In mild cases, application of cool compresses and topical antihistamines and decongestants can provide symptomatic relief. Oral antihistamines and topical corticosteroids may be helpful in more severe cases. Mast cell stabilizers are particularly useful in preventing recurrences with a known seasonal course and can be used alone or in combination with antihistamines or corticosteroids. Again, the best treatment is prevention by avoiding the allergen altogether.

VERNAL AND ATOPIC CONJUNCTIVITIS

Subjective

Vernal and atopic conjunctivitis are allergic reactions most commonly found in young people, particularly males. Vernal conjunctivitis is characterized by seasonal bouts of severe itching, usually in the spring and fall. Atopic conjunctivitis does not show seasonality. Although these two conditions are sometimes considered separately, a large percentage of patients with vernal conjunctivitis also have a history of atopic conjunctivitis.

Objective

Both vernal and atopic conjunctivitis are characterized by marked papillary reaction of the palpebral conjunctiva. A white, ropy discharge is often present. White Horner-Trantas' dots within limbal papillae and shield corneal ulcers are occasionally seen in association with vernal conjunctivitis. Conjunctival scrapings prepared with Giemsa or Diff-Quik stains reveal numerous eosinophils in vernal conjunctivitis. Atopic conjunctivitis is usually accompanied by eczema on the face, trunk, or extremities.

Plan

Application of cool compresses and topical antihistamines and decongestants can provide symptomatic relief in mild cases. Mast cell stabilizers, oral antihistamines, and topical corticosteroids may be helpful in more severe cases. Sometimes the only effective treatment for patients with severe vernal conjunctivitis is moving to a different climate.

GIANT PAPILLARY CONJUNCTIVITIS RELATED TO CONTACT LENS WEAR

Subjective

Giant papillary conjunctivitis is a condition most commonly associated with contact lens wear, although it is occasionally seen in patients wearing ocular prostheses. Symptoms include itching, burning, fluctuating vision, and generalized contact lens intolerance.

Objective

Giant papillary conjunctivitis is characterized by papillary hypertrophy, especially in the superior tarsal region. It is often associated with a stringy, mucoid discharge.

Plan

Giant papillary conjunctivitis is thought to be an inflammatory reaction to protein buildup on the contact lens; therefore, initial treatment usually involves cleaning or replacing the lens. Changing lens materials, cleaning solutions, or wearing schedule, or placing the patient on a frequent lens replacement program can also be helpful. Mast cell stabilizers and topical corticosteroids may be helpful in treating especially symptomatic patients. In particularly recalcitrant cases, discontinuance of contact lens wear is the treatment of choice.

SUTURE BARB CONJUNCTIVITIS

Subjective

One source of itching is a loose or exposed suture after intraocular surgery. It is anticipated that this problem will be encountered less frequently as the use of sutureless techniques in cataract surgery increases.

Objective

Close examination of the superior limbal area enhanced with fluorescein stain typically reveals a loose suture or exposed suture barb. The adjacent palpebral conjunctiva may be hyperemic or show a papillary response.

Plan

The offending suture should be removed with forceps when appropriate, and the area should be treated prophylactically with a topical antibiotic.

DEMODICOSIS

Subjective

Demodicosis is caused by an overabundance of the *Demodex* mites normally found in small numbers on the eyelids. This condition most commonly occurs in older adults and persons with diabetes. It is characterized by chronic itching and burning of the eyelids.

Objective

A cuffing or "tenting" of epithelial cells around the base of the cilia is sometimes observable through the slit lamp in patients with demodicosis. Madarosis is occasionally present. A particularly helpful diagnostic technique is to epilate several cilia and examine them through a clinical microscope for the presence of the mite larvae.

Plan

Management of demodicosis involves frequent lid scrubs and heavy application of an ophthalmic ointment on the lid margins at bedtime. This treatment is thought to trap the mites during their nocturnal migration.

PHTHIRIASIS

Subjective

Phthiriasis is an infestation of the lids usually by the pubic louse, *Phthirus pubis*. Phthiriasis is usually transmitted through sexual contact. The lids are less commonly infested by the head louse, *Pediculus humanis capitis*. Both types of louse infestation are associated with poor hygiene. Patients with this condition tend to complain of chronic itching of the lids.

Objective

In phthiriasis, adult lice may be observed through the slit lamp clinging to the cilia. Egg cases or nits attached to the cilia and reddish-brown debris at the base of the lashes may also be observed.

Plan

Treatment of phthiriasis initially involves removing the adult lice and nits with forceps. Heavy application of ophthalmic ointment twice a day is somewhat effective in smothering remaining parasites. Washing the head and body with a pediculicidal shampoo such as lindane may also be of benefit. Laundering clothing and bedding in very hot water and avoiding infested hosts can help prevent reinfestation.

SUGGESTED READING

Bartlett JD, Jaanus SD. Clinical Ocular Pharmacology (3rd ed). Boston: Butterworth–Heinemann, 1995.

Cullom RD, Chang B. The Wills Eye Manual: Office and Emergency Room Diagnosis and Treatment of Eye Disease (2nd ed). Philadelphia: Lippincott, 1994.

Fraunfelder FT, Roy FH. Current Ocular Therapy 4. Philadelphia: Saunders, 1995.

van Heuven WÅJ, Zwaan JT. Decision Making in Ophthalmology. St. Louis: Mosby–Year Book, 1992.

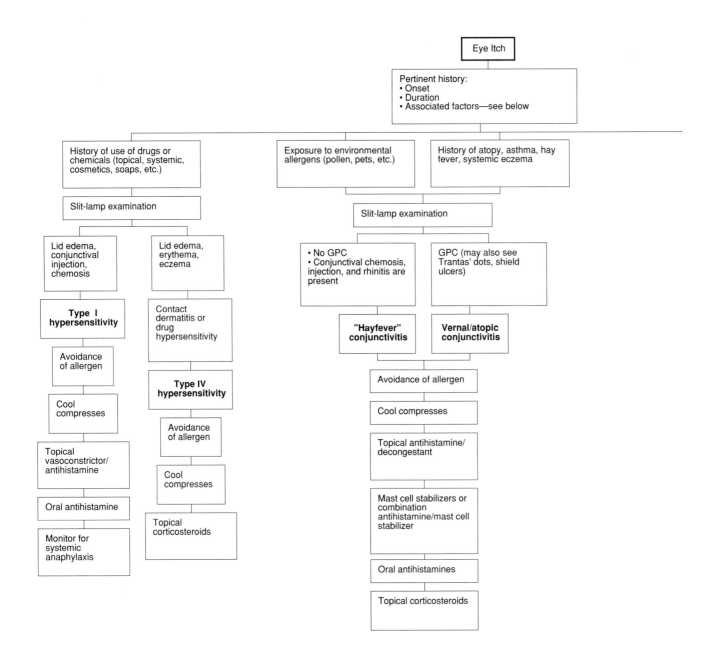

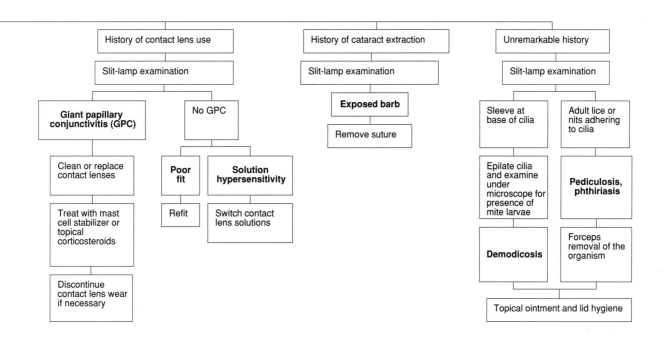

11

Eye Pain

Frank P. LaRussa

EYE PAIN AT A GLANCE

Scratchy or foreign body sensation
   Bacterial keratoconjunctivitis
   Viral keratoconjunctivitis
   Dry-eye syndrome
   Exposure keratitis
   Entropion and trichiasis
   Foreign body
   Abrasion
   Recurrent erosion
   Corneal ulcer
   Ultraviolet keratitis
   Toxic keratitis
   Contact lens overwear
   Episcleritis
   Pinguecula
   Inflamed pterygium
Ache or throbbing pain
   Hordeolum
   Preseptal cellulitis
   Orbital cellulitis
   Uveitis
   Angle-closure glaucoma
   Scleritis
   Accommodative dysfunction
   Uncorrected refractive error
   Wound leak
   Benign neuralgia
   Endophthalmitis
   Optic neuritis
   Migraine
   Herpes zoster
   Trigeminal neuralgia
   Benign neuralgia
   Sinusitis

Secondary to dental work
Use of miotics

When a patient presents with the complaint of pain in the eye, the first step is to determine the type of sensation. Eye pain can generally be divided into two categories: (1) scratchy or foreign body sensation, and (2) deep ache or throbbing pain. Once this initial determination is made, the clinician can narrow down the possible diagnoses.

SCRATCHY OR FOREIGN BODY SENSATION

Bacterial Keratoconjunctivitis

Subjective
Patients with bacterial keratoconjunctivitis usually complain of sticky, irritated, red eyes. They often mention that their eyelids are mattered in the morning. More severe pain may indicate a bacterial or acanthamoebal corneal ulcer.

Objective
Biomicroscopy reveals conjunctival injection, papillary hypertrophy, and superficial punctate keratitis. Mucopurulent discharge is often present. Culturing and Gram's staining are recommended in severe cases or in cases in which the purulent discharge is significant. If an infiltrate with an overlying epithelial defect is present, the diagnosis is ulcerative keratitis.

Plan
Bacterial conjunctivitis is initially treated with instillation of a topical broad-spectrum antibiotic such as gentamicin, tobramycin, or trimethoprim–polymyxin B. Subsequent therapy may be modified based on the results of culturing and sensitivity testing. If ulcerative keratitis is present, Gram's stain and a culture are advised. Ocuflux and/or

fortified antibiotics are advised until cultures definitively identify the organism.

Viral Keratoconjunctivitis/Adenovirus

Subjective
Patients with adenovirus usually complain of eye discomfort and significant tearlike discharge, but no mucus or purulence. The patient often has a history of a recent upper respiratory tract infection or contact with someone with a red eye. In some cases, the patient complains of blurred vision.

Objective
Biomicroscopy reveals a hyperemic bulbar conjunctiva and tarsal follicles. Palpable preauricular nodes are often present. In some adenoviral infections, subepithelial infiltrates may develop after the first week of infection. Small subconjunctival hemorrhages also may be noted in some forms of viral keratoconjunctivitis.

Plan
If visual acuity is not affected by infiltrates, instillation of artificial tears and application of cool compresses are recommended for treatment. Vasoconstrictor antihistamines such as naphazoline hydrochloride–pheniramine maleate give symptomatic relief. Topical steroids may be used if visual acuity is significantly reduced secondary to infiltrates or if pseudomembranes develop. Pseudomembranes may be gently peeled off before administration of topical steroids. The clinician should monitor carefully for recurrence of infiltrates when tapering a steroid.

Dry-Eye Syndrome

Subjective
Patients with dry eyes often complain of scratchy, burning eyes or a foreign body sensation. Dry-eye problems are most common among the elderly.

Objective
Patients with dry eyes have an interpalpebral keratitis that is easily detected with fluorescein stain. Rose bengal may also stain the cornea or interpalpebral conjunctiva. Patients with dry eye often have a decreased tear meniscus, reduced tear break-up time, and diminished Schirmer strip wetting.

Plan
Patients with dry eyes should be prescribed artificial tears for daytime use and bland ointments for nighttime use. Medications counseling and the use of room humidifiers may also be helpful. In more severe cases, punctal plug or laser punctal occlusion should be considered. Lateral tarsorrhaphy should be considered only as a last resort.

Exposure Keratitis

Subjective
Patients with exposure keratitis often complain of scratchy eyes. The sensation of sand in the eyes is common.

Objective
Patients with exposure keratitis have interpalpebral keratitis visible with fluorescein staining. They may have an incomplete blink, nocturnal lagophthalmos, or exophthalmos.

Plan
Patients with exposure keratitis should initially be treated with artificial tears and bland ointments. Taping the lids closed at night may be considered for nocturnal lagophthalmos. In extreme cases of damaging exposure, a partial or total tarsorrhaphy should be considered. When exophthalmos exists, underlying conditions such as thyroid disease should be ruled out.

Entropion and Spastic Entropion

Subjective
Patients with entropion often complain of a scratchy eye due to trichiasis. Entropion is most commonly found in the elderly.

Objective
Entropion is characterized by an inward turning of the lower lid, which allows lashes to touch the cornea. In spastic cases, this may occur only with a hard blink. Fluorescein staining reveals a tracking pattern of keratitis secondary to the lash trauma.

Plan
Lash epilation, gluing or taping the lid lightly to the cheek, or bandage contact lenses may provide temporary relief, but the best treatment for persistent entropion is surgical intervention.

Foreign Body

Subjective
Patients with a corneal or conjunctival foreign body usually complain of a scratchy eye. They are often aware of a recent foreign body insult. The clinician should carefully document the mechanism of injury: whether it was work related, whether safety glasses were being worn at the time of injury, and what first aid measures were taken.

Objective
Biomicroscopy usually reveals a foreign body on the cornea or conjunctiva. The lid should be everted to look for for-

eign bodies on the superior tarsal conjunctiva. If the foreign body did not become imbedded in the corneal or conjunctival tissue, fluorescein staining only reveals an abrasion.

Plan

The clinician must first determine the depth of the foreign body. A Seidel test and dilated fundus examination should be performed to rule out a perforating foreign body. High-velocity particles, such as metal thrown from a metal grinder, have an increased likelihood of causing a perforation.

Superficial foreign bodies can be removed with a spud or needle. Antibiotic drops or ointments should be prescribed, and the eye should be patched or bandaged with a contact lens if necessary. Topical nonsteroidal anti-inflammatory agents, cyclopegics, and oral analgesics can be used to reduce pain. If the foreign body is metallic and leaves a metallic rust ring, this ring should be removed with an Alger brush or Orthobur. If the foreign body is deep, is on the visual axis, or has perforated the globe, the patient should be referred to an ophthalmic surgeon.

Recurrent Corneal Erosion

Subjective

Patients with recurrent corneal erosion typically complain of a sharp, scratchy pain on awakening. The patient often has a past history of a sharp corneal insult, epithelial basement membrane disease, other corneal dystrophy, refractive surgery, or metaherpetic keratitis.

Objective

Biomicroscopy reveals an area of positive fluorescein staining within an area of negative staining.

Plan

The patient with recurrent corneal erosion may be treated initially with prophylactic topical antibiotic, cycloplegic, pressure patching, or bandage contact lenses, followed by administration of topical hyperosmotic drops and ointments for several months once the epithelium has healed. In persistent cases, needle stromal puncture or excimer laser phototherapeutic keratectomy should be considered.

DULL ACHE OR THROBBING PAIN

Anterior Uveitis

Subjective

The patient usually complains of a dull, aching pain in the eye and photophobia. The patient may have a history of similar episodes.

Objective

Slit-lamp biomicroscopy reveals cells, flare, or fibrin in the anterior chamber, and circumlimbal hyperemia. The affected pupil is often miotic. The presence of keratic precipitates should be noted. Fine precipitates are associated with non-granulomatous uveitis, and large mutton-fat precipitates are associated with granulomatous uveitis. Posterior synechiae may be present in more severe or chronic cases.

Plan

Mild to moderate cases may be treated with a topical cycloplegic agent such as homatropine and a steroid such as prednisolone acetate. The dosage of the steroid should be modified depending on the severity of the condition. Systemic or periorbital steroids may be administered in nonresponsive cases. In recurrent, severe, bilateral or granulomatous cases, laboratory or radiologic evaluation is indicated to rule out underlying systemic disease such as ankylosing spondylitis, inflammatory bowel disease, syphilis, sarcoidosis, or tuberculosis. Systemic evaluation is also indicated in cases of pediatric uveitis not associated with trauma. A dilated fundus examination should be performed on all patients with anterior uveitis to rule out posterior uveitis.

Hordeolum

Subjective

Patients with a hordeolum usually complain about dull pain in the lid region. Often the patient mentions an area of redness or swelling, or a lump in the affected lid.

Objective

The external examination reveals a well-circumscribed eyelid nodule. The nodule is red, warm, and tender to the touch.

Plan

Application of warm compresses and light massage are often the initial treatment. Topical antibiotics do not penetrate the lesion well but may be used to reduce the incidence of conjunctivitis secondary to a draining hordeolum. The point of a hordeolum may be punctured to initiate drainage. Oral antibiotics such as dicloxacillin or doxycycline may be used in persistent cases. Intralesional steroid injection or incision and curettage should be considered once the lesion is no longer tender and has become a chalazion.

Preseptal Cellulitis

Subjective

Patients with preseptal cellulitis often complain of a sore eye but do not have the severe pain and restricted motility on attempted eye movement or the proptosis associated with orbital cellulitis. Patients with preseptal cellulitis often complain of a swollen lid. They may have a history of a nonresolving hordeolum, trauma to the lid, or sinus infection.

Objective
External examination reveals a diffuse area of swelling on the lid. The lid also is hyperemic and warm to the touch. The patient does not show proptosis or restricted eye movements.

Plan
Mild cases may be treated with oral antibiotics such as amoxicillin-clavulanate or cefaclor. More severe cases or pediatric cases require hospitalization and intravenous administration of antibiotics.

Accommodative Dysfunction
Subjective
Patients with accommodative dysfunction often complain of dull pain in the eyes. This complaint is also common in early presbyopes or uncorrected hyperopes or astigmats. The pain is usually associated with prolonged near work.

Objective
Tests of accommodative function such as the push-up amplitude or plus/minus flippers reveal reduced ability or facility.

Plan
Correction of refractive error, prescription of a near add, or vision therapy usually provides symptomatic relief.

Angle-Closure Glaucoma (Primary Pupil Block)

Subjective
Patients with acute angle-closure glaucoma complain of dull pain in and above the eye. They often note blurry vision and the appearance of haloes around lights. They may also be nauseated.

Objective
Pupillary testing reveals a fixed, mid-dilated pupil. Biomicroscopy reveals corneal edema and conjunctival injection. The intraocular pressure is usually elevated above 30 mm Hg, and gonioscopy reveals a closed angle.

Plan
The initial management of angle closure consists of attempting to lower intraocular pressure through the instillation of topical beta blockers, pilocarpine (1% or 2%), or alpha-agonists, and oral administration of carbonic anhydrase inhibitors or hyperosmotics. Pilocarpine is not effective until the intraocular pressure is below approximately 50 mm Hg and should be avoided in patients with aphakic, pseudophakic, or mechanical angle closure. Once the intraocular pressure is under reasonable control, laser iridotomy is indicated.

Benign Neuralgia
Subjective
Patients with benign neuralgia complain of occasional sharp, brief, stabbing pain in the eye.

Objective
A comprehensive examination—including measurement of visual acuity, pupillary responses, and extraocular motilities, as well as perimetry, biomicroscopy, tonometry, and ophthalmoscopy—reveals no abnormal findings.

Plan
If the patient has had recent dental work, he or she should be referred to his or her dentist. Otherwise, the patient should be reassured, and a follow-up examination should be performed in 1 week. If the condition persists, refer the patient to a neurologist.

Postsurgical Wound Leak
Subjective
The patient with postsurgical wound leak may complain of an intensely throbbing eye. There is usually a history of recent intraocular surgery.

Objective
The characteristic signs of this condition are reduced visual acuity, low intraocular pressure, and a positive Seidel's sign. The pupil may be peaked pointing to the wound leak. The lids, anterior chamber, and vitreous should be examined carefully to rule out endophthalmitis.

Plan
The patient should be immediately referred to the surgeon for wound repair.

SUGGESTED READING

Bartlett JD, Jaanus SD. Clinical Ocular Pharmacology (3rd ed). Boston: Butterworth–Heinemann, 1995.

Cullom RD, Chang B. The Wills Eye Manual: Office and Emergency Room Diagnosis and Treatment of Eye Disease (2nd ed). Philadelphia: Lippincott, 1994.

Roy FH. Ocular Differential Diagnosis (5th ed). Philadelphia: Lea & Febiger, 1993.

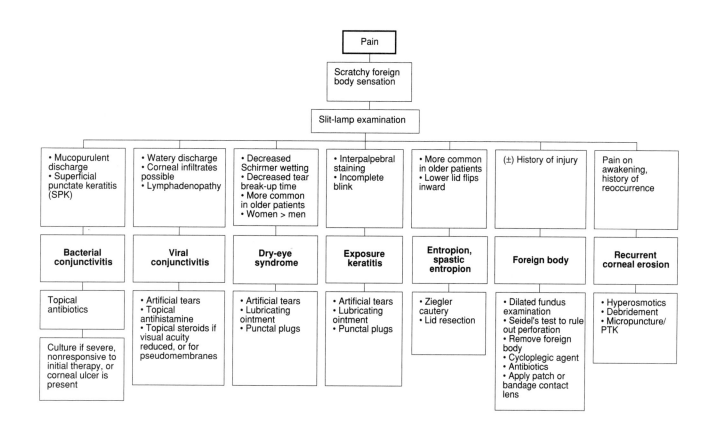

Pain

Scratchy foreign body sensation

Slit-lamp examination

• Mucopurulent discharge • Superficial punctate keratitis (SPK)	• Watery discharge • Corneal infiltrates possible • Lymphadenopathy	• Decreased Schirmer wetting • Decreased tear break-up time • More common in older patients • Women > men	• Interpalpebral staining • Incomplete blink	• More common in older patients • Lower lid flips inward	(±) History of injury	Pain on awakening, history of reoccurrence
Bacterial conjunctivitis	**Viral conjunctivitis**	**Dry-eye syndrome**	**Exposure keratitis**	**Entropion, spastic entropion**	**Foreign body**	**Recurrent corneal erosion**
Topical antibiotics	• Artificial tears • Topical antihistamine • Topical steroids if visual acuity reduced, or for pseudomembranes	• Artificial tears • Lubricating ointment • Punctal plugs	• Artificial tears • Lubricating ointment • Punctal plugs	• Ziegler cautery • Lid resection	• Dilated fundus examination • Seidel's test to rule out perforation • Remove foreign body • Cycloplegic agent • Antibiotics • Apply patch or bandage contact lens	• Hyperosmotics • Debridement • Micropuncture/ PTK
Culture if severe, nonresponsive to initial therapy, or corneal ulcer is present						

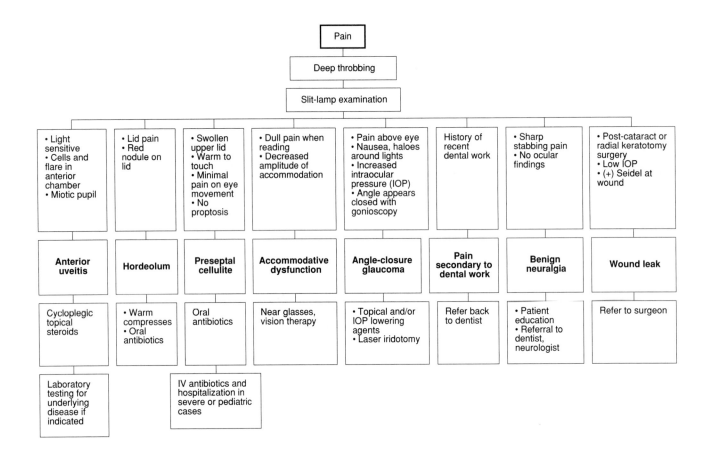

12

Photophobia

David P. Sendrowski

Abnormal visual intolerance of light is common in lightly pigmented persons. Usually it is without significance and may be relieved by wearing dark glasses. It is an important but nondiagnostic symptom in such entities as keratitis, uveitis, acute glaucoma, traumatic corneal epithelial abrasions, and after ocular surgery.

A new or sudden onset of photophobia should alert the clinician to look for an underlying ocular disease. Of particular concern to the clinician is a careful evaluation of the corneal epithelium, anterior chamber, and posterior segment of the eye.

ANIRIDIA

Subjective

Aniridia is the underdevelopment of the iris. This condition may be associated with many anterior segment anomalies. The patient with aniridia may or may not present with the initial complaint of photophobia.

Aniridia occurs bilaterally and has an autosomal dominant mode of inheritance. The history should focus on any family history of ocular diseases. The parents or patient should be asked if there are any other associated systemic abnormalities concurrent with the aniridia. The clinician should also determine whether other siblings in the family may also be affected by ocular or systemic diseases. Aniridia can arise spontaneously, but such spontaneous occurrence is usually in association with Wilms' tumor.

Objective

The entrance testing should include a complete examination of the anterior segment. Gonioscopy should be performed, because the condition is usually associated with glaucoma. The occurrence of glaucoma correlates with the adhesion of the peripheral iris to the trabecular meshwork. Examination of the cornea may reveal central scarring, hazy appearance, and superficial vascularization, which develop during the first and second decades of life. The corneal changes are usually associated with a very diminished tear break-up time and a deficiency of tears. These problems may be revealed with sodium fluorescein staining and Schirmer tear testing. Congenital lens opacities are frequently found.

A fundus examination should be performed using a high plus lens to evaluate the optic nerve head and the macula. Macular aplasia is present at birth in patients with hereditary aniridia, and it correlates with the diminished vision and nystagmus. Visual fields should be tested using a tangent screen, especially if there is diminished visual acuity and a searching type of nystagmus.

Plan

If signs of corneal involvement are found, the patient should be referred to a corneal specialist for an evaluation. If there is evidence of glaucoma, the patient may respond to topical beta blockers and oral carbonic anhydrase inhibitors (e.g., timolol maleate and acetazolamide). The use of custom opaque contact lenses may be helpful to the patient, both for refractive correction and for glare reduction. Cataract extraction may be indicated in some cases.

The patient should be followed at intervals of every few months or sooner, depending on the severity and type of associated ocular disease that is being monitored. When aniridia is diagnosed in a patient without a family history of the disorder, the patient should be referred to an internist or gastroenterologist for thorough evaluation of the abdomen to rule out Wilms' tumor. It is also recommended that the parents be advised about genetic counseling, especially if they have plans for future offspring.

MACULAR DYSTROPHIES AND ACHROMATOPSIA

Subjective

There are a number of different types of macular dystrophy. The patient with macular dystrophy typically presents with a complaint of slowly progressive bilateral vision loss with associated photophobia and color vision loss. The vision is usually better at night than during the day.

The family history is important for the diagnosis of ocular hereditary disorders. The patient should be asked specifically about any previous diagnoses of age-related macular degeneration, Stargardt's disease, central areolar choroidal atrophy, congenital color blindness, retinitis pigmentosa, optic neuropathies, vitelliform dystrophy (Best's disease), progressive cone-rod dystrophy, familial drusen, and butterfly pigment dystrophy of the fovea.

The patient's medication list should be thoroughly evaluated, and the patient should be asked specifically about the use of chloroquine.

Objective

Entrance testing should include a pupil examination to rule out optic nerve involvement, and color vision test-

ing. An Amsler grid test is useful in screening for central field loss. A more formalized visual field test (e.g., macular threshold, or central 10-2) can be very helpful in revealing a decrease in macular sensitivity.

A dilated fundus examination with a high plus lens examination of the macula and optic nerve head should be performed in both eyes. The entire retina should be evaluated with indirect ophthalmoscopy to rule out tapetoretinal degenerations.

Additional testing should include electrodiagnostics. An electro-oculogram is particularly useful in the diagnosis of Best's disease, and an electroretinogram is useful in ruling out certain other retinal diseases. Blood testing should be considered if a medication (e.g., chloroquine) is believed to be the cause of the dystrophy. Fluorescein angiography may provide additional information about the extent of macular involvement.

Plan

There is no treatment for a macular dystrophy. If the condition is secondary to use of a medication (e.g., chloroquine), the internist should be contacted and the medication reduced or changed if indicated.

The photophobia can be somewhat reduced through the use of solar shields or tinted spectacles. The use of miotic drops has been suggested to help reduce the photophobia and glare, especially during the day. A vision rehabilitation evaluation is recommended to determine whether the patient's remaining vision may be enhanced with low vision aids.

CORNEAL FOREIGN BODY

Subjective

The patient with a corneal foreign body should have some history of a traumatic event. Commonly, the patient can relate an event during which a foreign body is suspected to have entered the eye. It is important to gather as much information as possible about the foreign body and the event. If the patient was working near high-velocity projectiles at the time, penetration of the globe should be suspected. The patient should also be asked if any protective eyewear was being worn at the time of the injury. The patient may also have associated symptoms of photophobia, tearing, blurry vision, and foreign body sensation. These symptoms will be reported to varying degrees. It is important that the clinician rule out the presence of a vegetational foreign body, as contact with such material may lead to the development of a fungal keratitis.

Objective

The external adnexa should be evaluated for signs of penetrating injury before the internal examination is begun. The anterior chamber should be well-formed, and the pupillary responses should be normal. Visual acuity should be documented before and after any corneal procedure.

Sodium fluorescein staining is very helpful in locating the corneal foreign body. The upper lid should be everted to rule out the presence of any additional foreign bodies. This step is especially important if the sodium fluorescein stain reveals a linear type of epithelial damage to the cornea. Biomicroscopy is helpful in locating the corneal foreign body. In the event that no biomicroscope is available, a high plus loop worn over the examiner's spectacles can be useful in locating the foreign body. The anterior chamber angle should be evaluated for any sign of reaction (e.g., cells and flare).

Once the foreign body is located, the eye should be anesthetized and the foreign body removed. After the foreign body is removed, it should be evaluated under the biomicroscope to ascertain the composition of the material. Rust rings may develop from metallic foreign bodies. If a rust ring is present, it should be removed with an Alger brush or similar instrument. The size of the epithelial defect should be measured so that the healing process can be followed over time.

The eye should be dilated and the retina examined for any sign of perforating injury (e.g., retinal hemorrhage) or intraocular foreign body.

Plan

After removal of the foreign body, a broad-spectrum topical antibiotic ointment (e.g., bacitracin–polymyxin B) and a topical cycloplegic agent (e.g., homatropine) should be instilled into the eye. A pressure patch is then put over the eye for 24 hours to allow healing. In many cases, a bandage contact lens may be used as an alternative to patching. The patch should be removed in 24 hours, and the epithelial defect should be evaluated. If initial healing is good, a prophylactic topical antibiotic solution (e.g., ofloxacin) may be prescribed. The patient should be followed every 2–3 days after removal of the patch or until the corneal defect is completely healed.

CONJUNCTIVAL OR CORNEAL ABRASION

Subjective

Patients with a conjunctival or corneal abrasion are usually in pain. The patient may have associated symptoms of photophobia, tearing, and foreign body sensation, and a history of trauma. Common traumatic events include contact lens–related abrasions and blunt trauma to the anterior segment.

Objective

Depending on the severity of the abrasion, the periocular tissues should be evaluated for any signs of laceration or abrasion. Testing of the pupillary reactions may show a slightly miotic pupil in the affected eye.

Biomicroscopic evaluation with sodium fluorescein staining is the best method to locate the abrasion and assess its size and extent. The abrasion should be well-documented. The upper lid should be everted to make sure there are no additional foreign bodies.

Plan

If the abrasion is large, the patient should be given a broad-spectrum topical antibiotic (e.g., tobramycin) and a topical cycloplegic agent (e.g., homatropine), and pressure patched for 24 hours. The patient should be seen within 24 hours to have the patch removed and the size of the abrasion evaluated. If the abrasion is unchanged or the patient is still in pain, the patient should be pressure patched for another 24-hour period with additional antibiotic and cycloplegic agents. In many cases, a bandage contact lens can be used as an alternative to pressure patching. The use of a topical analgesic (e.g., diclofenac sodium) may eliminate the need for patching or bandage contact lens. As the defect begins to heal and the symptoms subside, the patient may only need a topical antibiotic solution (e.g., tobramycin) for prophylaxis.

If the patient is a contact lens wearer, the patient should not be patched and should be watched very closely for development of a corneal ulcer.

The patient should be followed every 2–4 days until the area has healed and there are no signs of infection or epithelial defects.

TRAUMATIC IRITIS

Subjective

Trauma to the eye can result in abrasion, laceration, or perforation of the lids, cornea, conjunctiva, or globe. Iritis can result from blunt trauma through irritation of the trigeminal nerve (cranial nerve V). The patient may complain of pain and photophobia, typically several days after blunt trauma to the eye. The patient may also complain of tearing and blurred vision.

Objective

The external examination may show evidence of the blunt trauma, such as ecchymosis, subconjunctival hemorrhage, and abrasions to the periocular tissues. The pupil examination often reveals pupillary miosis resulting from inflammation or trauma to the sphincter muscle of the iris. At first, the intraocular pressure may be low due to damage to the ciliary body and compression of aqueous fluid out of the eye. After several days, the intraocular pressure may be elevated due to trabecular inflammation or the clogging of the trabecular meshwork by inflammatory debris. Later, the chamber angle should be evaluated with a gonioscopic lens to look for evidence of angle recession.

Biomicroscopic examination of the anterior chamber may show evidence of cells and possibly flare. The anterior chamber should also be evaluated for hyphema. A dilated examination should be performed to rule out traumatic retinal detachment, commotio retinae, choroidal rupture, and other types of posterior segment involvement.

Plan

Initial treatment for traumatic iritis is the use of a long-acting cycloplegic agent (e.g., homatropine). If the anterior chamber reaction is severe or if the cells do not diminish within a few days of initiating cycloplegic therapy, a topical steroid (e.g., prednisolone acetate 1%) should be added. The frequency of the steroid drops is varied depending on the severity of the reaction. The patient may also benefit from the use of an oral nonsteroidal anti-inflammatory medication (e.g., ibuprofen) to relieve or reduce the ocular pain. The patient should be followed every 2 or 3 days to evaluate the resolution of the anterior chamber reaction.

The patient should be referred to an ophthalmic surgeon if there is any evidence of posterior segment involvement.

IDIOPATHIC ANTERIOR UVEITIS

Subjective

The patient with acute idiopathic iritis complains of a sudden onset of eye pain, redness, and photophobia without history of trauma. The condition is almost always unilateral. The patient is commonly between the ages of 18 and 50. Other associated signs that the patient may have are decreased vision and tearing.

The medical and ocular histories are usually unrelated to an idiopathic uveitis, although thorough medical and ocular histories should be obtained. The ocular history should not include the occurrence of a previous attack of iritis. If it does, the clinician should become suspicious of a systemic etiology.

Objective

The first goal of the examination is to rule out an infectious or inflammatory conjunctivitis and acute glaucoma. The entrance testing should include a pupil examination. In iritis, the pupil in the affected eye is miotic, whereas in acute glaucoma, it is fixed and dilated. Conjunctivitis does not affect pupillary response. Externally, the vasculature in the limbal area is engorged and reddened so that there is circumlimbal flush. The patient may also have a ptosis in the affected eye secondary to the blepharospasm. Confrontation fields usually suffice for field testing.

The biomicroscope with conical beam illumination should be used to evaluate the inflammatory reaction in the anterior chamber. In idiopathic iritis, the clinician may note cells and flare. Cells are usually more prominent than flare in the early stages of the inflammation. The intraocular pressure is initially lowered secondary to ciliary body inflammation and may rise as time passes.

A binocular indirect ophthalmoscopic fundus examination should be performed to rule out the possibility of a posterior inflammatory etiology for the anterior chamber reaction.

Plan

The patient should be put on a long-acting cycloplegic agent (e.g., homatropine) to reduce synechia formation. The inflammation should be treated with topical steroids (e.g., prednisolone acetate) every 1–4 hours depending on the severity of the reaction. A topical beta blocker (e.g., timolol maleate) can be used to reduce the intraocular pressure if it is elevated.

The follow-up should occur between 24 and 48 hours after the initial examination so that the clinician can evaluate the effect of the topical steroid and make sure the patient is complying well with the treatment schedule. The intraocular pressure and cornea should be checked at each follow-up visit. The administration of topical steroids should be based on the anterior chamber reaction. If the anterior chamber reaction shows improvement, the steroids can be slowly tapered. The patient should be seen several months after the inflammation has resolved to document residual ocular effects.

POSTERIOR SEGMENT INFLAMMATION

Subjective

If the posterior segment is affected by inflammation, the patient may complain about photophobia. It will not be the only complaint and is likely to be accompanied by several other complaints.

In retrobulbar neuritis and papillitis, the photophobia may be accompanied by orbital pain with eye movements, loss of color vision, reduced perception of light intensity, or vision loss. The vision loss may be exacerbated with exercise or increase in body temperature (Uhthoff syndrome).

In posterior scleritis, the patient may also complain of severe boring eye pain, which can radiate to the forehead, brow, or jaw and can awaken the patient from sleep. A loss of color vision, decreased visual acuity, and a deeply injected red eye may also be present.

In posterior uveitis, the photophobia may be accompanied by an increase in vitreous floaters, loss of vision, glare, and occasional redness and pain.

Photophobia is part of the complaint for each condition, but the associated symptoms help to delineate the etiology.

Objective

The patient should be given a thorough examination. This examination should include pupil testing to rule out an afferent pupillary defect, which suggests an optic nerve problem. Color vision testing and motility testing can also help to localize an optic nerve disorder.

The pupil should be dilated, and the optic nerve head, peripheral retina, macula, and vitreous should be examined with binocular indirect ophthalmoscopy and high plus fundus lenses. The clinician should look for cells in the vitreous, inflammatory lesions of the retina, blurring of the disc margins, white blood cells in front of the optic nerve head, and macular integrity. Threshold visual field testing may be of some help in the diagnosis.

Plan

Treatment varies widely depending on the cause of the condition. In the case of retrobulbar neuritis and papillitis, the patient may benefit from intravenous administration of methylprednisolone for 3–4 days followed by oral administration of prednisone as used in the optic neuritis treatment trial.

In cases of posterior scleritis and uveitis, the patient should be referred for laboratory testing, which may include Lyme immunofluorescent assay and enzyme-linked immunosorbent assay, and measurement of *Toxoplasma* titer, angiotensin-converting enzyme level, rapid plasma reagin level, fluorescent treponemal antibody absorption rate, erythrocyte sedimentation rate, antinuclear antibody level, levels of HLA-B5 and HLA-B27, *Toxocara* titer, and titers for cytomegalovirus and herpes simplex. A computed tomographic or magnetic resonance imaging scan may also be performed. A retinal specialist as well as a rheumatologist may need to be consulted.

SUGGESTED READING

Easty DL, Smolin G. External Eye Disease. Oxford, UK: Butterworth, 1985.

Nussenblatt RP, Palestine AG (eds). Uveitis, Fundamentals and Clinical Practice (2nd ed). St. Louis: Mosby–Year Book, 1996.

Yanoff M, Fine B. Ocular Pathology: A Text and Atlas (4th ed). Philadelphia: Lippincott, 1995.

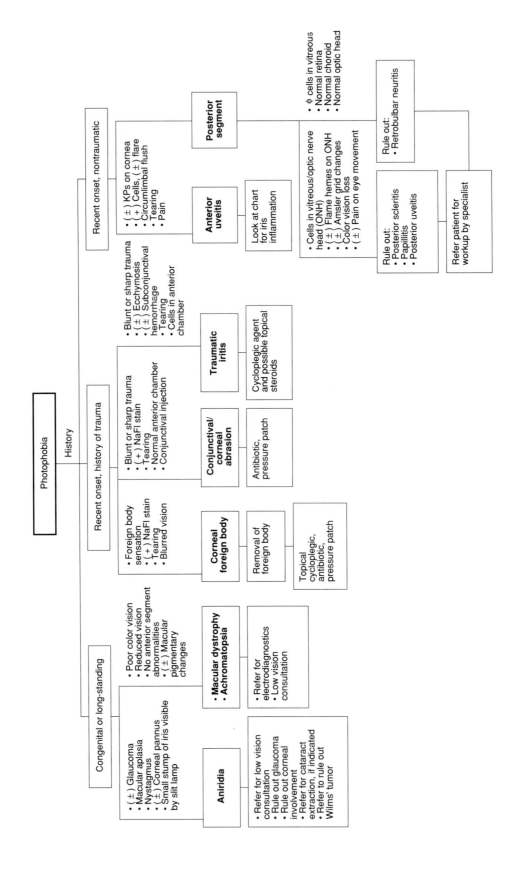

13

Headache

DAVID P. SENDROWSKI

HEADACHE AT A GLANCE

Acute, rapid onset
  Subarachnoid hemorrhage
  Cerebrovascular disease
  Meningitis
  Encephalitis
  Dietary headache
  Febrile headache
  Altitude headache
  Angle-closure glaucoma
Acute, more insidious onset
  Giant cell arteritis
  Intracranial mass
  Pseudotumor cerebri
  Trigeminal neuralgia
  Postherpetic neuralgia
  Hypertensive encephalopathy
  Dental inflammation
  Caffeine withdrawal
Chronic or recurrent
  Tension headache
  Asthenopia
  Migraine
  Cluster headache
  Sinusitis
  Cervical spine disease

Physicians and patients worry about headaches that are persistent, severe, or sudden in onset. Tumor is a common concern when the headache persists. However, only the rare patient has a worrisome cause for headache; thus, it is wasteful to subject all patients to extensive radiologic investigation.

In taking the history, the clinician should question the patient regarding the onset, frequency, severity, location, and duration of the headache, as well as associated symptoms, especially neurologic deficits and fever. A previous history of headaches and head trauma should also be noted. In all patients with headaches, the blood pressure and temperature should be checked for any elevations, the scalp should be examined for cranial artery tenderness, and the sinuses should be checked for tenderness to percussion.

SUBARACHNOID HEMORRHAGE

Subjective

Subarachnoid hemorrhages can occur spontaneously from a ruptured aneurysm or arteriovenous malformation, or can be a result of trauma. The headache caused by a subarachnoid hemorrhage is usually described by the patient as the worst headache the patient has ever had; therefore, the absence of a headache precludes the diagnosis. The headache occurs suddenly and with transient or complete loss of consciousness. Additional symptoms include vomiting and neck stiffness. Hemiparesis and aphasia may also result from the hemorrhage. The headache is not always severe, especially if it is caused by an arteriovenous malformation.

Objective

Before the hemorrhage, an aneurysm of the posterior communicating artery may cause pupillary dilation due to compression of the oculomotor nerve. The pupillary dilation may be in association with ptosis and motility problems of the eyes. Therefore, external examination of pupils, motility, and lid position are very important.

After the hemorrhage has occurred, the intracranial pressure may rise. The optic nerves may show insult from the subarachnoid bleeding or elevated intracranial pressure in the form of papilledema, peripapillary and nerve head hemorrhages, and venous engorgement. Bilateral preretinal or vitreous hemorrhages may also be present.

Plan

The patient should be transported immediately to a medical emergency care facility for evaluation by a neurologist or emergency medical personnel, and a lumbar puncture and diagnostic imaging should be performed.

If there are early signs of pupillary involvement without evidence of optic nerve head changes, the patient should be evaluated to rule out benign causes for the problem and should be referred immediately if indicated.

MENINGITIS OR ENCEPHALITIS

Subjective

Headache is the prominent feature of encephalitis and meningitis. The headache is usually throbbing in nature, bilateral, and occipital or nuchal in location. The headache is worsened by sitting upright, moving the head, and performing a Valsalva maneuver. The patient may also complain of photophobia. The headache usually develops over hours or days and is not sudden in onset.

Stiffness of the neck must be evaluated with care, because it may not be obvious early in the course of the illness. Lethargy and confusion may also be associated with the headache.

Objective

The entrance testing should include pupillary and motility testing. Attention should be paid to the lateral rectus muscles, because meningitis and encephalitis may cause diffuse cerebral edema that forces compression on the abducent nerve. Confrontation visual field testing and red cap testing are also useful in the differential diagnosis.

The dilated fundus examination should help in evaluating the optic nerve heads for evidence of papilledema, which may result from the cerebral edema. The use of high magnification may be of great benefit in detecting early signs of increased intracranial pressure.

Additional testing should include a lumbar puncture for cerebrospinal fluid examination and an imaging series done by a neurologist.

Plan

Because the cause of the inflammation must be determined, the patient should be referred immediately for further evaluation and treatment.

THROMBOTIC OR EMBOLIC STROKE

Subjective

Headache may be associated with a thrombotic or embolic stroke, but it is not the usual presenting sign. The headache is mild to moderate in nature and ipsilateral to the ischemic event. The location is variable based on the location of the thrombus or embolus. Transient ischemic attacks are associated with the headaches in up to half of the cases. Although it is unusual, the headache may precede the other symptoms in some cases. If the thrombosis or embolus occurs in the retinal artery or posterior cerebral artery, the headache may be mistaken for a migraine because of the visual aura associated with the attack. The physical impairment varies depending on the area of cerebral involvement.

Objective

The entrance testing should include pupillary response and motility testing. Confrontation field testing is helpful in localizing the area of thrombosis or embolic event. If formalized threshold field testing can be performed, it can be very informative. Stereopsis testing and optokinetic drum testing can be helpful in isolating parietal involvement. Auscultation of the internal carotid arteries and ophthalmodynamometry may be helpful in identifying the presence of carotid occlusive disease.

The dilated fundus examination is useful in visualizing evidence of embolic plaques in the retinal vasculature. If plaques are present, carotid occlusive disease should be suspected.

Additional testing could include Doppler ultrasonography of the carotid arteries and a magnetic resonance imaging (MRI) or computed tomographic (CT) scan series to localize the area of involvement.

Plan

If there are signs of visual field involvement, the patient should be referred to a neurologist immediately for evaluation and an imaging series. If evidence of retinal emboli is seen, the patient should be referred to a neurologist or cardiologist for evaluation and treatment. The treatment may take the form of oral anticoagulants or surgery.

After treatment, the patient should be seen for visual field testing, carotid evaluation, and dilated fundus examination every 3–4 months until the symptoms are stable. The patient can then be followed twice a year.

ACUTE ANGLE-CLOSURE GLAUCOMA

Subjective

In acute angle-closure glaucoma, the ocular complaints are related to a sudden increase in intraocular pressure. The complaints can include blurred vision, severe ocular pain or frontal headache, colored halos around lights, nausea, and vomiting.

The patient is usually older and female. Aging is associated with enlargement of the crystalline lens, and females have smaller chamber angles.

The attack can occur after retinal laser surgery that causes choroidal swelling or after a scleral buckling procedure. Tumors of the ciliary body may also precipitate an angle-closure attack. Peripheral anterior synechiae caused by uveitis and trabeculitis can also lead to an attack.

Objective

The clinician should note the appearance of the corneal reflex. A dull reflex can indicate an edematous cornea. The pupils are usually fixed and dilated. This finding is an excellent clue that the cause of the red eye is not an iritis or conjunctivitis. A biomicroscopic examination should be performed to look for keratitic precipitates, posterior synechiae, cells and flare, iris neovascularization, and a shallow chamber angle.

Gonioscopy is an important test in the diagnosis of angle closure. However, gonioscopy should be avoided on very edematous corneas because it predisposes the eye to corneal abrasion. If significant corneal edema is present, then gonioscopy should be performed after clearing the corneal epithelial edema with the topical application of glycerin. The procedure can confirm the lack of visible angle structures. Gonioscopy may be performed on the uninvolved eye to assess the angle approach and should be performed in cases of suspected iritic neovascularization or peripheral anterior synechiae to help determine the cause of the angle-closure attack.

Elevated intraocular pressure is the final confirmatory test to make the diagnosis of angle-closure glaucoma.

Plan

Before therapy is begun, the patient's systemic health—including cardiovascular status, presence of other systemic diseases such as diabetes, and any electrolyte imbalance—should be considered. If the intraocular pressure is above 50 mm Hg, the following sequence may be followed: oral carbonic anhydrase inhibitor (e.g., acetazolamide), topical alpha-adrenergic agonist (e.g., apraclonidine), and topical beta blocker (e.g., timolol maleate). As the pressure drops below 50 mm Hg, a topical parasympathomimetic (e.g., pilocarpine) should be initiated, and the intraocular pressure should be monitored every 15–30 minutes. Instillation of pilocarpine in the uninvolved eye should be considered to reduce the likelihood of an attack.

If the attack is of recent onset and there is no corneal edema, corneal compression with a gonioprism may help to open the angle and reduce the intraocular pressure.

After the intraocular pressure has been reduced to a satisfactory level, the patient should undergo a laser peripheral iridotomy. The patient should have baseline visual field testing and disc photography and should be followed on a regular basis.

TEMPORAL ARTERITIS

Subjective

The patient with temporal arteritis (arteritic anterior ischemic optic neuropathy [AION]) is usually 65 years or older. The complaints include a sudden, painless, initially unilateral vision loss. There may be antecedent headache, jaw claudication, scalp tenderness, joint ache, weight loss, fever, and depression occurring before the vision loss.

Medical history should include questions about present illness such as arthritis, polyarteritis, scleroderma, and other rheumatoid disorders.

Objective

The entrance testing should evaluate pupillary responses; the presence of a relative afferent pupillary defect should especially be noted. Other significant findings include loss of color vision, palpable tender and nonpulsable artery, and impaired ocular motility. Perimetry may reveal an altitudinal loss, which is a very useful diagnostic sign in these cases.

The dilated examination may reveal a pale, swollen disc, sometimes with flame hemorrhages. The macula is normal. There is no evidence of white blood cells in front of the optic nerve head.

Additional testing should include blood pressure measurement, a complete blood count, immediate measurement of a Westergren method erythrocyte sedimentation rate (ESR), and temporal artery biopsy, if indicated.

Plan

Arteritic AION is a true ocular emergency. Systemic steroids (e.g., prednisone) should be given immediately once the diagnosis of arteritic AION is suspected. This therapy should be initiated before obtaining a biopsy.

After the diagnosis is confirmed, the initial steroid dose should be maintained for 2–4 weeks or until symptoms reverse and the Westergren ESR normalizes. Treatment dosage should be adjusted according to the Westergren ESR. The treatment may last from 3 months to 1 year. The patient should be followed every 2–4 weeks during treatment, and intraocular pressure and lenticular clarity should be assessed.

INTRACRANIAL MASS

Subjective

Complaints of a new onset of a headache in middle to later life should raise concern about a mass lesion. The headache is usually nonspecific and is mild or moderate in severity. The headache is generally dull and steady and increases in intensity with change in position or maneuvers that increase intracranial pressure (e.g., Valsalva maneuver). The headache is worse on awakening in the morning and may be associated with nausea and vomiting. Some patients may complain about diplopia or transient obscuration of vision. The headache usually increases in severity over time and may be associated with drop attacks or altered consciousness.

Objective

The entrance testing should include pupillary, motility, cranial nerve, and confrontation field testing. Threshold visual field testing should also be performed to check for involvement of the visual pathway. Stereopsis and response to the optokinetic drum may be affected if the lesion is in the parietal lobe.

Phorometry may reveal a divergence insufficiency due to an abducent nerve palsy caused by an increase in intracranial pressure. A dilated fundus examination allows the clinician to use a high plus lens to examine the nerve heads for evidence of papilledema.

Plan

The patient should be referred to a neurologist for examination. Suspicion of an intracranial mass lesion demands prompt evaluation, preferably with CT scan or MRI. Lumbar puncture is not used as a diagnostic screening test, because the results are nonspecific, and the procedure may aggravate the symptoms of the intracranial mass.

PSEUDOTUMOR CEREBRI

Subjective

The patient with pseudotumor cerebri, or benign intracranial hypertension (BIH), is typically a female in her third decade. Obesity has been associated with the disease.

Diffuse headache is almost always a symptom, and diplopia and blurred vision occur in about two-thirds of cases. Patients may report brief or transient obscuration of vision that may also be described as visual blackouts. Nausea and vomiting may also be reported.

The medical history should include questions regarding intracranial venous drainage obstruction, endocrine dysfunction, pregnancy, congestive heart failure, chronic hypercapnia, chronic meningitis, otitis media, and head trauma. Medications such as vitamin and drug therapies should be reviewed, because they may also be a factor in the etiology of the disorder.

Objective

The objective assessment of a patient with suspected pseudotumor cerebri is the same as for intracranial mass.

Plan

The patient should be referred immediately to a neurologist for evaluation. The patient should be evaluated initially as if he or she had an intracranial mass. After an imaging series and lumbar puncture are completed, the diagnosis of pseudotumor cerebri is made by excluding other diseases. Methods of treatment include weight loss if the patient is overweight, prescription of diuretics (e.g., acetazolamide), and discontinuation of any oral medications that may be contributing to the condition. The use of systemic steroids in the treatment of BIH is controversial.

Surgical intervention is initiated in cases in which intractable headaches or visual field or acuity loss occurs. Optic nerve decompression surgery is performed for visual field or acuity loss, and a lumboperitoneal shunt procedure is performed for intractable headaches.

ASTHENOPIA

Subjective

Patients with asthenopia complain of chronic pulling or drawing sensations around the eyes and fatigue or reduced stamina with near visual tasks. Severity of the discomfort typically increases throughout the day. Asthenopia is precipitated by prolonged near work. In addition, the annoying ocular sensations are often aggravated by illness, physical exertion, emotional stress, or a combination of factors, such as one might experience when studying for exams.

The medical history is usually unremarkable with regard to associated systemic diseases. If the patient is taking prescribed or over-the-counter medications, these medications should be assessed for possible ocular side effects. Antianxiety medications are of a particular concern because they may affect accommodation.

Objective

Visual acuity, ocular motility, and pupillary responses are normal. Refraction should be performed to rule out refractive errors such as hyperopia and astigmatism. Visual analysis of the accommodative and binocular systems should be performed. Commonly, the patient manifests poor accommodative facility or a binocular dysfunction.

The ocular health assessment, including tonometry and dilated fundus examination, typically reveals no abnormal findings.

Plan

If refractive error is present, the patient may find relief from spectacle correction. If there are accommodative and binocular dysfunctions, the patient may be referred to a vision training specialist for evaluation and management. Alternatively, the patient may be prescribed a series of ocular exercises to be performed at home. The patient should be seen on a regular basis to assess the effectiveness of the treatment.

TENSION HEADACHE

Subjective

Patients with tension headaches complain of daily attacks of nonthrobbing, bilateral occipital head pain that are not associated with nausea, vomiting, or a prodromal visual disturbance. The pain is usually described as a tight band around the head. More women than men tend to be affected, and the headaches begin usually after age 20. The headaches occur more frequently toward the end of the day and are not present early in the morning.

Medication history is usually positive for the use of aspirin, acetaminophen, or a nonsteroidal anti-inflammatory drug taken to help dissipate the pain. There are no systemic illnesses that predispose individuals to tension headaches; however, the patient's occupation and daily routine can contribute to the development of the headache.

Objective

The clinician should look to rule out more serious causes for the headache. Entrance testing should include tests of pupillary response, ocular motility, confrontation visual fields, and color vision. All entrance tests should be normal. Transillumination of the sinuses should also be performed. A biomicroscopic examination can aid in evaluating the anterior angle chamber depth and inflammatory status. The chamber angle should be open, and there should be no signs of inflammation in the anterior chamber.

Dilation allows examination of the optic nerve heads, which should appear normal. A screening visual field test can be performed to evaluate the integrity of the visual pathways, which should also be normal.

Plan

The patient should be educated about the origin of the headaches. Acute attacks may respond to aspirin, acetaminophen, or other nonsteroidal anti-inflammatory medications. If these drugs offer no relief, the patient should be referred to an internist for additional treatment for relief of the headache. Psychotherapy, physical therapy, or relaxation techniques may also be of benefit for certain cases.

MIGRAINE

Subjective

A patient with a migraine attack is typically a female in the early decades of life. Most migraine attacks (about 90%) occur before the age of 40. A family history of migraine attacks is present in many cases.

The headache itself is generally unilateral but can be bilateral, and the pain is described as throbbing. The headache may be preceded by a variety of neurologic symptoms, the most common of which is a visual aura. Scalp tenderness and muscle contraction can compound the symptoms. Associated symptoms that occur during the headache include nausea, vomiting, and photophobia. Migraine attacks can be precipitated by certain foods (e.g., tyramine-containing cheeses or meat with nitrates) or food additives (e.g., monosodium glutamate). Fasting, menses, oral contraceptive agents, and bright lights may also trigger migraine attacks.

Objective

The clinician should suspect migraine when the patient's age, sex, and headache characteristics match the profile given above. The examination should help rule out any other possible causes of headache.

The entrance tests should include pupillary testing. The findings should be normal, but after a migraine attack an individual may manifest Horner's syndrome due to involvement of the carotid plexus. Additional testing should include ocular motility testing, confrontation field testing, and color vision testing. Transillumination of the sinus is also recommended. If the patient is having a migraine attack during the examination, a useful diagnostic test for common and classic migraine is to compress the ipsilateral carotid or superficial temporal artery. If the severity of the headache is reduced by this maneuver, then a vascular cause for the attack is demonstrated.

A dilated fundus examination to observe the optic nerve heads for papilledema and a threshold visual field test to rule out a lesion along the visual pathway are recommended.

Plan

Acute migraine attacks may be eased with simple oral analgesics (e.g., acetaminophen). If these medications provide no relief, the patient should be referred to an internist, who may prescribe ergot derivatives (e.g., ergotamine tartrate–caffeine [Cafergot]) or other medications. Migraine attacks can be very incapacitating to patients; if the patient has not seen a physician, he or she should be referred to one.

Patients should be educated as to the cause of their headache pain, trigger factors, and the visual phenomena that occur with it.

CLUSTER HEADACHE

Subjective

Cluster headaches are seen more commonly in men than in women. They usually occur in patients who are in their mid-20s. The condition appears as a brief, unilateral, constant,

very severe, nonthrobbing headache that lasts from minutes to hours. The attacks occur at night and will wake the patient from sleep. They can recur daily for periods of weeks or months and then suddenly stop for months or years.

The headache begins as a burning or tingling sensation over the lateral aspect of the nose or as a pressure behind the eye. The attack is accompanied by lacrimation, nasal stuffiness, and Horner's syndrome. The headaches can be triggered by alcohol or vasodilating drugs.

Objective

The clinician should suspect cluster headaches based on the age and sex of the patient and the description of the headache. The examination should rule out any other cause for the pain.

Entrance testing should include assessment of pupillary responses. The clinician should keep in mind that Horner's syndrome has been reported after an attack due to the involvement of the carotid plexus. Testing of ocular motility, confrontation fields, and color vision should also be performed to rule out other conditions. The sinuses should be transilluminated, and the lid position measured.

A dilated examination allows for observation of the optic nerve heads, which should be normal in the cluster headache patient. Threshold field testing can help rule out any lesions along the visual pathways.

Plan

Because cluster headaches are usually very severe, the patient should be referred to an internist for prescription of one or more drugs (e.g., ergotamine, dihydroergotamine, methysergide, or calcium channel antagonists).

Patients should be educated about the etiology of the headaches and the associated ocular effects. The patient should be encouraged to avoid trigger factors that may initiate an attack.

SINUSITIS

Subjective

The patient with a sinus disorder may refer to the pain as headache. The pain is usually located over the maxillary or frontal sinuses. If the inflammation is in the ethmoidal or sphenoidal sinus, it produces a deep midline pain behind the nose. The pain is usually increased by bending forward, sneezing, and coughing.

The medical history may be positive for atopic disease, sinus inflammation, or other sinus disorders. If the sinusitis is from an atopic disease, then the headaches are usually seasonal.

Objective

The examination should rule out other causes of headache that are more serious. Entrance testing should include pupillary response, ocular motility, confrontation fields, and color vision testing. All of these tests should be within normal limits. Tenderness and accentuation of pain on percussion over the frontal or maxillary area are very suggestive of sinus involvement. Transillumination of the frontal ethmoidal maxillary sinus may show involvement if the sinus areas are inflamed from infection. If infection is present, the illumination should not be clear and may show some turbidity.

Dilated fundus examination allows observation of the optic nerve heads to rule out papilledema. A threshold field test may also be performed to rule out any lesion along the visual pathway.

Plan

Sinusitis is best treated with vasoconstrictor nose drops (e.g., phenylephrine hydrochloride), oral antihistamines, oral decongestants, or oral antibiotics. If there is no relief from any of these treatments, the patient should be referred to an internist; allergist; or ear, nose, and throat specialist for further evaluation and management.

SUGGESTED READING

Bajandas FJ, Kline LB. Neuro-Ophthalmology Review Manual (4th ed). Thorofare, NJ: Slack, 1996.

Burde RM, Savino PJ, Trobe JD. Clinician Decisions in Neuro-Ophthalmology (2nd ed). St. Louis: Mosby, 1992.

Lance JW. Mechanism and Management of Headache (5th ed). Oxford, UK: Butterworth–Heinemann, 1993.

Raskin NH. Headache (3rd ed). New York: Churchill Livingstone, 1993.

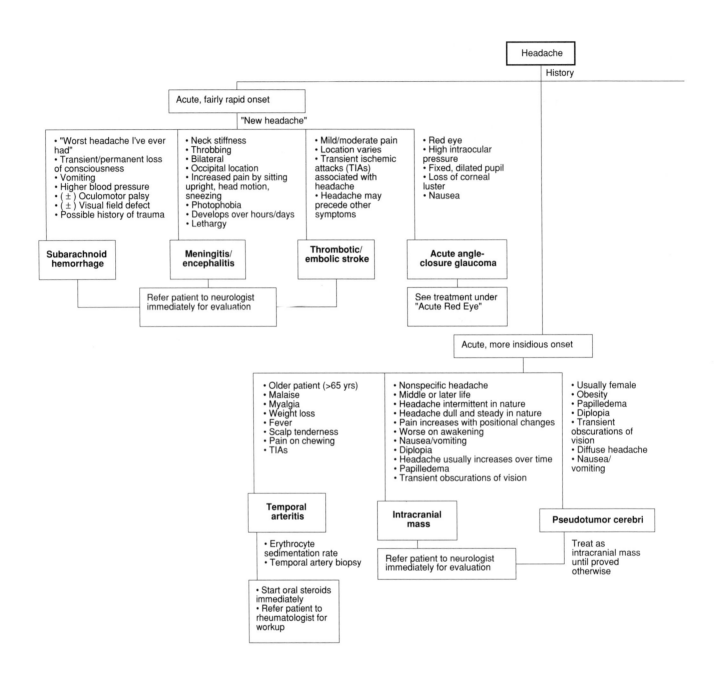

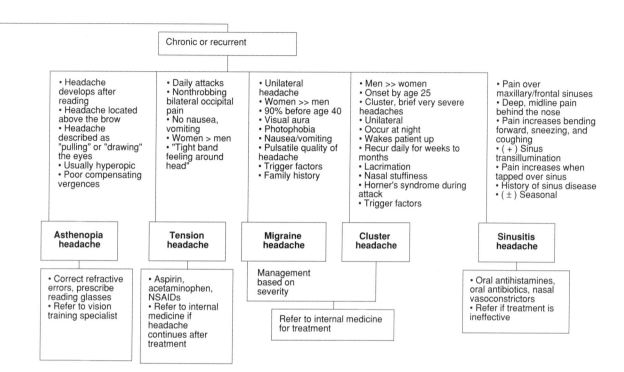

Chronic or recurrent

Asthenopia headache
- Headache develops after reading
- Headache located above the brow
- Headache described as "pulling" or "drawing" the eyes
- Usually hyperopic
- Poor compensating vergences

- Correct refractive errors, prescribe reading glasses
- Refer to vision training specialist

Tension headache
- Daily attacks
- Nonthrobbing bilateral occipital pain
- No nausea, vomiting
- Women > men
- "Tight band feeling around head"

- Aspirin, acetaminophen, NSAIDs
- Refer to internal medicine if headache continues after treatment

Migraine headache
- Unilateral headache
- Women >> men
- 90% before age 40
- Visual aura
- Photophobia
- Nausea/vomiting
- Pulsatile quality of headache
- Trigger factors
- Family history

Management based on severity

Refer to internal medicine for treatment

Cluster headache
- Men >> women
- Onset by age 25
- Cluster, brief very severe headaches
- Unilateral
- Occur at night
- Wakes patient up
- Recur daily for weeks to months
- Lacrimation
- Nasal stuffiness
- Horner's syndrome during attack
- Trigger factors

Sinusitis headache
- Pain over maxillary/frontal sinuses
- Deep, midline pain behind the nose
- Pain increases bending forward, sneezing, and coughing
- (+) Sinus transillumination
- Pain increases when tapped over sinus
- History of sinus disease
- (±) Seasonal

- Oral antihistamines, oral antibiotics, nasal vasoconstrictors
- Refer if treatment is ineffective

Signs

14

Acute Red Eye

DAVID P. SENDROWSKI

ACUTE RED EYE AT A GLANCE

Conjunctivitis (allergic, bacterial, viral)
Iritis
Acute angle-closure glaucoma
Trauma
Subconjunctival hemorrhage
Foreign body
Postoperative
Toxic reaction
Drug induced
Abrasion
Hordeolum
Orbital cellulitis
Caustic injuries
Keratitis
Episcleritis
Scleritis
Corneal ulcer
Cavernous sinus thrombosis

Inflammation is a protective response of tissues to injury that is designed to destroy, delete, eliminate, or wall off an infectious agent. Classically, inflammation is described in terms of five clinical signs: redness, heat, increase in tissue mass, pain, and loss of function.

To evaluate the acute red eye, the clinician should take a thorough history and look for systemic signs such as fever and preauricular node involvement. Biomicroscopy with the use of vital stains such as sodium fluorescein and rose bengal is very helpful in diagnosing the etiology of the inflammation.

ANGLE-CLOSURE GLAUCOMA

Subjective

The patient with angle-closure glaucoma is usually older and female. Aging is associated with enlargement of the crystalline lens, and females tend to have smaller chamber angles than males do. The attack can occur after retinal laser surgery due to choroidal swelling or after a scleral buckling procedure. Tumors of the ciliary body may also precipitate an angle-closure attack. In addition, peripheral anterior synechiae can cause angle closure.

The ocular complaints are related to a sudden increase in intraocular pressure. The complaints can include blurred vision, severe ocular pain or frontal headache, colored haloes around lights, nausea, and vomiting.

Objective

The clinician should note the appearance of the corneal reflex. A dull reflex indicates an edematous cornea. The pupil in the affected eye is usually fixed and dilated. This finding is an excellent clue that the cause of the red eye is not an iritis or conjunctivitis. The biomicroscopic examination should be used to look for keratic precipitates, posterior synechiae, iris neovascularization, cells and flare, and a shallow chamber angle.

Gonioscopy should be performed. However, gonioscopy should be avoided on very edematous corneas, because it is more likely to cause a corneal abrasion in these cases. If significant corneal edema is present, gonioscopy should be done after clearing the corneal epithelial edema with topical glycerin. The procedure confirms the lack of visible angle structures. Gonioscopy may be performed on the uninvolved eye to assess the angle approach and should be considered in cases of suspected iris neovascularization and peripheral anterior synechiae to help determine the cause of the attack.

Elevated intraocular pressure is the final confirmatory test to make the diagnosis of angle-closure glaucoma.

Plan

Before therapy is started, the patient's systemic health should be considered, including cardiovascular status and presence of other systemic diseases such as diabetes or any electrolyte imbalance. If the intraocular pressure is above 50 mm Hg, the following sequence may be followed: oral carbonic anhydrase inhibitor (e.g., acetazolamide), topical alpha-adrenergic agonist (e.g., apraclonidine), and topical beta blocker (e.g., timolol maleate). As the pressure drops below 50 mm Hg, a topical parasympathomimetic (e.g., pilocarpine) should be initiated and the intraocular pressure should be monitored every 15–30 minutes. Instillation of pilocarpine in the uninvolved eye should be considered to reduce the likelihood of an attack.

If the attack is of recent onset and without corneal edema, corneal compression with a gonioprism may help open the angle and reduce the intraocular pressure.

After the intraocular pressure has been reduced to a satisfactory level, the patient should have a laser peripheral iridotomy. The patient should have baseline visual field testing and disc photography and should be followed on a regular basis.

CHLAMYDIAL CONJUNCTIVITIS

Subjective

Patients with chlamydial conjunctivitis are usually young, sexually active adults. It is possible for elderly patients to contract the disease as well, but this occurs much less frequently. The disease may also occur in neonates and adolescents. In adolescents, sexual abuse or contact with an infected adult is a possible means of transmission of the disease.

Patients with chlamydial infection have a mucopurulent conjunctivitis that may have already been treated without success. The conjunctivitis takes 4–10 days to develop fully, after which time it becomes a more chronic conjunctivitis.

Frequently, when asked, the patient admits having acquired a new sexual partner within the last 1 or 2 months. The patient should be asked about a concomitant vaginitis, urethritis, or cervicitis.

Objective

The patient with chlamydial conjunctivitis presents with associated signs that are not seen in bacterial conjunctivitis. For example, positive lymphatic adenopathy, follicles on the upper palpebral conjunctiva, marginal and possibly central corneal infiltrates, and superior limbal pannus all occur in chlamydial infections. In addition, the conjunctiva is very hyperemic, with numerous papillae and mucopurulent discharge in the lower palpebral conjunctiva.

Additional testing may help in confirming the diagnosis. Giemsa stain of conjunctival scrapings may reveal basophilic intracytoplasmic inclusion bodies in the acute phase of the disease. MicroTak direct fluorescent antibody testing of scrapings is far more reliable than the Giemsa stain. An enzyme immunoassay or chlamydial culture of conjunctival scraping can be very helpful as well.

Plan

To manage the systemic infection, the patient should be given oral tetracycline or, alternatively, doxycycline or erythromycin for a 3-week period. If the patient is noncompliant or has difficulty with a prolonged treatment regimen, azithromycin can be given as treatment. The patient's sexual partners should be treated as well. Tetracycline or erythromycin ointment should be prescribed for 3 weeks to treat the concurrent conjunctivitis.

The patient should be followed on a weekly basis until the condition is resolved. Referral to an internist or family practitioner to rule out other sexually transmitted diseases is also indicated.

ALLERGIC CONJUNCTIVITIS

Subjective

Patients with allergic conjunctivitis usually present with a bilateral complaint of red, itching eyes. Itching is a very important complaint because it strongly suggests an allergic etiology. The patient may have a history of atopic diseases such as hay fever, atopic dermatitis, or allergic rhinitis. If there is no history of atopic disease, the clinician should consider other causes such as animal dander, dust, molds, environmental pollutants, and pollens. The conjunctivitis is usually a seasonal complaint if caused by an atopic disease.

Objective

The examination should reveal conjunctival chemosis, and the conjunctiva should have a glassy or gelatinous appearance. The conjunctiva may become so chemotic that it bulges over the lid margin or limbal area. Hyperemia is usually less marked than the chemotic response. A mucoid discharge is seen in the inferior fornix, more so in individuals with chronic disease. The lids should be examined for signs of edema, urticaria, or angioneurotic edema. The cornea usually shows no staining with sodium fluorescein. The pupillary and intraocular pressure readings are normal.

Conjunctival scraping may be ordered to evaluate the number of eosinophils, which should predominate over other inflammatory cells.

Plan

The first approach to treatment is to interrupt histaminic activity. This goal can be accomplished with the use of a topical antihistamine (e.g., levocabastine hydrochloride), combination antihistamine–mast cell stabilizer (e.g., olopatadine hydrochloride), or combination antihistamine-decongestant (e.g., naphazoline hydrochloride–pheniramine maleate). A topical antiprostaglandin (e.g., ketorolac tromethamine) can also provide symptomatic relief. Lid edema and itching may be further reduced with oral antihistamines (e.g., chlorpheniramine maleate). The clinician should be careful to ask the patient about cardiovascular disorders and check the angle chambers before prescribing oral antihistamines.

Mast cell stabilizers (e.g., lodoxamide tromethamine) are extremely useful for chronic allergy sufferers and should be taken 3–4 weeks in advance of allergy season to minimize the ocular reaction. They are effective alone or in combination with other ocular allergy drugs.

Cool compresses can be applied as supportive therapy to reduce chemosis through a vasoconstrictive activity. Preservative-free artificial tears may also be used to help remove allergens in the tear film.

Topical steroids are generally not recommended unless the reaction is severe enough to incapacitate the patient. In nonsevere cases, avoidance of steroids is recommended to reduce overuse and ocular complications.

The patient should be followed up every 1–2 weeks to evaluate for reduction of symptoms.

VIRAL CONJUNCTIVITIS

Subjective

A patient with epidemic keratoconjunctivitis (EKC) or adenoviral variant of EKC usually complains of a rapid onset of eye redness and irritation. Other complaints may include watery discharge, foreign body sensation, photophobia, fullness of the lids, glare, and slight blurring of vision.

The medical history should concentrate on early cold symptoms such as malaise, mild fever, and headache. There may be no symptoms associated with the ocular findings.

The clinician should ask whether coworkers, family members, or other close associates may have also recently had an eye infection. This infection is by nature very contagious.

Objective

Initially, EKC may be very hard to distinguish from a nonspecific viral conjunctivitis. Several signs that aid in the diagnosis are tender and visible preauricular nodes, diffuse subepithelial infiltrates (these usually do not appear until day 16 of the disease course), formation of a membrane (true vs. pseudomembrane) on the upper palpebral conjunctiva, and petechial hemorrhages. Other, less specific findings are a follicular response in the palpebral conjunctiva, mild lid edema, and mild superficial punctate keratitis (SPK).

Plan

Treatment is supportive, as EKC is a self-limiting disease. Application of artificial tears and cool compresses are the mainstay of treatment for EKC. Vasoconstrictor drops (e.g., phenylephrine hydrochloride–zinc) may be used along with oral analgesics (e.g., acetaminophen) to relieve the pain.

If there is a considerable degree of SPK, the clinician may consider a topical antibiotic (e.g., norfloxacin) to reduce the likelihood of secondary infection. A cycloplegic agent (e.g., homatropine) can also be used to reduce the likelihood of secondary iritis from corneal irritation.

The use of topical steroids to treat EKC is very controversial. In the case of dramatic loss of acuity from subepithelial infiltrates or scar formation from membrane development, a steroid may be of benefit. A steroid should not be used to reduce mild symptoms.

The patient should be seen every 3–5 days to evaluate the corneal involvement and the anterior chamber. The patient should also be advised of the contagious nature of this infection and instructed in the importance of frequent hand washing and the use of separate linens, towels, and bedding. The clinician should consider advising that infected individuals be quarantined from coworkers and classmates to control the spread of this infection.

BACTERIAL CONJUNCTIVITIS

Subjective

There are no age- or race-related predispositions to staphylococcal infection of the conjunctiva. Patients with this condition usually complain of eye redness, irritation, or foreign body sensation. The onset is 2–3 days after exposure, and the second eye is infected 1–3 days after the first eye. The patient may complain that the lids are stuck together on awakening in the morning. The astute clinician does not confuse this finding with normal mild crusting or scaling at the canthi that occurs on awakening.

The patient should be asked about recent colds, upper respiratory tract infections, sinus disease, and chronic ocular inflammations such as blepharitis. The medical history should also include a review of diseases that compromise the immune system, such as diabetes. Regimens of topical and oral medications that may alter the normal ocular resistance to infection, such as long-term use of steroids, should also be investigated.

Objective

The examination should begin with a visual observation of the patient to rule out any ongoing surface disease around the periocular tissue that might be causing the infection.

Visual acuity is minimally affected by the conjunctivitis. The intraocular pressure, anterior chamber, and pupils should be normal, and there should be no preauricular or submandibular lymphatic adenopathy.

Biomicroscopic examination reveals a mild to very pronounced hyperemia of the conjunctiva. Evaluation of the bulbar conjunctiva should reveal engorged vessels but no evidence of petechial hemorrhages. If such hemorrhages are present, the clinician should consider additional causes for the infection, such as *Streptococcus pneumoniae* and *Haemophilus influenzae*, especially in children. The palpebral conjunctiva may show a predominance of papillae.

After sodium fluorescein staining, there may be a punctate stain on the inferior one-third of the corneal epithelium. The stain may be present on the bulbar conjunctiva as well. The lids may be edematous and the lashes matted. *Staphylococcus aureus* infections may be associated with blepharitis and the presence of phlyctenules and marginal sterile infiltrates.

Conjunctival samples for routine culture and sensitivity testing using Gram's stain should be ordered for more severe cases or cases that show resistance to topical medications.

Plan

A topical broad-spectrum antibiotic (e.g., polymyxin B sulfate–trimethoprim, ciprofloxacin, or bacitracin) should be prescribed for 7–10 days. Artificial tears and warm compresses may also be used to hasten the recovery.

Recovery should be fairly rapid. If topical therapy is ineffective, conjunctival scrapings should be cultured to identify the causative agent.

SUBCONJUNCTIVAL HEMORRHAGE

Subjective

A subconjunctival hemorrhage is usually unilateral and sudden in onset. It often causes great alarm to the patient. Commonly, the patient calls requesting to see the doctor immediately because of "blood in the eye" or a "broken blood vessel in the eye." Although subconjunctival hemorrhages can occasionally cause mild irritation, the cosmetic appearance is the major subjective complaint.

The clinician must first rule out underlying systemic causes before diagnosing the case as idiopathic. The history should include questions regarding heavy lifting or performance of Valsalva maneuvers, acute or chronic cough, bleeding disorders, clotting problems, eating disorders, constipation, blood-borne diseases (e.g., acquired immunodeficiency syndrome), recent surgeries, and trauma. The use of oral medications (e.g., aspirin, warfarin) should be thoroughly evaluated as a potential cause of the hemorrhage.

Objective

The clinician should use simple observational techniques to evaluate the patient. Under direct light, the periocular tissues, conjunctiva, cornea, and anterior chamber should be grossly observed.

If there is a history of recent trauma, Seidel's test should be performed to rule out perforation of the globe. A slit-lamp evaluation can help to isolate the ruptured vessel and evaluate the size and extent of the hemorrhage, which accumulates toward the limbus with a clear zone between the hemorrhage and the cornea. The anterior chamber should be clear, and in trauma cases a hyphema should be ruled out. Finally, the blood pressure should be evaluated. If the hemorrhaging is recurrent, laboratory testing (i.e., prothrombin time, partial thromboplastin time, and a complete blood count) can help to rule out a systemic cause.

Plan

In most cases, the patient can be reassured of the benign nature of the hemorrhage. Patient education should include description of the color changes that the hemorrhage will go through during the reabsorption.

Artificial tears and cool compresses may be used initially to reduce ocular irritation. Application of warm compresses after 1–2 days may hasten the blood reabsorption process. The patient should be advised to return in 1–2 weeks for evaluation of the hemorrhage. If recurrence is noted, the patient should be referred to a family practitioner or internist for evaluation.

RUPTURED GLOBE DUE TO TRAUMA

Subjective

The patient with a ruptured globe must have a history of severe trauma or penetrating injury to the globe. A patient with a penetrating injury may have experienced a sharp pain while working on a grinding wheel or hammering on a piece of metal. Ocular complaints can vary greatly depending on the degree of trauma and size of the penetrating object.

Objective

Evaluation should concentrate on confirming the rupture of the globe and preparing the patient for transport to an ophthalmic surgeon.

External examination may reveal periocular abrasions and lacerations. Ocular ductions may be decreased. The biomicroscope should be used to evaluate the conjunctiva and look for subconjunctival edema and hemorrhage. There may be signs of corneal abrasion and hyphema. The anterior chamber is abnormally shallow after rupture of the globe, and the pupils may also be sluggish in response to light.

Three very important diagnostic signs of a ruptured globe are hypotony, shallow anterior chamber, and positive Seidel's test. The clinician should attempt to perform ophthalmoscopy but may find it difficult if vitreous hemorrhage or hyphema obscures the view.

Plan

The patient should have a Fox (protective) shield placed over the ruptured globe and be referred immediately to an ophthalmic surgeon. The ophthalmic surgeon should be apprised of the examination data, including location of the perforation and condition of the globe.

IDIOPATHIC ANTERIOR UVEITIS

Subjective

The patient with acute idiopathic iritis complains of a sudden onset of pain and redness in the eye, as well as pho-

tophobia, but with no history of trauma. The condition is almost always unilateral and commonly occurs in patients between the ages of 18 and 50. Increased lacrimation may cause a decrease in vision as well.

The medical and ocular histories are usually unremarkable. If there is a history of a previous attack of iritis, the clinician should become suspicious of an underlying systemic etiology.

Objective

The first objective of the examination is to rule out an infectious or inflammatory conjunctivitis and acute glaucoma. The entrance testing should include a pupillary examination. In iritis, the pupil in the affected eye is miotic, whereas in acute glaucoma, it is fixed and dilated. Conjunctivitis does not affect pupillary response. Externally, the vasculature in the limbal area is engorged and reddened, so that there is circumciliary flush. The patient may also have a ptosis in the affected eye secondary to the blepharospasm. Confrontation field testing usually suffices for initial peripheral vision testing.

The biomicroscope should be used with conical beam illumination to evaluate the inflammatory reaction in the anterior chamber. In idiopathic iritis, the clinician may note cells and flare. Cells are usually the more prominent feature in the early stages of the inflammation. The intraocular pressure is lowered secondary to ciliary body inflammation and may rise as time passes.

A binocular indirect ophthalmoscopic fundus examination should be performed to rule out the possibility of a posterior inflammatory cause for the anterior chamber reaction.

Plan

The patient should be prescribed a long-acting cycloplegic agent (e.g., homatropine) to reduce synechia formation. The inflammation should be treated with topical steroids (e.g., prednisolone acetate) every 1–4 hours depending on the severity of the reaction. A topical beta blocker (e.g., timolol maleate) can be used to reduce the intraocular pressure if it is elevated.

The follow-up examination should occur within 24–48 hours so that the clinician can evaluate the effect of the topical steroid and assess the patient's compliance with the treatment schedule. The intraocular pressure and cornea should be checked at each follow-up visit. Administration of the topical steroids should be based on the anterior chamber reaction. If the anterior chamber reaction shows improvement, the steroids can be slowly tapered. The patient should be seen several months after the inflammation has resolved to document residual ocular effects.

EPISCLERITIS

Subjective

Patients with episcleritis are usually young adults. Patients may or may not have a history of systemic diseases. The history should include questions about gout, herpes zoster attacks, syphilis, Crohn's disease, hepatitis B infection, rheumatoid arthritis, systemic lupus erythematosus, polyarteritis, and Lyme disease. Women are affected more often than men are, and the disorder typically occurs between the second and fourth decades.

Patients complain of a rapid onset of mild pain or irritation in one or both eyes. There may be tenderness over the area of redness. The vision is rarely affected, and there is no circumlimbal injection as seen in uveitis. The symptoms usually progress in the first 3–5 days and then spontaneously resolve in 7–10 days. Recurrence is frequent.

Objective

If possible, the area of redness should be viewed in natural light to evaluate for the bluish hue associated with scleritis. Biomicroscopy shows a segmented, nodular, or diffuse vascular engorgement and edema of the episclera. One drop of 2.5% phenylephrine hydrochloride causes the episcleral vessels to blanch after 15–20 minutes and the area of redness to disappear. The area may also be moved with a moistened cotton-tipped applicator after topical anesthesia. Nodular episcleritis manifests non-tender movable nodules. The cornea is clear and does not stain with sodium fluorescein. The anterior chamber is also deep and quiet.

If a systemic etiology is suspected, laboratory and blood testing might include determination of antinuclear antibody level, erythrocyte sedimentation rate, serum uric acid level, and fluorescent treponemal antibody absorption rate and testing for rheumatoid factor.

Plan

Mild cases can usually be treated with topical artificial tears or a topical vasoconstrictor–antihistamine combination (e.g., naphazoline hydrochloride–pheniramine maleate). In more severe cases, a topical steroid (e.g., fluorometholone) may be needed. This treatment will rapidly reduce the symptoms and redness.

Patients may also benefit from instillation of a topical antiprostaglandin (e.g., ketorolac tromethamine), but the results vary widely. Oral antiprostaglandins (e.g., ibuprofen) can also be helpful in reducing symptoms.

Patients on steroids should be checked weekly for intraocular pressure changes; patients treated with other medications need not be seen for several weeks.

SUGGESTED READING

Easty DL, Smolin G. External Eye Disease. Oxford, UK: Butterworth, 1985.
Tabbara KF, Hynduik RA. Infections of the Eye. Boston: Little, Brown, 1986.
Yanoff M, Fine B. Ocular Pathology: A Text and Atlas (4th ed). Philadelphia: Lippincott–Raven, 1996.

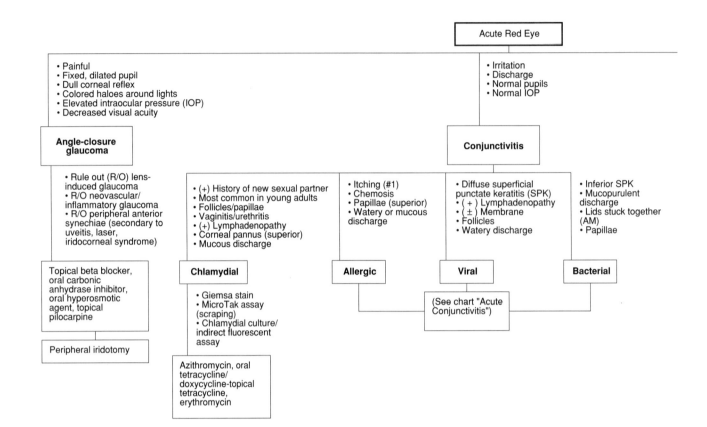

Acute Red Eye

• Painful
• Fixed, dilated pupil
• Dull corneal reflex
• Colored haloes around lights
• Elevated intraocular pressure (IOP)
• Decreased visual acuity

• Irritation
• Discharge
• Normal pupils
• Normal IOP

Angle-closure glaucoma

Conjunctivitis

• Rule out (R/O) lens-induced glaucoma
• R/O neovascular/inflammatory glaucoma
• R/O peripheral anterior synechiae (secondary to uveitis, laser, iridocorneal syndrome)

• (+) History of new sexual partner
• Most common in young adults
• Follicles/papillae
• Vaginitis/urethritis
• (+) Lymphadenopathy
• Corneal pannus (superior)
• Mucous discharge

• Itching (#1)
• Chemosis
• Papillae (superior)
• Watery or mucous discharge

• Diffuse superficial punctate keratitis (SPK)
• (+) Lymphadenopathy
• (±) Membrane
• Follicles
• Watery discharge

• Inferior SPK
• Mucopurulent discharge
• Lids stuck together (AM)
• Papillae

Topical beta blocker, oral carbonic anhydrase inhibitor, oral hyperosmotic agent, topical pilocarpine

Chlamydial

Allergic

Viral

Bacterial

• Giemsa stain
• MicroTak assay (scraping)
• Chlamydial culture/indirect fluorescent assay

(See chart "Acute Conjunctivitis")

Peripheral iridotomy

Azithromycin, oral tetracycline/doxycycline-topical tetracycline, erythromycin

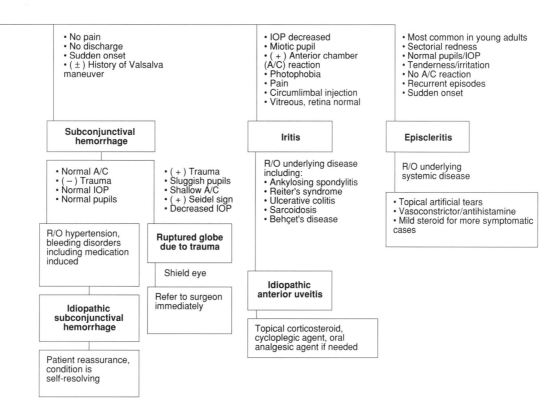

15

Acute Conjunctival Inflammation

David P. Sendrowski

ACUTE CONJUNCTIVAL INFLAMMATION AT A GLANCE

Allergic conjunctivitis
Bacterial conjunctivitis
Viral conjunctivitis
Toxic conjunctivitis
Herpes simplex conjunctivitis
Epidemic keratoconjunctivitis
Pharyngoconjunctival fever
Oculoglandular syndrome
Direct irritations (e.g., foreign body)
Chemical irritants
Trauma
Chemical burns
Acute glaucoma
Acute iritis
Inclusion conjunctivitis
Herpes zoster conjunctivitis
Fungal conjunctivitis
Superior limbal keratoconjunctivitis
Exposure keratopathy
Behçet's syndrome
Reiter's disease
Ocular pemphigoid
Stevens-Johnson syndrome

The location of the conjunctiva exposes it to many microorganisms and other stressful environmental factors. Common pathogens that can cause conjunctivitis include *Streptococcus pneumoniae*, *Haemophilus influenzae*, *Staphylococcus aureus*, human adenovirus strains, and sexually transmitted agents such as *Chlamydia trachomatis* and *Neisseria gonorrhoeae*. Allergic antigens can also react with the conjunctiva, creating an acute inflammatory response.

The clinical signs exhibited by the conjunctival inflammatory response usually depend on the nature of the causative agent. The most common signs exhibited during conjunctival inflammations are hyperemia, chemosis, discharge, papillae, and follicles. The patient history is very important in helping to determine the causative agent in each case.

ALLERGIC CONJUNCTIVITIS

Subjective

Patients with allergic conjunctivitis usually present with a bilateral complaint of red, itching eyes. Itching is a very important complaint, since it strongly suggests an allergic cause. The patient may have a history of atopic diseases such as hay fever, atopic dermatitis, or allergic rhinitis. The conjunctivitis is usually a seasonal complaint if it is caused by an atopic disease. If there is no history of atopic disease, the clinician should consider other causes, such as animal dander, dust, molds, environmental pollutants, and pollens.

Objective

The examination often reveals conjunctival chemosis, and the conjunctiva may have a glassy or gelatinous appearance. The conjunctiva may become so chemotic as to bulge over the lid margin or limbal area. Hyperemia is usually less marked than the chemotic response. A mucoid discharge is seen in the inferior fornix, more so in individuals with a chronic disease. The lids should be examined for signs of edema, urticaria, or angioneurotic edema. The cornea usually shows no staining with sodium fluorescein. The pupillary and intraocular pressure findings are normal.

Conjunctival scraping may be ordered to evaluate the number of eosinophils, which should predominate over other inflammatory cells.

Plan

The first approach to treatment is to interrupt histaminic activity. This goal is accomplished with the use of topical antihistamine-decongestants (e.g., naphazoline hydrochloride–pheniramine maleate), which help reduce the conjunctival reaction. Topical antihistamines (e.g., levocabastine hydrochloride) or topical antiprostaglandins (e.g., ketorolac tromethamine) may also provide rapid relief for the symptomatic patient. The lid edema is reduced using oral antihistamines. The clinician should be careful to ask the patient about cardiovascular disorders and check the angle chambers before prescribing oral antihistamines.

Cool compresses can be applied to reduce chemosis through vasoconstriction. Preservative-free artificial tears may also be given to help remove allergens in the tear film.

Mast cell stabilizers (e.g., lodoxamide tromethamine) are extremely useful for chronic allergy sufferers and should be taken 3–4 weeks in advance of allergy season to minimize the ocular reaction. They are effective alone or in combination with other ocular allergy drugs.

Recently, a new topical preparation, Alrex (loteprednol etabonate), has been approved by the U.S. Food and Drug Administration for treatment of ocular allergies. The exact role of the drug in ocular allergy therapy will not be known for several years.

Topical steroids (e.g., prednisolone acetate) are not recommended unless the reaction is severe enough to incapacitate the patient and other treatments are ineffective. In nonsevere cases, avoidance of steroids is recommended to reduce overuse and secondary ocular complications.

The patient should be followed up every 1–2 weeks to evaluate for reduction of symptoms.

VERNAL CONJUNCTIVITIS

Subjective

Vernal conjunctivitis occurs more frequently in males than in females. It rarely starts before the age of 3 or after the age of 25. The condition usually develops by the age of 14 or younger. Vernal conjunctivitis generally occurs during spring and fall.

The patient complains of a severe itching around the eyes. The itching may be exacerbated by exposure to dust,

wind, or bright lights, or by physical exertion. The patient may also complain of photophobia, irritation, discomfort, and "hot lids." The patient may have to remove thick, ropy strings of mucus throughout the day. The condition may be a very disabling one in which the patient is confined to home or bed.

The medical history is important to help determine whether the patient has an atopic disease such as asthma, allergic rhinitis, eczema, or hay fever.

Objective

The cornerstone of the diagnosis is the severe hypertrophy of tarsal papillae in the upper lid (cobblestone papillae). The clinician may note a ptosis of the upper lid secondary to the swelling. The conjunctiva is usually very chemotic, and a thick, ropy mucus may be noted in the inferior fornix.

Another possible finding is corneal staining in the superior one-third of the cornea, which is referred to as *keratitis of Togby*. If the papillae cause erosion of the corneal epithelium, the result could be a sterile shield ulcer. Whitish dots around the corneal limbal area or on the palpebral conjunctiva are calcified eosinophils and are referred to as *Horner-Trantas' dots*.

The pupils and intraocular pressures are normal. There should also be no evidence of palpable or tender preauricular or submandibular lymph nodes.

If necessary, a conjunctival scraping may be ordered to confirm the presence of eosinophils, which should be very predominant in the scraping. The diagnosis, however, is usually a clinical one.

Plan

If the patient is incapacitated by the allergic reaction, a steroid pulse may be necessary to rapidly reduce the symptoms. The use of a topical steroid (e.g., prednisolone acetate) every 2 hours during waking hours for 2–3 days, then reduction to four times a day for the next 3–4 days usually reduces the allergic response. When the patient's symptoms are approximately two-thirds resolved, the steroids should be discontinued. The steroids should be used for no longer than 1 week. If steroid therapy is given for longer than 1 week, the steroids should be tapered before discontinuance.

If the patient is only moderately or mildly affected, the clinician should consider using a combination of topical antihistamine–decongestant (e.g., naphazoline hydrochloride–pheniramine maleate) and a topical mast cell stabilizer (e.g., lodoxamide tromethamine). Alternate therapies include a topical antihistamine (e.g., levocabastine hydrochloride) or a topical antiprostaglandin (e.g., ketorolac tromethamine). The patient may also be instructed to apply cool compresses several times a day, instill artificial tears for symptomatic relief, and wear sunglasses to reduce glare and photophobia.

The patient should be followed up every 1–2 weeks so the clinician can monitor for reduction in symptoms and corneal complications. It would be advisable for patients with seasonal exacerbation of the condition to start the mast cell stabilizer several weeks before the time symptoms usually occur. A referral to an allergist may be recommended for more severe cases.

If the patient has a shield ulcer, a topical steroid pulse should be initiated immediately, along with a topical broad-spectrum antibiotic (e.g., polymyxin B sulfate–trimethoprim) four times a day to reduce the chance of secondary infection. A cycloplegic agent (e.g., homatropine) and a topical mast cell stabilizer (e.g., cromolyn sodium) should be prescribed. Cool compresses may provide additional relief. The patient should be followed every 1–3 days to check for the reduction of the shield ulcer. The topical medications should be reduced in response to the resolution of the ulcer. If there is progression of the ulcer after 48 hours, the patient should be referred to a corneal specialist immediately.

STAPHYLOCOCCAL CONJUNCTIVITIS

Subjective

There are no age- or race-related predispositions to staphylococcal infection of the conjunctiva. Patients with this condition usually complain of eye redness, irritation, or foreign body sensation. The onset is 2–3 days after exposure, and the second eye is infected 1–3 days after the first eye in about half the cases. The lids may be stuck together when the patient awakens in the morning. The astute clinician does not confuse this finding with normal crusting or scaling at the canthi that occurs on awakening.

The patient should be asked about recent colds, upper respiratory tract infections, sinus disease, and chronic ocular inflammations such as blepharitis.

The medical history should include a review of diseases that compromise the immune system, such as diabetes. Regimens of topical and oral medications that may alter the normal ocular resistance to infection, such as steroids, should also be investigated.

Objective

The examination should begin with a visual observation of the patient to rule out any ongoing surface disease around the periocular tissue that might be causing the infection.

Visual acuity is minimally affected by the conjunctivitis. The intraocular pressure, anterior chamber, and pupils should be normal, and there should be no preauricular and submandibular lymphadenopathy.

Biomicroscopic examination reveals a mild to very pronounced hyperemic conjunctiva. Evaluation of the bulbar conjunctiva should reveal engorged vessels but no evidence of petechial hemorrhages. If such hemorrhages are present, the clinician should consider additional causes for the infection, such as *S. pneumoniae* and *H. influenzae*, especially in children. The inferior palpebral conjunctiva may show a predominance of papillae.

After sodium fluorescein staining, there may be a punctate stain on the inferior one-third of the corneal epithelium. The stain may be present on the bulbar conjunctiva as well. The lids may be edematous and the lashes matted. *S. aureus* infections may often be associated with blepharitis and the presence of phlyctenules and marginal sterile infiltrates.

Conjunctival samples for routine culture and sensitivity testing using Gram's stain should be ordered in the more severe cases or those cases with resistance to topical medications.

Plan

A topical broad-spectrum antibiotic (e.g., polymyxin B sulfate–trimethoprim, ciprofloxacin, or bacitracin) should be instilled every 3 hours to four times a day, depending on severity, for 7–10 days.

Artificial tears and warm compresses may also be used for symptomatic relief and to hasten the recovery. Recovery should be fairly rapid. If topical therapy is ineffective, laboratory investigation is indicated to identify the causative agent.

STREPTOCOCCAL CONJUNCTIVITIS

Subjective

In cases of conjunctivitis due to *S. pneumoniae*, the complaints are similar to those for staphylococcal conjunctivitis with a few exceptions. Streptococcal infection is more common in children and in institutional settings. The patient's medical history may include a history of upper respiratory tract infection. The conjunctivitis reaches its peak at day 2 or 3 and lasts 7–10 days.

Objective

The findings are similar to those for staphylococcal conjunctivitis, except that petechial subconjunctival hemorrhages may be present. Cultures with Gram's stain are helpful for confirming the diagnosis, and sensitivity testing aids in making appropriate therapeutic decisions.

Plan

A topical antibiotic (e.g., bacitracin, erythromycin, ciprofloxacin, or polymyxin B sulfate–trimethoprim) is the first line of defense. It is usually given every 3 hours to four times a day depending on the severity of the infection. If there is a coexisting upper respiratory tract infection, the patient should be referred to an internal medicine specialist for evaluation and treatment. Application of artificial tears and warm compresses, in addition to the topical antibiotics, is good supportive therapy.

HAEMOPHILUS INFLUENZAE CONJUNCTIVITIS

Subjective

Conjunctivitis due to *H. influenzae* occurs more frequently in children, particularly those residing in warmer climates. It may be associated with fever, sinusitis, upper respiratory tract infections, and leukocytosis. The symptoms are similar to those of staphylococcal conjunctivitis and reach their peak at day 3 or 4.

Objective

The examination findings are also similar to those for staphylococcal conjunctivitis except that petechial subconjunctival hemorrhages may be present. The petechial hemorrhages are more common in *H. influenzae* than in *S. pneumoniae*. Accompanying an acute infection is the presence of inferior corneal limbal infiltrates. The infiltrates are a manifestation of the toxicity of the gram-negative bacteria.

Definitive diagnosis is achieved through culture and staining.

Plan

A topical antibiotic (e.g., bacitracin, polymyxin B sulfate, polymyxin B sulfate–bacitracin, or ciprofloxacin) is given every 3 hours to four times a day depending on the severity of the infection. Ointment is preferred over solution for the pediatric population because it is easier to administer.

Warm compresses are a good supportive therapy to accompany the topical antibiotic.

PRIMARY HERPES SIMPLEX CONJUNCTIVITIS

Subjective

Primary herpes simplex conjunctivitis usually occurs in young children. The main subjective complaints include watery discharge, mild pain, photophobia, and foreign body sensation. The child may also have a concurrent fever along with malaise.

Objective

The key clinical sign is small, pinhead-sized vesicular eruptions around the lids, especially near the lid margins. They may be hidden between eyelashes, and careful slit-lamp examination is warranted.

Other signs include a follicular conjunctivitis, tender preauricular or submandibular lymph nodes, mild to moderate lid edema, and diffuse superficial punctate keratitis (SPK). The SPK may follow the conjunctivitis by 1 or 2 weeks. Careful examination of the cornea with sodium fluorescein and rose bengal stains is vital to define dendritic or geographic patterns of herpes simplex.

The pupils, intraocular pressure, and anterior chamber should all be normal in these cases.

Plan

The skin lesions are treated with an oral antiviral (e.g., acyclovir) and topical antibiotic ointment (e.g., bacitracin) three times a day. Warm soaks to the skin lesions should also be used. If there are skin lesions near the eyelid margin, a topical ocular antiviral medication (e.g., trifluridine) should be started.

The conjunctivitis is treated with topical antiviral medication (e.g., trifluridine) five times a day. The medication is usually given for 7–14 days until the conjunctivitis has resolved.

If corneal involvement is present, topical antiviral medication (e.g., trifluridine) is indicated every 2 hours for 7–14 days or until resolution of the epithelial defect is noted. A cycloplegic agent (e.g., homatropine) instilled three times a day should also be used if corneal involvement is present to reduce the likelihood of an anterior chamber reaction.

Topical steroids should be avoided because of the potential for proliferation of the virus.

The patient should be followed every 1–3 days to check on the response to treatment and then every 3–5 days depending on the clinical findings.

The clinician should be aware that topical antivirals may cause a toxic reaction. If such a reaction occurs, reducing the frequency of medication or switching to another topical antiviral medication is recommended.

PHARYNGOCONJUNCTIVAL FEVER CONJUNCTIVITIS

Subjective

Pharyngoconjunctival fever (PCF) is most common among children. The ocular complaints can include watery eyes, irritation, photophobia, and foreign body sensation. A recent history of an associated sore throat and fever is helpful in the diagnosis. The conjunctivitis usually occurs after the sore throat and fever. The associated complaints may also include malaise, myalgia, headache, diarrhea, and gastrointestinal distress.

This virus is shed from the conjunctiva for 14 days but remains in fecal matter for 30 days. It is commonly passed on to other individuals through infected swimming pools. Therefore, the history should include questions regarding recent swimming and contact with other family members or coworkers with eye infections.

Objective

Confirmation testing should include evaluation of oral temperature and palpation of the preauricular and submandibular nodes for inflammation and tenderness.

The slit-lamp examination should reveal a follicular conjunctivitis, mild to moderate hyperemia, and chemosis. The cornea may show subepithelial infiltrates, but these are much less common than in epidemic keratoconjunctivitis (EKC). More commonly, sodium fluorescein staining reveals a diffuse SPK. The pupils, intraocular pressure, and anterior chamber should all be normal.

Plan

This infection is self-limiting. Supportive therapy could include topical lubricants, used as frequently as needed; vasoconstrictor drops (e.g., naphazoline) four times a day; and application of cool compresses. The clinician should be aware of the possible overuse of lubricants with preservatives, which can cause a topical medicamentosa.

If the SPK is severe, a cycloplegic agent (e.g., homatropine) may be given three times a day to reduce the likelihood of a secondary anterior chamber reaction. A topical antibiotic (e.g., polymyxin B sulfate–trimethoprim) may be given four times a day to reduce the chance of secondary bacterial infection. Topical antivirals are of no proven value to these patients.

The patient should be told to meticulously avoid sharing bedding, towels, and linen as this may potentiate the spread of the virus. It is also important to inform the patient of the potential for spreading the infection and to suggest that avoidance of school or work may be necessary for several days to weeks. The patient should be followed every 5–7 days to rule out corneal or anterior chamber reaction. The clinician should also take care to use universal precautions in equipment cleaning to avoid contamination and possible spread of the virus.

EPIDEMIC KERATOCONJUNCTIVITIS

Subjective

A patient with EKC usually complains of a rapid onset of eye redness and irritation. Complaints may include watery discharge, foreign body sensation, photophobia, fullness of the lids, glare, and slight blurring of vision.

The medical history should concentrate on early cold symptoms such as malaise, mild fever, and headache. There may be no systemic symptoms associated with the ocular findings.

The clinician should ask whether coworkers or family members may have also recently had an eye infection. This infection is by nature very contagious.

Objective

Initially, EKC may be very hard to distinguish from other types of viral conjunctivitis. Several signs that may be diagnostic to the clinician are tender and visible preauricular nodes, diffuse subepithelial infiltrates (but these usually do not appear until around day 16 of the disease course), formation of a membrane (true vs. pseudomembrane) on the upper or lower palpebral conjunctiva, and petechial hemorrhages.

Other findings that may not be as diagnostic are a follicular response in the palpebral conjunctiva, mild lid edema, and mild SPK.

Plan

Treatment is supportive because EKC is a self-limiting disease. Application of artificial tears and cool compresses is the mainstay of treatment for EKC. Vasoconstrictor drops (e.g., naphazoline) may be used along with oral analgesics (e.g., acetaminophen) to relieve the pain.

If there is a considerable degree of SPK, the clinician may consider a topical antibiotic (e.g., norfloxacin) to reduce the likelihood of secondary infection. A cycloplegic agent (e.g., homatropine) can also be used to reduce the likelihood of secondary iritis from corneal irritation.

The use of topical steroids is very controversial. If there is dramatic acuity loss from subepithelial infiltrates or scar formation from membrane development, a steroid may be of benefit. In mild cases, the use of steroids should be avoided.

The patient should be seen every 3–5 days to evaluate the corneal involvement and to rule out anterior chamber reaction. The patient should also be advised of the contagious nature of this infection and told to meticu-lously avoid sharing linens, towels, and bedding. The clinician should consider advising that infected individuals be quarantined from coworkers or classmates, because this infection can spread very rapidly.

SUGGESTED READING

Bartlett JD, Jaanus SD. Clinical Ocular Pharmacology (3rd ed). Boston: Butterworth–Heinemann, 1995.

Catania LJ. Primary Care of the Anterior Segment (2nd ed). Norwalk, CT: Appleton & Lange, 1996.

Mannis MJ. Bacterial Conjunctivitis. In TD Duane (ed), Clinical Ophthalmology, Vol 4. New York: Harper & Row, 1989.

Pavan-Langston D (ed). Manual of Ocular Diagnosis and Therapy (4th ed). Boston: Little, Brown, 1995.

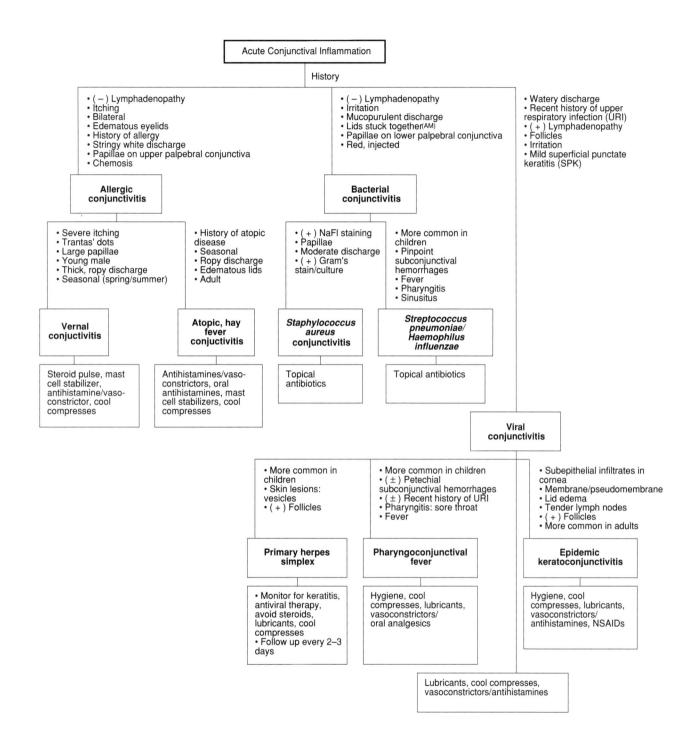

Acute Conjunctival Inflammation

History

• (−) Lymphadenopathy
• Itching
• Bilateral
• Edematous eyelids
• History of allergy
• Stringy white discharge
• Papillae on upper palpebral conjunctiva
• Chemosis

• (−) Lymphadenopathy
• Irritation
• Mucopurulent discharge
• Lids stuck together(AM)
• Papillae on lower palpebral conjunctiva
• Red, injected

• Watery discharge
• Recent history of upper respiratory infection (URI)
• (+) Lymphadenopathy
• Follicles
• Irritation
• Mild superficial punctate keratitis (SPK)

Allergic conjunctivitis

Bacterial conjunctivitis

• Severe itching
• Trantas' dots
• Large papillae
• Young male
• Thick, ropy discharge
• Seasonal (spring/summer)

• History of atopic disease
• Seasonal
• Ropy discharge
• Edematous lids
• Adult

• (+) NaFl staining
• Papillae
• Moderate discharge
• (+) Gram's stain/culture

• More common in children
• Pinpoint subconjunctival hemorrhages
• Fever
• Pharyngitis
• Sinusitus

Vernal conjuctivitis

Atopic, hay fever conjuctivitis

Staphylococcus aureus conjunctivitis

Streptococcus pneumoniae/ Haemophilus influenzae

Steroid pulse, mast cell stabilizer, antihistamine/vaso- constrictor, cool compresses

Antihistamines/vaso- constrictors, oral antihistamines, mast cell stabilizers, cool compresses

Topical antibiotics

Topical antibiotics

Viral conjunctivitis

• More common in children
• Skin lesions: vesicles
• (+) Follicles

• More common in children
• (±) Petechial subconjunctival hemorrhages
• (±) Recent history of URI
• Pharyngitis: sore throat
• Fever

• Subepithelial infiltrates in cornea
• Membrane/pseudomembrane
• Lid edema
• Tender lymph nodes
• (+) Follicles
• More common in adults

Primary herpes simplex

Pharyngoconjunctival fever

Epidemic keratoconjunctivitis

• Monitor for keratitis, antiviral therapy, avoid steroids, lubricants, cool compresses
• Follow up every 2–3 days

Hygiene, cool compresses, lubricants, vasoconstrictors/ oral analgesics

Hygiene, cool compresses, lubricants, vasoconstrictors/ antihistamines, NSAIDs

Lubricants, cool compresses, vasoconstrictors/antihistamines

16

Conjunctivitis in Neonates

DAVID P. SENDROWSKI

CONJUNCTIVITIS IN NEONATES AT A GLANCE

Chemical conjunctivitis
Neisseria gonorrhoeae
Chlamydia trachomatis
Herpes simplex
Corynebacterium diphtheriae
Inclusion conjunctivitis
Moraxella
Neisseriae meningitis
Pneumococcus
Staphylococcus
Streptococcus
Trichomonas vaginalis
Pseudomonas pyocyanea
Impatent lacrimal drainage system

Neonatal conjunctivitis (ophthalmia neonatorum) is described as inflammation of the conjunctiva during the first month of life. It is very important to understand that this conjunctival inflammation is frequently a manifestation of a potentially serious systemic infection.

Several factors should be considered in all cases of neonatal conjunctivitis, including trauma, organisms harbored in the birth canal, integrity of the ocular tissues, type and adequacy of topical prophylaxis, duration of exposure of the infant to infectious agents, and the time of onset of the conjunctivitis. There is no subjective history for these types of conjunctivitis. Therefore, a time line is the best starting point in isolating the conjunctivitis.

The objective testing is similar for all types of conjunctivitis in neonates. The ocular examination is usually conducted with a penlight or transilluminator. Close attention should be paid to the cornea for any signs of involvement. Sodium fluorescein can be instilled, and a blue filter used over the light source should help with the corneal examination. Conjunctival scrapings should be ordered for Gram's and Giemsa staining. Cultures should also be ordered. Blood and chocolate culture agar are good media with which to begin. If a viral infection is believed to be the cause of the conjunctivitis, then a viral culture may be ordered.

CHEMICAL CONJUNCTIVITIS

Subjective

A chemical conjunctivitis usually starts within hours after the instillation of a prophylactic agent such as silver nitrate.

Objective

The conjunctiva is mildly to moderately injected, usually without mucopurulent discharge. All laboratory testing is negative with a chemical conjunctivitis.

Plan

No treatment is necessary. The eyes should be re-evaluated within 24 hours.

NEISSERIAL CONJUNCTIVITIS

Subjective

This type of neonatal conjunctivitis is caused by maternal transmission of the organism *Neisseria gonorrhoeae*. Neisserial conjunctivitis starts between days 2 and 7 after birth. If it is suspected, the mother should be questioned about a history of gonorrhea or other sexually transmitted disease. The incidence of neonatal conjunctivitis caused by *N. gonorrhoeae* has decreased markedly since the introduction of Credé's silver nitrate prophylaxis in 1881. With the institution of silver nitrate use, the incidence decreased almost immediately to less than 0.4%. Alternative prophylactic treatments include topical erythromycin, tetracycline, or povidone-iodine.

Objective

A neisserial infection usually starts in one eye and quickly moves to the other. There is generally a copious amount of mucopurulent discharge. If the discharge is cleared away, much more is produced within several minutes. The conjunctiva is severely inflamed, and the lashes are matted from the discharge. The lids are very edematous to the point of ballooning. The cornea is also at risk for ulceration. *Neisseria* is one of the organisms that can penetrate an intact corneal epithelium. Gram's stain reveals gram-negative diplococci. Culture and sensitivity testing should also be ordered.

Plan

In the case of *N. gonorrhoeae*, an intravenous antibiotic should be initiated (e.g., ceftriaxone sodium). A topical antibiotic (e.g., bacitracin or ciprofloxacin ointment) should also be instilled. Topical lavage is recommended to remove the discharge and should be done on an hourly basis. After approximately 1 week, the intravenous antibiotic can be changed to an oral antibiotic such as penicillin or cefaclor if the condition is significantly improving. There may be a secondary iritis, particularly if the cornea is involved. In this event, a topical cycloplegic agent helps to reduce secondary complications.

Some practitioners recommend that all neonates with gonorrhea should also be treated for chlamydial infection, usually with erythromycin syrup. Neonates should be treated in consultation with a pediatrician. The parents should have cultures performed and should be treated for gonorrhea infection as well.

CHLAMYDIAL CONJUNCTIVITIS

Subjective

Conjunctivitis due to *Chlamydia trachomatis* occurs roughly in the same time frame as gonorrheal conjunctivitis. It can occur between days 2 and 15. The mother should be questioned regarding a history of venereal disease.

Objective

The eyes may show purulent, mucopurulent, or mucous discharge as with gonorrhea. There is marked conjunctival injection, chemosis, and eyelid edema. A membranous conjunctivitis may develop and result in conjunctival scarring and a superficial corneal vascularization.

Chlamydia causes the production of intracytoplasmic inclusion bodies in the conjunctiva. These are seen very well on Giemsa-stained conjunctival scrapings. Inclusions appear in the Giemsa-stained preparations as particulate, dark purple or blue cytoplasmic masses that cap the nucleus of the epithelial cells.

Newer diagnostic procedures, including fluorescent antibody stains and enzyme immunoassay tests, have somewhat superseded the Giemsa stain.

Plan

A 3-week course of oral antibiotics (e.g., erythromycin or azithromycin) and topical antibiotics (e.g., tetracycline ointment or 10% sodium sulfacetamide solution) is usually effective in eradicating the *Chlamydia*. The parents should be evaluated for chlamydial infection and should be treated if indicated.

HERPES SIMPLEX CONJUNCTIVITIS

Subjective

The primary herpes simplex conjunctivitis typically manifests between days 5 and 28 after birth.

Objective

There is a watery discharge from the eyes and a mild injection. It is very important to evaluate the periocular skin tissue for vesicles. These vesicles may appear on the eyelids and lid margins. They are usually associated with severe edema of the lids. There may also be a tender and palpable preauricular node.

Rose bengal stain may reveal a dendritic pattern on the cornea. It should be noted that corneal involvement is less common in primary than in recurrent ocular herpes simplex.

A moistened cotton-tipped applicator may be rolled along the palpebral conjunctiva and put into a viral transport medium for further diagnostic testing. Cultures and stains are usually negative, although intranuclear inclusion bodies can be seen when Papanicolaou's stain is used. An enzyme-linked immunosorbent assay test for herpes simplex is also available.

Plan

If corneal involvement is seen or suspected, a topical antiviral (e.g., trifluridine) should be prescribed. The patient should be evaluated every 24 hours for regression of corneal lesions. It should be noted that, with prolonged treatment, the antiviral agent can produce a toxic punctate keratopathy. In some cases, systemic acyclovir may be of benefit. A pediatrician should be consulted before prescribing this medication.

SUGGESTED READING

Jarvis VN, Levine R, Asbell PA. Ophthalmia neonatorum: study of a decade of experience at the Mount Sinai Hospital. Br J Ophthalmol 1987;71:295.

Phillips G, Forsyth JS, Harper IA. Diagnosis of neonatal conjunctivitis. Arch Dis Child 1990;65:894.

Sandstrom EG, Knapp KS, Reller LB. Microbial causes of neonatal conjunctivitis. J Pediatr 1984;105:706.

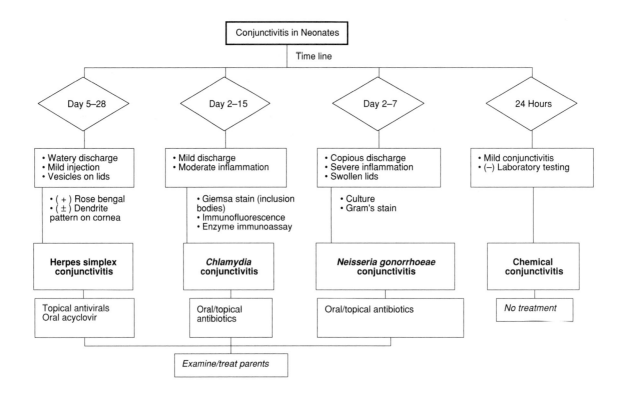

17

Lesions of the Conjunctiva

David P. Sendrowski

LESIONS OF THE CONJUNCTIVA AT A GLANCE

Tumors
  Keratoacanthoma
  Papilloma
  Epithelioma
  Adenoma
  Lymphoma
  Angioma
  Lymphangioma
  Melanoma
  Nevus
  Neurofibroma
  Kaposi's sarcoma
  Carcinoma in situ
  Pinguecula
  Pterygia
  Pyogenic granuloma
  Amyloid nodules
  Sarcoid granuloma
Cysts
  Retention
  Traumatic
  Muscle inclusion
  Lymphatic
  Dermoid
Pigmentation
  Melanin pigment (brown)
  Blood pigment (red)
  Bile pigment (yellow)
  Nevus of Ota
  Argyrosis (silver)
  Iron (siderosis)
  Copper (chalcosis)
  Gold (chrysiasis)

Drug induced
Neoplasms (see Tumors)

Conjunctival lesions may be classified as congenital or acquired, elevated or flat, pigmented or nonpigmented. Conjunctival pigmentation alone is a normal racial variant in African- and Asian-Americans. Also, the various forms of acquired melanosis must be distinguished from ocular melanocytosis, melanosis oculi, and congenital pigmentation that is not associated with conjunctival melanoma but may increase the risk of choroidal and orbital melanoma. Conjunctival pigmentation may result from conjunctival inflammation, chemicals or toxins (i.e., argyrosis, radiation, chlorpromazine hydrochloride [Thorazine], topical epinephrine), pregnancy, and Addison's disease, and is not malignant.

The clinician needs to take a thorough history and closely evaluate the location, color, and morphology of a conjunctival lesion before making a proper diagnosis.

CONGENITAL OCULAR MELANOSIS

Subjective

Congenital ocular melanosis is usually present at birth or shortly thereafter. It is very common in African-Americans, Asian-Americans, and other darkly pigmented patients and less common in whites. It is usually bilateral and may increase with age. The patient is probably aware of the pigmented area on the conjunctiva and generally has no complaints other than a cosmetic one.

Objective

Ocular melanosis is a nonprogressive condition. The pigment is actually on the episclera rather than the conjunctiva. This is demonstrated by the fact that the conjunctiva can be moved without a corresponding movement of the lesion. The affected area looks grayish brown to black. (The pigment is flat and irregular and usually located near the limbal area.) Heterochromia of the iris may also be present in the involved eye. If the dermal tissue around the orbit is involved, the condition is usually referred to as a *nevus of Ota*.

Plan

Patient reassurance is the best management. Patients should be followed yearly with dilated fundus examinations, because there is a very slight predisposition to malignant melanoma of the uveal tract, orbit, and brain. The risk is greater for patients with a nevus of Ota.

PRIMARY ACQUIRED MELANOSIS

Subjective

Primary acquired melanosis usually appears in middle-age adults and almost always occurs in whites. Any portion of the conjunctiva may be affected. There is a mild to moderate chance that these lesions will develop into a malignant melanoma. Benign acquired melanosis may also occur from the use of Thorazine or from metabolic by-products caused by Addison's disease or pregnancy. This pigment buildup is usually benign.

The patient may be alarmed by the sudden appearance of irregular, flat, brown patches on the conjunctiva and present with that as the chief complaint. Primary acquired melanosis is otherwise asymptomatic.

Objective

The lesion is a unilateral, flat, brownish pigmented area that moves freely over the sclera when the conjunctiva is moved. The area does not stain with sodium fluorescein. Pupils, intraocular pressure, and anterior chambers are all normal.

Plan

Management of the patient should begin with photodocumentation of the lesion. Frequent follow-ups should be scheduled to evaluate the lesion for changes in size and position. If changes are noted, the patient should be sent for a biopsy of the area. The entire conjunctival area of the eyes should be evaluated for changes. The progression is variable.

The patient should be educated about the risk of the condition becoming malignant. Use of sunglasses that provide protection from UV radiation should also be considered.

CONJUNCTIVAL NEVI

Subjective

Nevi of the conjunctiva are lesions that may not appear clinically until the second or third decade of life. The patient may complain of a recent onset of the pigmentation or of increasing pigment. This increase in pigment is especially prominent during puberty or pregnancy. The patient is usually otherwise asymptomatic.

Objective

The clinician should look for and ask about other nevi on the face, neck, and head. A key sign in the diagnosis is the presence of small cysts within the lesion. Greater than one-half of conjunctival nevi contain islands or small cysts of surface epithelium, which can easily be observed with the biomicroscope. Nevi on the palpebral conjunctiva are rare, and additional investigations should be performed on lesions in this location. Unlike the lesions in congenital melanosis, most nevi move with movement of the conjunctiva. Nevi have varying degrees of vascularization.

Plan

The nevi should be photodocumented and should be re-evaluated every 6–12 months. Any variation in size or color change over this period should arouse suspicion. The patient should also be told to monitor for changes and return immediately if changes are noted. The use of glasses or sunglasses with UV radiation protection may be beneficial, especially for those patients whose occupations or avocations expose them to sunlight for extended periods.

DERMOID

Subjective

Children or adults may present with dermoids, epidermoids, and dermolipomas. A parent may bring in a child with the complaint that the globe is malpositioned. Cystic dermoids may occasionally originate from the conjunctiva and extend posteriorly into the orbit, producing proptosis and orbital enlargement. The dermoid does not usually cause complaints unless it becomes large enough to cause diplopia or is of cosmetic concern to the parent.

In adults complaints are either cosmetic or functional, because a larger dermoid may impair vision by causing secondary diplopia. Additional complaints are usually of a dry-eye nature, such as irritation, burning, and foreign body sensation.

Objective

A thorough biomicroscopic evaluation of the lesion is a good starting point. Conjunctival dermoids are usually located at the limbus, whereas dermolipomas are most often located near the temporal canthus. Dermoids appear as round, yellow-white, smooth, elevated masses that may have hairs (cilia) protruding from them. There is usually no vascularization such as might be expected from an inflammatory mass.

The dermoid may enlarge the width of the vertical palpebral fissure. The fissure should be measured with a ruler and compared with that of the other eye. A clear plastic ruler may be helpful in measuring the distance between the separation of the Hirschberg reflexes. The dermoid may alter its symmetric position.

Plan

The dermoid should be evaluated for size, elevation, and location. Photodocumentation is an excellent means to follow the dermoid for changes over time. If the dermoid is cosmetically unacceptable to the patient or affects visual function, a surgical consultation should be sought.

CONJUNCTIVAL MELANOMA

Subjective

Patients who develop conjunctival melanomas are typically middle-aged to elderly individuals. The patient usually presents with a previously known pigmented lesion on the conjunctiva (e.g., primary acquired melanosis) and may report a change in the size or shape of the lesion. Most melanomas arise from pre-existing acquired melanosis. Patients may also present with a complaint that they have discovered a newly acquired lesion on their conjunctiva.

There are very few ocular complaints unless the lesion is quite large. The cosmetic appearance is what usually brings the patient to the office.

Objective

The lesion appears as a nodular brown mass. The lesion is usually well-vascularized and may have a large conjunctival vessel (feeder vessel) entering into the mass.

Gonioscopy and fundus examination should be performed on the dilated eye to check for an underlying ciliary body melanoma or intraocular extension of the tumor. The pupil may show distortion if there is ciliary body involvement, so pupil shape should be evaluated and documented.

The intraocular pressure is usually unaffected. A ciliary body melanoma may cause an anterior chamber seeding phenomenon to occur. If the clinician sees cells in the anterior chamber, meticulous biomicroscopic examination should be performed to delineate white blood cells from pigment cells.

Not all conjunctival melanomas are pigmented; melanomas with little or no pigment can resemble squamous and sebaceous gland carcinomas, papillomas, and even pterygia. B-scan ultrasonography can provide additional information on the size and location of the melanoma.

Plan

The patient with a suspected melanoma should be referred to an ophthalmologist or ophthalmologic oncologist for excisional biopsy. If the biopsy is positive for cancerous cells, the surgeon usually discusses the treatment options with the patient.

Because conjunctival melanomas behave very similarly to melanomas of the skin, the patient should be educated regarding growths on other areas of the skin exposed to the sun. Sunglasses with UV radiation protection would be an excellent recommendation to the patient postsurgically.

PAPILLOMA

Subjective

Papillomas found in children and young adults are usually of viral origin. Papillomas that occur in older patients are typically of a nonviral origin and should be considered precancerous.

The younger patient with papillomas of the conjunctiva usually complains of the cosmetic appearance of the lesion. Papillomas may cause dry-eye symptoms if they become large enough, but most of the time patients are asymptomatic.

Objective

The papilloma arises from a broad base at or near the limbus. It may be located on the palpebral or bulbar conjunctiva. It has a stalk; is raised; has smooth, nonkeratinized surfaces; and is highly vascularized.

Plan

Papillomas of viral origin are usually benign, and, if cosmetic appearance is not a concern, they are left alone. They may resolve spontaneously and tend to have a high recurrence rate if removed surgically. Cryotherapy has been used to treat some cases successfully.

Papillomas of nonviral origin that occur in the elderly population may have a cancerous potential and therefore warrant an excisional biopsy. The patient should be referred for evaluation and biopsy.

PYOGENIC GRANULOMA

Subjective

The pyogenic granuloma is a lesion usually found at a site of prior traumatic insult. The patient may develop a pyogenic granuloma over a site of surgical entry, or penetrating trauma. The patient should be asked about recent cataract, retinal, or anterior segment surgery. Questions concerning prior trauma to the eye or history of chalazion removal are also important.

Objective

A pyogenic granuloma occurs over the site of surgery or trauma or previous chalazion and appears as a deep, red, pedunculated mass. If the injury or surgery is close to the limbal area, some corneal haze may be associated with the lesion.

Findings from evaluation of the pupils, intraocular pressure, and anterior chambers may vary depending on the type of injury.

Plan

A pyogenic granuloma may respond to a steroid-antibiotic combination (e.g., prednisolone-gentamicin) given four times a day. The drops should be given for 1–2 weeks.

The patient should be evaluated every 3–5 days, and the intraocular pressure checked along with the granuloma. If the granuloma persists after 2 weeks, the patient may require surgical excision.

SARCOID GRANULOMA

Subjective

Sarcoid granulomas may be found in patients with a history of sarcoidosis. These patients are usually African-American and in the third or fourth decade of life; often they are females.

The granulomas may be seen as a confirmatory sign while assessing a patient for iridocyclitis, because iridocyclitis frequently occurs in patients with sarcoidosis. An African-American patient who has a history of sarcoidosis and who is in the third to fourth decade of life should have a thorough examination of the superior and inferior palpe-bral conjunctivas. Patients with sarcoid granulomas are asymptomatic unless there is an associated uveitis or posterior segment involvement.

Objective

Sarcoid granulomas appear as discrete yellow nodules that are generally less than 2 mm in diameter. They can occur on the skin of the lids but may also occur in the tarsal conjunctiva, the fornices, the bulbar conjunctiva, and the conjunctiva overlying the lacrimal gland. The position of these granulomas should be noted, because many are easily biopsied if needed for confirmation of the disease.

The anterior chamber may show signs of inflammatory disease (e.g., posterior synechiae, endothelial keratitic precipitates, and iris nodules), or it may be normal. The intraocular pressure may be elevated if the drainage angle is involved, or it may be normal. The posterior segment should be evaluated for signs of sarcoidosis, such as vitritis or clumps of cells ("snowballs") in the vitreous body. Retinal periphlebitis in the midperiphery is highly suggestive of sarcoidosis. Small exudates near retinal veins ("candle-wax drippings"), choroidal granulomas (Dalen-Fuchs nodules), and neovascularization of the disc may also be present in these patients.

Plan

If the patient has no other ocular signs except for the sarcoid granuloma, the patient should be sent to an internist for an evaluation that may include one or several of the following tests: chest radiography; gallium scan of the head and neck; measurement of angiotensin-converting enzyme, serum lysozyme, and serum calcium levels; and a biopsy of the conjunctiva granuloma. These are a few diagnostic tests that could help confirm the suspicion of sarcoidosis.

Patients should be told to return immediately if they experience eye redness, irritation, or photophobia, as this could indicate the onset of iridocyclitis. If the patient presently has an ongoing iridocyclitis, the patient should be treated with a topical cycloplegic agent (e.g., homatropine) twice a day and a topical steroid (e.g., prednisolone acetate) every 1–4 hours depending on the severity of the anterior chamber reaction.

The patient should be followed closely, especially during periods of exacerbation of the disease.

AMYLOIDOSIS

Subjective

Amyloidosis may be a localized process or a manifestation of a systemic disease state. Amyloidosis is an accumulation of various insoluble fibrillin proteins in the tissues.

Manifestations of the disease are nonspecific. Complaints are variable depending on the organ or system that has been affected. The nodules produced by the disorder may be restricted to the conjunctiva and orbit. The clinician usually suspects this condition based on clinical signs rather than specific complaints.

Objective

Smooth, yellow, waxy masses are seen in the conjunctiva, especially in the lower fornix. There are usually small hemorrhages around the masses. Pupils, intraocular pressure, and anterior chamber are normal.

Plan

The patient should be referred for biopsy of the nodules. The biopsy results should provide the definitive diagnosis. The patient should be referred to an internist for systemic evaluation and treatment if indicated. The patient should be followed closely for involvement of other ocular structures such as the extraocular muscles, vitreous, and sclera.

PTERYGIUM

Subjective

Pterygia are most common in males who have been chronically exposed to UV radiation or the elements (e.g., wind). Pterygia may cause the patient to complain of irritation, redness, decreased visual acuity, foreign body sensation, photophobia, or the cosmetic appearance of the lesion. Decreased vision or diplopia may be a complaint if the lesion becomes large enough to affect the visual axis.

Objective

A pterygium is a triangular band of fibrovascular tissue growth. There is a broad band on the nasal or temporal bulbar conjunctiva, and the apex of the triangle is on the cornea. An iron line (Stocker's line) may be seen in the cornea preceding the growth. Tear break-up time may be affected by the lesion. Corneal dellen may develop in front of the pterygia. Pterygia are variable in their growth patterns; some are much more aggressive than others.

Refraction may show increasing amounts of astigmatism, and keratometry can reveal irregular mires if the visual axis is being compromised by the lesion.

Plan

The eyes should be protected from sun, dust, and wind with sunglasses providing UV radiation protection. Artificial tears or a mild vasoconstrictor (e.g., naphazoline) may be given four to five times a day. A mild topical steroid (e.g., fluorometholone) may be used in more severe cases.

If an adjacent corneal dellen is present, topical lubrication with artificial tears or a bland ophthalmic ointment helps to resolve it.

Pterygia are removed surgically. The pterygium should be excised down to the bared sclera. Mitomycin C, either in a single application at surgery or given several days postoperatively, significantly reduces recurrence.

PINGUECULA

Subjective

Pingueculae are the result of aging and environmental factors. Patients with pingueculae are generally asymptomatic. Most patients are unaware of the lesion, and it is commonly found during ocular examinations. Occasionally, a patient may complain of the cosmetic appearance. A pinguecula may become inflamed and cause mild ocular irritation.

Objective

Pingueculae appear as yellow-white, flat or slightly elevated lesions on the bulbar conjunctiva. They occur more commonly in the medial bulbar conjunctiva. They do not directly involve the cornea; however, they can cause the formation of a dellen.

Plan

Management consists primarily of reassuring the patient about the benign nature of the lesion. If environmental factors are a concern, the patient should be educated about the use of UV-filtering sunglasses for protection against sun and wind. Artificial tears are usually given as needed.

In the case of pingueculitis, a mild topical vasoconstrictor (e.g., naphazoline) or steroid (e.g., fluorometholone) is prescribed and usually reduces the ocular irritation.

SUGGESTED READING

Easty DL, Smolin G. External Eye Disease. Oxford, UK: Butterworth, 1985.

Miller S. Clinical Ophthalmology. Bristol, UK: IOP Publishing, 1987.

Hornblass A (ed). Oculoplastic, Orbital and Reconstruction Surgery, Vols 1 & 2. Baltimore: Williams & Wilkins, 1989.

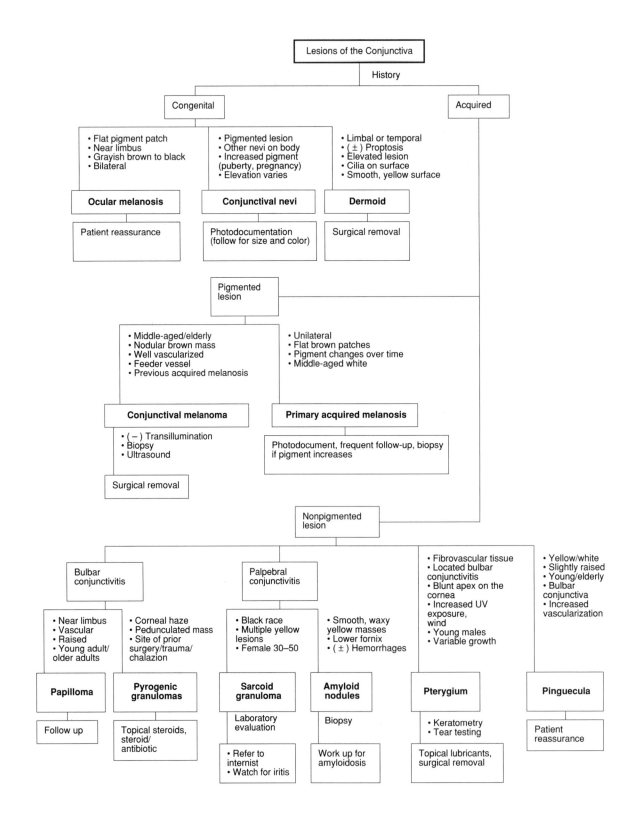

18

Punctate Keratopathy

John H. Nishimoto

PUNCTATE KERATOPATHY AT A GLANCE

Bacterial keratoconjunctivitis
Staphylococcal blepharokeratoconjunctivitis
Lagophthalmos (exposure keratitis)
Trichiasis
Keratoconjunctivitis sicca
Ultraviolet radiation keratitis
Thygeson's superficial punctate keratitis
Contact lens induced keratopathy
Viral keratoconjunctivitis
Toxic reaction
Superior limbic keratoconjunctivitis
Limbal vernal keratoconjunctivitis
Trachoma/inclusion keratoconjunctivitis
Anterior basement membrane dystrophy
Fuchs' endothelial/epithelial dystrophy
Verruca
Molluscum contagiosum
Rosacea

Damage to the corneal epithelium can cause punctate keratopathy, which consists of discrete areas of epithelial loss that stain with sodium fluorescein. Staining can occur in various patterns depending on the etiology. Generally, punctate staining is categorized into five major patterns: (1) inferior, (2) interpalpebral, (3) central, (4) superior, and (5) diffuse.

In managing patients with punctate keratopathy, the clinician should always be alert to the possibility of secondary infection. Epithelial disruption allows a route of access for pathogens that normally cannot penetrate the epithelium. Organisms such as *Pseudomonas aeruginosa* cannot invade a healthy, intact cornea; but once the organ-ism has reached the corneal stroma, collagenase can rapidly degenerate the cornea.

This chapter discusses some of the causes of punctate corneal staining as well as treatment and management of these conditions.

INFERIOR CORNEAL STAINING

Bacterial Keratoconjunctivitis

Subjective
Most bacterial keratoconjunctivitis results from the organism *Staphylococcus aureus*. The punctate staining is due to the release of exotoxins that break down the epithelium. *S. aureus* resides predominantly at the lid margin and fornix region of the conjunctiva. Because the inferior portion of the cornea is closest to these structures, this area is the most affected. Patients with bacterial keratoconjunctivitis often experience irritation or pain with slight photophobia. The symptoms of pain and photophobia are due to disruption of the corneal surface, which causes nerves to be exposed. The patient may also complain that the lids are matted shut in the morning.

Objective
In addition to inferior punctate staining of the corneal epithelium, due to the formation of fine papillae, the palpebral conjunctiva have a red, velvetlike appearance. Hyperemia is usually greatest toward the fornix region of the bulbar conjunctiva. The clinician also should look for mucopurulent discharge. Accumulation of this discharge often is greatest in the morning, causing the lids to be matted or even stuck shut. It should be noted that the patient

may have washed most of the discharge out of the eyes before coming to the eye doctor's office.

Plan

Treatment for bacterial conjunctivitis consists of topical antibiotic therapy. Because the cornea is compromised and is more susceptible to *Pseudomonas* infection, broad-spectrum antibiotics such as gentamicin, polymyxin B sulfate–trimethoprim, or ciprofloxacin are most appropriate. If broad-spectrum therapy is not effective, then a culture and antibiotic sensitivity evaluation is useful to determine the best treatment for the organism causing the problem.

Staphylococcal Blepharokeratoconjunctivitis

Subjective

Staphylococcal blepharitis is a bacterial infection of the lids, especially the lid margin. Because the organism that causes the problem is most commonly *S. aureus*, the exotoxins produced can create punctate corneal staining. Symptoms vary from none to irritation and pain about the lid margin. Occasionally, the patient mentions that pulling on the lashes seems to provide temporary relief. Patients may also have an associated bacterial conjunctivitis; thus, mucopurulent discharge with lid matting may be an associated complaint.

Objective

In acute staphylococcal blepharitis, red and scaly lid margins are the predominant sign. The scales are hard and brittle. They are found at the base of the lashes or surrounding individual cilia (collarettes). Because the lid margin is adjacent to the cornea, release of toxins can create punctate staining, especially of the inferior cornea. Conjunctival involvement with hyperemia, papillary hypertrophy, and mucopurulent discharge may be an associated finding. Staphylococcal infection of the lid margins also can give rise to internal or external hordeola. Chronic inflammation can give the lid margin a thickened, uneven appearance. Other signs of chronic blepharitis include madarosis, poliosis, rosettes, and trichiasis.

Plan

The goal of therapy for staphylococcal blepharokeratoconjunctivitis is to reduce the population of the bacteria, particularly at the lid margins. Mild cases of staphylococcal blepharitis can be treated by gentle cleansing with dilute, nonirritative shampoo or a specially formulated lid-cleansing agent. Warm soaks applied to the lids before cleansing can also help loosen debris and scales. If the meibomian glands are blocked or secretions are excessive, expression of the glands may be helpful.

In more severe cases, antibiotic ointment such as bacitracin, gentamicin, or a combination of bacitracin and polymyxin B sulfate should be applied to the lids. The moist soaks and cleansing should be performed before application of the ointment. If inflammation and hyperemia are substantial, an antibiotic-steroid combination can be useful in decreasing the inflammatory ocular reaction and making the lids less tender.

Lagophthalmos (Exposure Keratitis)

Subjective

Lagophthalmos is the inability to fully close the lids. It can be physiologic, nocturnal, orbital, mechanical, or paralytic. Common causes include Bell's palsy and Graves' disease. In true lagophthalmos, 2 mm or more of the inferior limbal cornea is exposed. The exposed portion of the cornea is susceptible to desiccation and other damage (exposure keratopathy). Patients with lagophthalmos may complain of a gritty, foreign body sensation due to epithelial damage and erosion.

Objective

The physical examination should confirm the presence of lagophthalmos. This confirmation is usually accomplished by instructing the patient to gently close the eyes. In cases of nocturnal lagophthalmos, lagophthalmos may not be noted until the patient is in a supine position and the closed eyelids are examined carefully with a penlight. Another simple way to determine if nocturnal lagophthalmos is occurring is to ask a family member if the patient sleeps with his or her eyes open. Vital stains with sodium fluorescein and rose bengal can be clinically useful in detecting epithelial defects that indicate exposure keratopathy. If the patient has a proptotic appearance, exophthalmometry should be performed. Proptosis of 3 mm or more above the normal range is suggestive of Graves' disease, and laboratory workup to rule out thyrotoxicosis is indicated. Other etiologies of proptosis such as tumor also should be considered.

Plan

When corneal exposure is mild, bland ocular lubricating ointment applied at bedtime is usually sufficient to eliminate symptoms. In addition, the eyelids can be taped closed at bedtime by applying the tape first to the cheek and then to the brow and forehead. In severe lagophthalmos, a moisture chamber can be placed over the eye at bedtime. Instillation of artificial tears, preferably preservative free, during the day may also be required depending on the severity of the exposure. Extended-wear bandage contact lenses may also be used along with antibiotic or lubricant therapy. Surgical correction may be necessary if these therapies fail and the condition is long-standing.

Trichiasis

Subjective
Trichiasis is a common clinical problem characterized by one or more in-turning lashes on the upper or lower lid. It can be idiopathic or associated with chronic blepharitis or entropion. Other less common causes include trachoma, Stevens-Johnson syndrome, ocular pemphigoid, and trauma. Patients with trichiasis may complain of irritation or foreign body sensation from the misdirected lash's rubbing against the cornea. In severe cases of trichiasis, vision loss secondary to corneal scarring can occur.

Objective
The diagnosis of trichiasis is made by careful examination with the biomicroscope. One or more in-turned lashes are observed, and conjunctival hyperemia or inferior corneal staining in the area of the in-turned lash may be evident. If the trichiasis is a result of inflammation, such as in trachoma or Stevens-Johnson syndrome, the conjunctiva may also have scarring and symblepharon formation.

Plan
Management involves removing the offending lashes as well as treating the compromised conjunctiva or cornea. When only a few lashes are involved, manual epilation is effective, but it usually must be repeated every few weeks or months, because it fails to destroy the lash follicle.

Electrolysis can be used to destroy the cilia follicles when only a few lashes are involved. Simple epilation or electrolysis is impractical when one-third or more of the eyelid margin is involved. In such cases surgical procedures such as cryosurgery or argon laser thermal ablation are indicated. If entropion is present, surgery to correct the lid position effectively eliminates trichiasis.

INTERPALPEBRAL CORNEAL STAINING

Keratoconjunctivitis Sicca (Dry Eyes)

Subjective
Keratoconjunctivitis sicca can be caused by a number of factors, including aging, collagen-vascular disease, environmental desiccation, reduced blink rate, inflammation, lid deformities, vitamin deficiencies, and certain medications. Patients with dry eyes frequently experience irritation, pain, and slight photophobia. Occasionally vision can be affected. The symptoms are usually more pronounced later in the day due to prolonged environmental exposure. In some case patients can experience paradoxical tearing from reflex lacrimation.

Determining the cause of dry eyes is important and often difficult. The clinician should question the patient about environmental factors, including smoke, fumes, air currents from air conditioning or heating ducts, and so forth, that can contribute to corneal desiccation and irritation. In addition, with prolonged concentrated near work, the blink rate is reduced, and thus proper tear production and lubrication are not provided. The clinician should also take a careful history of the use of medications such as antihistamines, beta blockers, and hormone supplements, as well as of systemic conditions such as Sjögren's syndrome.

Objective
In keratoconjunctivitis sicca, the predominant corneal staining pattern is interpalpebral. This area is most exposed to the environment, and ocular tissues can become damaged from desiccation. Punctate epithelial erosions can be detected with fluorescein staining. Sodium fluorescein staining indicates not only areas of epithelial defects and damage but also areas of tear-film instability. A tear-breakup time of less than 10 seconds can be considered abnormal. Rose bengal and lissamine green stains devitalized tissue of the cornea and conjunctiva. Another test helpful in diagnosing dry eyes is Schirmer's test (an evaluation to determine aqueous layer production). Schirmer's test may be performed with or without topical anesthesia. The practical clinical information obtained from the Schirmer I test is the confirmation of hyposecretion when less than 5 mm of strip wetting occurs. Greater than 15 mm of wetting could indicate decreased, normal, or increased compensatory (reflex) secretion. If this result occurs, one must try to differentiate between basal and reflex tearing. The difference in the results of Schirmer's tests with and without topical anesthetic is presumed to represent the reflex portion of the tear film. Of particular value is a finding of less than 5 mm of wetting on the basic secretion, which suggests a diagnosis of hyposecretion. The phenol red thread test is an alternate technique to Schirmer's test.

Another test available to the clinician is to determine the amount of lysozyme in the tears. Tear lysozyme level is a useful measure of aqueous tear secretion, because lysozyme constitutes nearly one-fourth of total tear protein. It is important to note that lysozyme levels are reduced because of dilution in cases of hypersecretion and are also reduced in aqueous-deficient conditions such as Sjögren's syndrome.

Plan
The initial treatment of dry eye consists largely of the use of artificial lubricants. The dosage varies with the severity of the condition. Preservative-free artificial tears are preferable for long-term use to reduce the risk of medicamentosa. If the corneal epithelium remains compromised,

supplementation with lubricating ointments can help moisten the ocular tissues.

In cases in which lubricating therapy is not sufficiently effective or noncompliance is suspected, punctal plugs can be implanted to reduce tear drainage. Other techniques that are less frequently used to manage dry eye include the use of moisture chambers and punctal cautery.

Ultraviolet Radiation Keratitis

Subjective
UV radiation is one of the most common causes of ocular injury. UV radiation causes an inhibition of mitosis and subsequent loosening of the epithelial layer. Sunlamps and welding arcs are common sources of this form of radiation. Improper protection of the eyes from UV radiation during recreational activities such as sunbathing, river rafting, water sports, and snow skiing also can result in enough UV-radiation exposure to cause corneal damage. Photophobia, pain, lacrimation, and blepharospasm are common symptoms. After exposure there is usually a lag time of about 6 hours before symptoms of the burn become evident.

Objective
Biomicroscopy reveals a keratoconjunctivitis with corneal staining that is most intense in the interpalpebral region. If sunlight or reflected light rays become intense, people tend to squint, so that there is damage only to the exposed areas of the cornea. Commonly associated findings include conjunctival hyperemia, periorbital edema, and associated burn of the face and eyelids. Secondary iridocyclitis also may be present.

Plan
If the keratitis is severe enough to cause extreme discomfort, then a pressure patch or bandage contact lens should be applied to promote re-epithelialization. Topical antibiotic ointments or drops should be used to prevent a secondary infection, and a cycloplegic agent such as 1% cyclopentolate hydrochloride or 5% homatropine should be used to relieve ciliary spasm. If the patient is only experiencing mild discomfort, patching may not be necessary. The symptoms tend to resolve within 24 hours.

CENTRAL CORNEAL STAINING

Thygeson's Superficial Punctate Keratitis

Subjective
Several theories have been postulated regarding the cause of Thygeson's superficial punctate keratitis (SPK). It was once thought to be virally based because of its clinical similarity to adenoviral infection. More recently, a hyperimmune mechanism has been suggested, although this explanation has not been proven. In Thygeson's SPK, patients often complain of symptoms associated with epithelial disruption, including photophobia, foreign body sensation, pain, and excessive tearing.

Objective
Thygeson's SPK is typically seen as a bilateral epithelial keratitis affecting the central cornea. The faint gray corneal lesions appear as coarse punctate epithelial defects. They are usually round or stellate and may resemble subepithelial infiltrates. The lesions may stain minimally with fluorescein, may stain with rose bengal, and can appear slightly elevated. When microerosions occur, these areas stain more brightly with sodium fluorescein. This disease is marked by the lack of significant findings elsewhere in the ocular tissues. The cornea appears to be the only structure involved. The defects can be slight, with only a few defects, or severe, with up to as many as 50 defects. The condition can also have exacerbations and remissions, with no residual findings between attacks. Exacerbations can be triggered by corneal trauma.

Plan
In mild cases ocular lubricants can provide symptomatic relief. The most successful treatment for moderate Thygeson's SPK is the prescription of mild topical steroids such as 0.12% prednisolone acetate or fluorometholone. The dosage depends on the severity of the condition and should be tapered slowly. In some cases long-term administration of a low dosage of topical steroids may be needed to control the disease. In severe cases soft bandage contact lenses may be used to provide proper corneal re-epithelialization.

Contact Lens–Induced Punctate Keratopathy

Subjective
Central corneal epithelial problems associated with contact lens wear may be due to several causes. If the patient wears rigid contact lenses and the fit of the lens is steep, there is little exchange with oxygenated tears; this lack can lead to corneal hypoxia and central punctate staining. Corneal damage can occur from overwear of either rigid or soft contact lenses. The history may reveal that the patient has increased wearing time dramatically or that the patient slept with the lenses on the eyes. Corneal damage can occur from contact lens overwear, either from soft or rigid lens wear. Improper soft contact lens removal techniques also can lead to changes causing central corneal staining. Symptoms include pain, burning dryness, photophobia, excessive lacrimation, and blepharospasm.

Objective

Contact lens–associated punctate keratopathy is best observed with slit-lamp biomicroscopy and the use of sodium fluorescein staining, which causes the affected areas to fluoresce. Signs vary from slight punctate stippling in the central region of the cornea to intense, coalesced epithelial damage similar in appearance to mechanical corneal abrasion. The condition may be severe enough to create a secondary anterior chamber reaction, which is indicated by a circumlimbal injection and cells in the anterior chamber. The clinician should also look for other signs of corneal hypoxia, including corneal clouding, thickening, and spectacle blur.

Plan

If central corneal staining is due to an improper contact lens fit, refitting the lens usually solves the problem. A rigid contact lens should not be refit too flat, because the lens can overbear on the central cornea and cause the epithelium to break down. Patients suffering from contact lens overwear need to reduce their wearing time or be deprived of their lenses until the cornea has re-epithelialized. Application of a topical antibiotic to prevent infection and a cycloplegic to prevent a secondary iritis may be indicated.

DIFFUSE CORNEAL STAINING

Viral Keratoconjunctivitis

Subjective

Viral keratoconjunctivitis is most commonly caused by the adenoviruses or herpes simplex. Herpes zoster and viruses shed from a lid lesion such as verruca or molluscum contagiosum also can cause keratopathy. Patients with viral keratopathy commonly present with complaints of pain, irritation, photophobia, and excessive tearing. They may have a recent history of sore throat or upper respiratory tract infection. Close associates to the patient may recently have had a similar condition. In some cases the patient has a history of swimming in a poorly disinfected pool. If the viral condition is suspected to be herpes simplex, the clinician should ask the patient whether similar episodes have occurred previously and whether the patient is prone to getting cold sores or fever blisters.

Objective

In all viral ocular conditions, the initial corneal presentation is diffuse punctate staining. Later the lesions develop a unique appearance based on the etiology. Common adenoviral diseases that can cause punctate keratopathy are pharyngoconjunctival fever and epidemic keratoconjunctivitis (EKC). In pharyngoconjunctival fever, besides slight diffuse punctate staining of the cornea, other signs include follicles in the palpebral conjunctiva, preauricular lymphatic adenopathy, sore throat, and fever. EKC presents in similar fashion except that there is more corneal involvement. After approximately 1 week from onset of the infection, the diffuse punctate staining appears. After another week, subepithelial infiltrates develop. These infiltrates can remain for several months to a year and can cause decreased vision.

Another viral condition causing keratopathy is herpes simplex. Later in this condition the diffuse punctate staining can give way to the appearance of dendritic lesions. These lesions stain brightly with rose bengal, lissamine green, and sodium fluorescein. A useful test in the diagnosis of herpes simplex keratitis is to evaluate corneal sensitivity with a cotton wisp or esthesiometer. In herpes simplex, the sensitivity is often reduced. In addition to keratopathy, there may be conjunctivitis and vesicular lesions of the lids, particularly in primary herpes simplex. Fever blisters or cold sores commonly occur in patients with secondary herpes simplex keratitis.

In herpes zoster conjunctivitis there are dendritic lesions; however, the ends of the lesions are not as bulbous as in herpes simplex conjunctivitis. These pseudodendrites are slightly elevated mucous plaques. They stain brightly with rose bengal but minimally with sodium fluorescein.

Verruca are multilobed, elevated skin lesions cause by papillomavirus. Molluscum contagiosum are round, elevated nodules with an umbilicated center. When either verruca or molluscum involves the lids, the virus-laden cells can be shed into the tear film and infect the cornea; the result is diffuse punctate staining.

Plan

Each viral condition mentioned here has a separate mode of treatment. There is currently no cure for adenoviral infections; however, EKC and pharyngoconjunctival fever can be managed with supportive therapy that includes the use of artificial tears, topical vasoconstrictors, and cold compresses. If the subepithelial infiltrates of EKC interfere with vision, topical corticosteroids such as prednisolone acetate or fluorometholone can be prescribed to improve vision and comfort. Tapering must be initiated carefully, because the chance of recurrence of the infiltrates is high if tapering is abrupt.

Topical antiviral medications such as trifluridine drops are used in the initial management of herpes simplex keratitis, especially if the lesions have developed into a dendritic ulcer. In conjunction with trifluridine, vidarabine ointment should be used at night. It should be noted that diffuse punctate staining is a relatively common toxic side effect of topical antiviral medications.

In herpes zoster, oral acyclovir and famciclovir have been used to suppress the virus and diminish the severity of the disease. If there is only diffuse punctate staining of the cornea, no treatment is necessary, although artificial tears may provide symptomatic relief. If corneal pseudodendrites are present, then topical debridement may be necessary.

The treatment of verruca is surgical excision or removal with a one-time application of dichloroacetic acid, a chemical cauterizing agent. Because the cause of the corneal staining has been removed, the punctate staining resolves. For molluscum contagiosum, the most successful method of treatment is surgical excision of the lesions, especially when the conjunctiva and cornea are involved. The conjunctivitis and keratitis usually resolve spontaneously after eradication of the lesions.

Toxic Reaction

Subjective
A toxic reaction of the cornea can occur from many sources. Common sources include ophthalmic medications such as aminoglycosides and antivirals, and the preservatives in ophthalmic solutions, including contact lens preparations and artificial tears. Toxicity can also occur from accidental instillation of a noxious chemical. The symptoms vary depending on the severity of the condition. If the toxic reaction is from ophthalmic medications or preservatives, the patient may experience mild discomfort, burning, and stinging. With continued use of the solution, the symptoms may become worse. Toxicity from nonophthalmic preparations may cause more pain, photophobia, and excessive tearing. Vision may be affected if there is significant epithelial disruption.

Objective
Signs of toxic reaction include diffuse punctate fluorescein staining of the cornea, palpebral, and bulbar conjunctiva, which is best viewed with a slit-lamp biomicroscope. Other findings, especially in acute cases, include conjunctival chemosis, diffuse injection, lid edema, punctal edema, and occlusion. In chronic conditions where exposure to the offending agent has occurred over a period of months, there may be conjunctival follicles and scarring.

Plan
In many cases removal of the offending agent solves the problem and, depending on the severity of the condition, reverses the damage and symptoms that occurred. If there is significant damage to the cornea and conjunctiva, the use of a prophylactic broad-spectrum antibiotic such as polymyxin B sulfate–trimethoprim drops prevents a secondary infection. Topical corticosteroids such as 1% pred-

nisolone acetate or rimexolone can provide symptomatic relief and reduce scarring. Unfortunately, if scarring of the conjunctiva or cornea has occurred, the damage is irreversible. Chronic dry eyes may become a secondary problem due to damage to the conjunctival goblet cells. Preservative-free artificial tears may provide symptomatic relief in these cases.

SUPERIOR CORNEAL STAINING

Superior Limbic Keratoconjunctivitis

Subjective
Superior limbic keratoconjunctivitis (SLK) is a bilateral disorder that affects the superior tarsal region and limbal region. The etiology is currently unknown; however, some cases of SLK have been associated with thyroid dysfunction. Patients with this condition typically present with symptoms of photophobia, foreign body sensation, and tearing. The symptoms are transient because the condition undergoes exacerbations and remissions.

Objective
Inflammation of the superior tarsal conjunctiva and limbal region is a prominent feature in SLK. In addition, there is hyperemia and chemosis in the affected area of the conjunctiva. Punctate staining in the superior region of the cornea may be seen with fluorescein and rose bengal. Approximately one-third to one-half of patients with SLK develop filamentary keratopathy. During remissions no signs may be present; however, in some chronic and progressive cases, pannus formation can occur.

Plan
Topical ocular lubricants and topical steroids may be used to provide temporary relief, but more aggressive treatment is needed to completely alleviate SLK. SLK may also be treated by pressure patching to eliminate the mechanical effect of globe movement and by protecting the cornea with a soft contact lens. A 0.5–1.0% silver nitrate solution followed by irrigation can be used to debride the degenerating keratinized epithelial cells. Surgical intervention with a conjunctival grafting may be needed for those patients who do not respond to topical treatment.

Limbal Vernal Keratoconjunctivitis

Subjective
Vernal keratoconjunctivitis is a bilateral inflammation affecting the palpebral conjunctiva and, infrequently, the limbal conjunctiva. It usually affects children and young

adults, and is more commonly found in males than in females. The limbal form of this disease tends to occur more often in African-Americans and Native Americans than in other races. Vernal keratoconjunctivitis is seasonal, occurring primarily from the months of April to September. Approximately 50% of patients with vernal conjunctivitis have asthma, eczema, and allergic rhinitis; hay fever; or a combination of these disorders. A positive family history of atopic disease is a common finding. Symptoms may include intense itching, tearing, discharge, photophobia, and swelling of the lids.

Objective

Patients with limbal vernal keratoconjunctivitis have papillary hypertrophy and thickening of the superior limbus, which can protrude over the cornea. Within the limbal papillae, whitish, chalky dots called *Horner-Trantas' dots* can occur; these represent calcification of eosinophils. Other signs associated with limbal vernal keratoconjunctivitis include thick, ropy discharge, ptosis, and large cobblestone papillae. Due to mechanical irritation from the large papillae, there may be areas of epithelial damage of the cornea that predominantly stain with fluorescein, particularly in the superior region. Areas of epithelial damage may coalesce, forming a round shield ulcer. Giemsa or Diff-Quik staining of conjunctival scrapings to show eosinophils is useful in the diagnosis of this condition.

Plan

Topical antihistamines such as levocabastine or vasoconstrictor-antihistamine combinations such as 0.05% naphazoline hydrochloride with 0.5% antazoline phosphate, along with application of cool compresses, can provide relief in mild cases. Preservative-free artificial tears can be used to help eliminate the offending allergen. Patients with more severe limbal vernal keratoconjunctivitis may benefit from a regimen of a topical corticosteroid such as 1% prednisolone acetate or rimexolone or a nonsteroidal anti-inflammatory agent such as ketorolac tromethamine. Mast cell stabilizers can be quite beneficial in preventing the allergic response. They are most effective if therapy is initiated just before allergy season.

Trachoma

Subjective

Trachoma is a disorder caused by the microorganism *Chlamydia trachomatis.* Trachoma and its complications still represent a serious public health problem in many underdeveloped areas of the world. In the United States, trachoma occasionally is seen among the Native American populations of the Southwest and among immigrants from areas where the disease is endemic. Symptoms include pain, photophobia, lacrimation, mucopurulent discharge, and severe dry eye due to goblet cell destruction. In later stages of the disease, corneal scarring can cause severe vision loss.

Objective

In the early stages, a follicular conjunctivitis is present, usually located in the upper palpebral conjunctiva. Corneal involvement is typically a superior epithelial keratitis with an associated marginal infiltration, superficial vascularization (pannus), and limbal edema. The pannus is usually more marked in the superior cornea, and a limbal cicatrization produces depressions known as *Herbert's pits.* As the disease progresses, conjunctival scarring with resultant cicatricial entropion and trichiasis occurs. Corneal desiccation, ulceration, and scarring can follow. Immunofluorescence tests can be used to confirm the presence of *Chlamydia.*

Plan

Trachoma usually responds to a 3-week course of oral tetracycline or doxycycline. In pregnant women and children younger than 8 years of age, tetracycline is contraindicated because it can discolor the teeth and depress bone growth in infants. Erythromycin should be prescribed in these cases. Topical tetracycline or erythromycin ointment can be used concomitantly with oral medications; however, studies have shown that topical preparations alone may provide only an incomplete cure, and subsequent transmission of the disease can occur.

SUGGESTED READING

Arffa RC, Grayson M. Grayson's Diseases of the Cornea (4th ed). St. Louis: Mosby–Year Book, 1997.
Bartlett JD, Jaanus SD. Clinical Ocular Pharmacology (3rd ed). Boston: Butterworth–Heinemann, 1995.
Catania LJ. Primary Care of the Anterior Segment (2nd ed). Norwalk, CT: Appleton & Lange, 1995.
Classé JG (ed). Corneal Disease Update. Norwalk, CT: Appleton & Lange, 1995.
Cullom RD, Chang B. The Wills Eye Manual. Office and Emergency Room Diagnosis and Treatment of Eye Disease (2nd ed). Philadelphia: Lippincott, 1994.
Smolin G, Thoft RA. The Cornea: Scientific Foundations and Clinical Practice. Boston: Little, Brown, 1994.

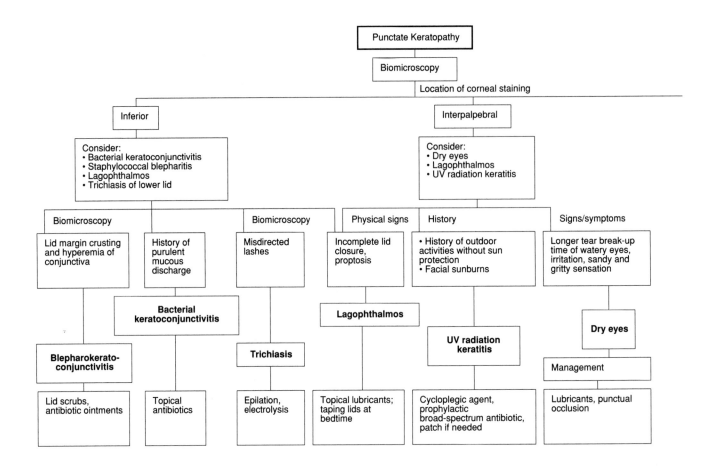

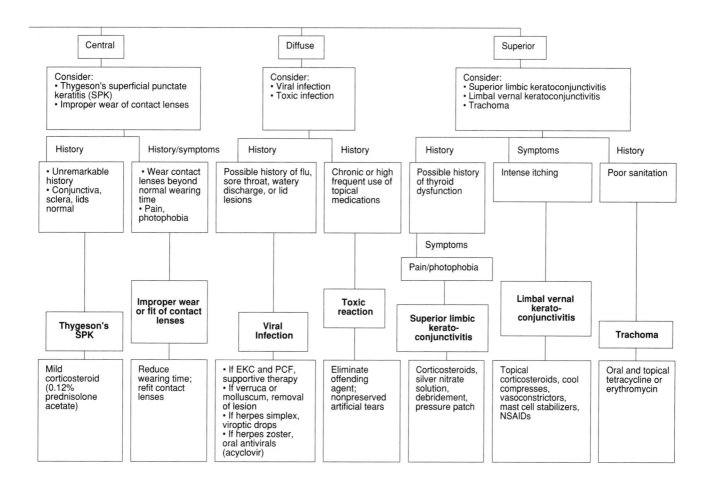

Central	

Consider:
• Thygeson's superficial punctate keratitis (SPK)
• Improper wear of contact lenses

History	History/symptoms
• Unremarkable history • Conjunctiva, sclera, lids normal	• Wear contact lenses beyond normal wearing time • Pain, photophobia

Improper wear or fit of contact lenses

Thygeson's SPK

Mild corticosteroid (0.12% prednisolone acetate)

Reduce wearing time; refit contact lenses

Diffuse	

Consider:
• Viral infection
• Toxic infection

History	History
Possible history of flu, sore throat, watery discharge, or lid lesions	Chronic or high frequent use of topical medications

Viral Infection

Toxic reaction

• If EKC and PCF, supportive therapy
• If verruca or molluscum, removal of lesion
• If herpes simplex, viroptic drops
• If herpes zoster, oral antivirals (acyclovir)

Eliminate offending agent; nonpreserved artificial tears

Superior	

Consider:
• Superior limbic keratoconjunctivitis
• Limbal vernal keratoconjunctivitis
• Trachoma

History	Symptoms	History
Possible history of thyroid dysfunction	Intense itching	Poor sanitation

Symptoms

Pain/photophobia

Superior limbic kerato-conjunctivitis

Limbal vernal kerato-conjunctivitis

Trachoma

Corticosteroids, silver nitrate solution, debridement, pressure patch

Topical corticosteroids, cool compresses, vasoconstrictors, mast cell stabilizers, NSAIDs

Oral and topical tetracycline or erythromycin

19

Corneal Filaments

JOHN H. NISHIMOTO

CORNEAL FILAMENTS AT A GLANCE

Keratoconjunctivitis sicca
Recurrent corneal erosion
Superior limbic keratoconjunctivitis
Neurotrophic keratitis
Keratoconus
Chemical trauma
Prolonged eye patching
Infectious corneal disease
Chronic bullous keratopathy

Corneal filaments are strands of epithelium and mucus that usually indicate that the epithelium is compromised or diseased. The formation of filaments starts when a small depression is created on the corneal surface. Lipid-containing mucus attaches to these areas, and, within a short time, epithelium grows down these mucous cores, creating a filament. This chapter reviews the most common ocular conditions associated with the formation of filaments.

KERATOCONJUNCTIVITIS SICCA

Subjective

Keratoconjunctivitis sicca is a condition characterized by dry eye. It is said to occur when the quantity or quality of the tear film is insufficient to maintain the integrity of the epithelial surface. Dry eye is caused by a deficiency in the aqueous, mucin, or lipid layers of the tears. It can also be caused by lid-surfacing disorders, neurologic disorders, epitheliopathies, and environmental factors.

The patient history is very important in the diagnosis of dry eye. Dry-eye patients are often quite sensitive to drafts and winds. They may state that they are intolerant to air conditioning or driving in the car with the windows rolled down. Reading may exacerbate the condition because the blink frequency decreases during tasks requiring concentration. The systemic health history provides useful information, because illnesses such as pemphigoid, Stevens-Johnson syndrome, rosacea, and rheumatoid arthritis cause dry-eye problems.

Investigating the patient's systemic medications, both prescription and over the counter, is also important, because numerous medications decrease tear production. Some of the commonly used medications in this group include chlorpheniramine, isotretinoin, hydrochlorothiazide, and propanolol hydrochloride.

Patients with keratoconjunctivitis sicca may report symptoms of irritation, redness, or a nonspecific ocular discomfort. Some patients with dry eyes complain of tearing or excessive secretion in the eyes. This symptom is due to reflex lacrimation triggered by ocular irritation. Patients with filamentary keratitis often experience pain when the filaments are pulled during blinking.

Objective

Formation of corneal filaments is commonly associated with severe keratoconjunctivitis sicca. The mucoid filaments stain with sodium fluorescein dye. The tear breakup time also is decreased. Rose bengal staining is another useful test in the diagnosis of keratoconjunctivitis sicca. Rose bengal stains devitalized epithelial cells, mucus, and filaments. Schirmer's, Sno-strip, and phenol red thread tests are useful in determining whether the filamentary keratitis is associated with very low tear production. Lissamine green dye has also been promising in staining filaments.

Plan

Artificial tears can be used as the initial treatment for filamentary keratitis secondary to dry eye. Lubricating ointments and punctal occlusion also can be helpful. In some instances, the filaments can be mechanically removed with forceps. In addition, the use of acetylcysteine drops can be beneficial for dissolving the mucus. Hypertonic saline drops and ointment then are used to promote proper re-epithelialization. Bandage contact lenses can be used to quickly promote the resolution of filaments and provide pain relief. The concurrent use of rewetting drops and prophylactic antibiotic drops is recommended.

RECURRENT CORNEAL EROSION

Subjective

Recurrent corneal erosion (RCE) is characterized by repeated episodes of epithelial breakdown due to poor adhesion between the epithelium and basement membrane. The patient with RCE may have a history of corneal trauma, epithelial basement membrane dystrophy, herpes simplex keratitis, or diabetes mellitus. Symptoms include pain and photophobia, which often occur upon awakening. Vision can be reduced if the visual axis is affected.

Objective

In anterior epithelial basement membrane dystrophy, lesions resembling maps, dots, or fingerprints can be observed in the anterior cornea under magnification. During an acute episode of RCE, one or more patches of epithelial sloughing that stain well with sodium fluorescein dye are noted. Other findings include epithelial microcysts, bullae, loosely adherent areas of epithelium, epithelial filaments, conjunctival injection, and occasionally anterior uveitis. As the cornea begins to re-epithelialize, the lesion may form a dendritic pattern similar to that seen in herpetic keratitis. Between attacks, epithelial cysts, surface irregularity, or subepithelial scarring may be observed.

Plan

The treatment of recurrent corneal erosion is directed toward re-establishing tight adhesion between the epithelium and basement membrane. The first goal is to heal the erosion through the use of a patch or bandage contact lens. Removal of loose epithelium may be needed to promote healing.

The simplest method of reducing recurrences is to lubricate the cornea well, especially at bedtime. Hypertonic

drops and ointment appear to be particularly beneficial in promoting proper basement membrane adhesion. One drop of 5% sodium chloride solution instilled four to five times daily and ointment instilled at bedtime typically are prescribed. Treatment should be continued for at least 3 months. If further treatment is necessary, other options include corneal debridement, bandage contact lens wear, anterior stromal puncture, and excimer laser phototherapeutic keratectomy.

SUPERIOR LIMBIC KERATOCONJUNCTIVITIS

Subjective

The specific cause of superior limbic keratoconjunctivitis (SLK) has not been determined, but in some cases it is associated with thyroid disease, keratoconjunctivitis sicca, or autoimmune disorders. Patients with SLK generally complain of irritation and redness, but there is minimal or no discharge from the eye. In some instances the irritation is more prominent when the patient looks upward. Less common symptoms include a burning or foreign body sensation, pain, photophobia, and blepharospasm. Corneal filaments occur in approximately one-third of cases of SLK and can cause significant pain. SLK is usually bilateral and often runs a chronic course with exacerbations and remissions.

Objective

The common clinical signs of SLK include papillary hypertrophy of the superior tarsal conjunctiva, thickening and hyperemia of the superior bulbar and limbal conjunctiva, and a fine epithelial keratitis of the superior cornea. The superior one-third of the corneal epithelium reveals punctate or blotchy staining with fluorescein or rose bengal dyes. Multiple corneal and conjunctival filaments often develop in the superior cornea, limbus, and palpebral conjunctiva at some point in the disease course. Microscopic analysis of superior conjunctival scrapings prepared with Giemsa or Papanicolaou's stains can be used to confirm the diagnosis.

Plan

In mild cases, artificial tears and ointments are satisfactory for relieving discomfort. Intermittent patching or prolonged therapy with topical 4% cromolyn sodium can be helpful in some cases. If filaments are present, 10% acetylcysteine drops may be used. In more severe cases, topical 0.5% or 1.0% silver nitrate solution applied to an anesthetized upper tarsus and followed by irrigation generally results in relief of symptoms for 4–6 weeks. A prophylactic antibiotic ointment should be applied for 1 week after this procedure. If this procedure does not give the patient sufficient relief, it may be repeated in 1 week. Other treatment modalities include mechanical debridement, cryotherapy, and thermal cauterization. Surgical resection or recession of the involved bulbar conjunctiva can provide long-term relief of symptoms. In addition to managing the ocular disease, the clinician should order a thyroid profile to rule out thyroid dysfunction in patients with SLK.

NEUROTROPHIC KERATITIS (NEUROPARALYTIC KERATITIS, TRIGEMINAL NEUROPATHIC KERATOPATHY)

Subjective

Patients with neurotrophic keratitis most commonly have a history of herpes zoster, herpes simplex, or trauma causing damage to the trigeminal nerve. In addition, trigeminal ganglionectomy for the management of tic douloureux can create corneal anesthesia and keratitis in 15–18% of patients. Other conditions causing neurotrophic keratitis include multiple sclerosis, tumor, aneurysms, and cerebrovascular accidents. Radiation therapy can also produce diffuse or segmental damage to the trigeminal nerve with resultant corneal anesthesia.

Patients with neurotrophic keratitis are surprisingly asymptomatic given their clinical appearance. They occasionally report a relative numbness of the affected side. They may also experience blurred vision due to epithelial erosions.

Objective

Once the corneal innervation from the ophthalmic branch of the trigeminal nerve becomes abnormal, epithelial cell death frequently occurs. This cell death may result in recurrent or persistent epithelial defects. Corneal sensitivity testing is useful in the diagnosis of fifth nerve dysfunction. Gross qualitative assessment of corneal sensation may be accomplished with a sterile cotton wisp; quantitative assessment is best performed with an esthesiometer. Early neurotrophic keratitis is characterized by diffuse punctate epithelial erosions that stain well with rose bengal dye. Excessive mucus production is common. Later the cornea develops larger areas of epithelial detachment with filamentary borders. Descemet's folds and anterior uveitis may be present. Stromal lysis is the primary sign of advanced neurotrophic keratitis. Regardless of the cause of neurotrophic keratitis, the longer the epithelial defect persists, the greater the risk for corneal ulceration.

Plan

While the underlying cause of neurotrophic keratitis is usually not treatable, the therapeutic goal of the clinician is to prevent disruption of the fragile corneal epithelium. Early pathologic changes of the epithelium can be treated with ocular lubricants. Nocturnal lagophthalmos, if present, should be treated by lid taping at bedtime. Soft lens therapy can be successful in treating early neurotrophic keratitis but should be monitored judiciously due to the increased risk of infection. Cycloplegics such as 1% cyclopentolate hydrochloride and prophylactic topical antibiotics such as 0.3% ciprofloxacin may be used in conjunction with a bandage contact lens. In more advanced cases, tarsorrhaphy or injection of botulinum toxin A into the levator palpebrae superioris to induce lid closure may be used to protect the cornea from trauma and desiccation.

SUGGESTED READING

Arffa RC, Grayson M. Grayson's Diseases of the Cornea (4th ed). St. Louis: Mosby–Year Book, 1997.

Bartlett JD, Jaanus SD. Clinical Ocular Pharmacology (3rd ed). Boston: Butterworth–Heinemann, 1995.

Cullom RD, Chang B. The Wills Eye Manual: Office and Emergency Room Diagnosis and Treatment of Eye Disease (2nd ed). Philadelphia: Lippincott, 1994.

Kanski JJ. Clinical Ophthalmology (3rd ed). Oxford, UK: Butterworth–Heinemann, 1994.

Fraunfelder FT, Roy FH. Current Ocular Therapy 4. Philadelphia: Saunders, 1995.

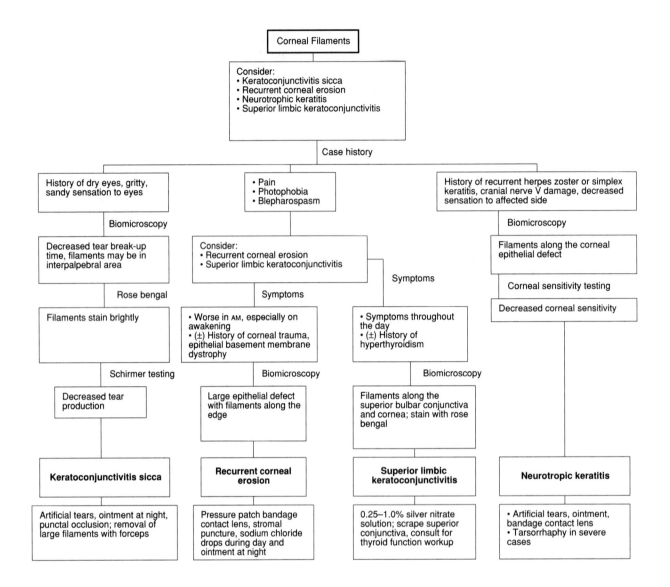

20

Infectious Corneal Disease

JOHN H. NISHIMOTO

INFECTIOUS CORNEAL DISEASE AT A GLANCE

Bacterial corneal ulcer
Marginal limbal ulcer
Herpes simplex
Herpes zoster
Acanthamoeba
Fungal keratitis
Tuberculosis
Variola
Acquired immunodeficiency syndrome

Corneal infections usually arise from bacterial, viral, or fungal inoculations. Patients with corneal infections often present with pain and photophobia. This chapter discusses the organisms and conditions that contribute to the development of infectious corneal disease.

BACTERIAL CORNEAL ULCER

Subjective

Trauma, poor hygiene, and contact lens wear (especially extended wear) may introduce bacteria that can cause infectious keratitis. Diabetes mellitus is another risk factor. In addition, the clinician should determine whether the patient is using topical corticosteroids. These drugs cause immunosuppression and can contribute to the development or exacerbation of corneal infections. Patients with bacterial corneal ulcers may complain of pain, photophobia, discharge, and decreased vision due to the involvement of the corneal visual axis and cells in the anterior chamber. Patients with mild keratitis, however, may have minimal subjective symptoms.

Objective

Signs of bacterial corneal ulcer include not only epithelial and stromal defects, but also corneal infiltration and edema. Corneal infiltrates are discrete clusters of inflammatory cells that have migrated throughout the cornea. They originate from the limbal vasculature or from the tears in response to chemotactic factors released from damaged tissues. Conjunctival edema and injection often accompany severe keratitis. An anterior chamber reaction, seen as flare and cells in the aqueous humor, is a common associated finding. Neovascularization, corneal thinning, and scarring may occur after episodes of acute or chronic keratitis. Culturing a corneal sample is helpful in identifying the infectious organism. *Staphylococcus*, *Streptococcus*, and *Pseudomonas* are some of the more common corneal pathogens.

Plan

Proper initial management of infectious keratitis includes prompt therapeutic intervention and identification of the causative organism. Culturing using blood agar, chocolate, and thioglycolate broth and Gram's staining are useful in identifying most organisms. Bacterial corneal ulcers should be presumed to be caused by *Pseudomonas* until proved otherwise, because of the prevalence of this organism and its potential for rapid sight-threatening damage unless appropriate intervention is instituted. Initial therapy of presumed bacterial keratitis should include broad-spectrum antibiotics with adequate gram-negative coverage. Presumed bacterial corneal ulcers are usually treated with fluoroquinolones such as ciprofloxacin, ofloxacin, and norfloxacin or fortified aminoglycosides such as gentamicin or tobramycin and cefazolin or vancomycin. Sensitivity testing can help the clinician evaluate and modify the initially selected therapeutic regimen.

FUNGAL KERATITIS

Subjective

Symptoms of fungal keratitis are similar to those of bacterial ulcer: decreased vision if the visual axis is involved, pain, and photophobia. There may be a history of corneal abrasion or other trauma involving some kind of vegetable matter. The clinician also should determine whether the patient has a history of contact lens wear, especially soft contact lens wear, because solutions can be contaminated and the contact lens itself may have fungal deposits. In addition, patients whose immune systems are compromised due either to acquired immunodeficiency syndrome (AIDS) or to the use of immunosuppressive agents such as corticosteroids are more susceptible to fungal infection.

Objective

Fungal ulcers often have a greenish white area of infiltration with an elevated, rough, textured surface. The margins of the lesion, which are irregular and feathery, extend into the adjacent stroma. Satellite lesions, or remote foci of infiltration, may be seen several millimeters away from the main area of involvement. In some cases, the epithelium can remain intact over the infiltrate. Conjunctival injection and purulent discharge may be present, even when the infiltrate appears minimal. The anterior chamber reaction may be quite severe and result in hypopyon formation.

Sabouraud agar should be used to culture samples from a suspected fungal ulcer. Microscopic evaluation of a scraping prepared with potassium hydroxide can provide additional useful information. Among the more commonly identified fungi from corneal ulcers are *Candida* and *Aspergillus*. It is important to note that fungi are sometimes difficult to culture.

Plan

Treatment of fungal keratitis is often difficult. In most cases, the lesion is initially treated as bacterial until proved otherwise. The available antifungal agents tend only to inhibit growth and allow the host to eradicate the infection. Among these agents are amphotericin B, natamycin, and miconazole. In addition, a cycloplegic with 0.25% scopolamine or 5% homatropine helps minimize secondary anterior chamber reaction.

HERPES SIMPLEX KERATOCONJUNCTIVITIS

Subjective

Herpes simplex infection can cause numerous symptoms and signs. Symptoms of epithelial disease include tearing, irritation, photophobia, and often blurring of vision. Patients with suspected herpes simplex keratoconjunctivitis should be asked about previous ocular trauma, corneal ulcers, and ocular inflammation (iridocyclitis). The clinician also should determine whether the patient is prone to developing nasal or oral cold sores or genital sores. Immune deficiency states associated with AIDS or drug therapy using corticosteroids or other immunosuppressive agents can predispose the patient to development of herpes simplex keratoconjunctivitis.

Objective

Herpes simplex keratoconjunctivitis typically involves the epithelium, stroma, or both. In rare cases the endothelium is affected. In epithelial disease, the initial presentation is often a diffuse superficial punctate keratopathy that can develop into dendritic (branchlike) ulcers with terminal bulbs or geographic (map-shaped) ulcers. These lesions stain brightly with sodium fluorescein and rose bengal dyes. If slit-lamp examination reveals dendritic or geographic ulceration, the clinician should assume the condition is herpes simplex keratoconjunctivitis until proved otherwise. Reduction of corneal sensitivity in the affected area as measured with a cotton wisp or esthesiometer is another useful sign. Trophic ulceration occurs in areas where the epithelium does not adhere properly to the basement membrane as a result of previous herpes simplex ulceration. Its clinical appearance is similar to that of a recurrent corneal erosion.

Stromal disease can cause edema, infiltration with pannus, and neovascularization. An antigen-antibody complement–mediated immune response to the herpes simplex infection is characterized by interstitial keratitis, immune rings, or limbal vasculitis. Multiple patches of infiltrates develop, with stromal neovascularization leading to the lesion. Disciform keratitis is a hypersensitivity reaction that presents as a focal, disc-shaped area of stromal edema. Other anterior segment signs associated with herpes simplex keratoconjunctivitis are conjunctival injection and iridocyclitis.

Plan

Several antiviral agents have proved effective in the treatment of herpes simplex keratitis: trifluridine, vidarabine, idoxuridine, and acyclovir. Currently, trifluridine is the initial drug of choice. It is prescribed in the amount of one drop every 2 hours, up to nine doses daily. This dosage is continued until the cornea has re-epithelialized; then it is reduced to one drop every 4 hours for another week.

Topical corticosteroids remain the primary mode of therapy for stromal disease. Antiviral drugs are used to treat concurrent epithelial disease or as a prophylactic against recurrent infectious disease. If the epithelium is ulcerated, topical steroids should be discontinued or used with extreme caution. Once the epithelium has healed, the reintroduction of steroids can reduce or eliminate the inflammation or hypersensitivity reaction. It should be noted that withdrawing from steroid treatment can be difficult. If the steroid therapy is stopped too abruptly, recurrence of the immune disease may occur. Tapering slowly is crucial for proper discontinuation.

HERPES ZOSTER OPHTHALMICUS

Subjective

The varicella virus causes both varicella (chickenpox) and herpes zoster (shingles). After the primary infection, the virus becomes latent, residing in the dorsal root ganglion of the spinal cord or the trigeminal ganglia. Months or decades later, the patient can develop zoster due to reactivation of the latent virus. Herpes zoster is most commonly found in people older than 50; the peak incidence is between the ages of 80 and 89. Herpes zoster in a young adult may be an indicator of an immune deficiency state such as AIDS. Systemic symptoms include headache, malaise, fever, and chills followed in 1–2 days by neuralgia. Depression is also common. Ocular symptoms include pain, photophobia, and reduced vision.

Objective

Herpes zoster affects the peripheral spinal nerves and cranial nerve V, the trigeminal nerve. The ophthalmic division of the trigeminal is the most commonly affected branch. Approximately 2–3 days after the onset of neuralgia, dermal signs develop. These include redness and painful edema of the involved dermatome. The skin of the affected dermatome erupts with multiple watery vesicles. It should be noted that a single dermatome does not cross the midline of the body. Vesicles on the tip of the nose (Hutchinson's sign) indicate that the nasociliary branch of the ophthalmic division is affected. This sign is highly suggestive of eye involvement as well. Later the vesicular lesions crust over and ultimately may form scars.

The corneal presentation is quite varied and can include one or more of the following signs: punctate keratitis, pseudodendrites, anterior stromal infiltrates, sclerokeratitis, keratouveitis-endotheliitis, peripheral ulcerative keratitis, disciform keratitis, neurotrophic keratitis, and exposure keratitis. Unlike the dendrites seen in herpes simplex keratitis, those seen in herpes zoster appear as heaped up, superficial, plaquelike lesions. They are coarser than herpes simplex dendrites, lack terminal bulbs, and stain poorly with sodium fluorescein. Corneal sensitivity testing provides additional useful information because the cornea often becomes markedly hypoesthetic, even in apparently mild cases of herpes zoster keratitis.

Stromal disease may be local or diffuse and may or may not have concurrent epithelial involvement. Interstitial inflammation and Wessely immune rings are signs of stromal involvement.

In addition to keratitis, anterior segment signs of herpes zoster ophthalmicus include lid retraction secondary to scarring, paralytic ptosis, follicular conjunctivitis, episcleritis, scleritis, Argyll-Robertson pupil, isolated pupillary paralysis, and iridocyclitis. Posterior segment signs include hemorrhagic retinitis, acute retinal necrosis, choroiditis, papillitis, and retrobulbar optic neuritis. Other ophthalmic manifestations include partial or complete third, fourth, or sixth nerve palsy; acute or chronic glaucoma; and sympathetic ophthalmia.

Plan

The first line of treatment for herpes zoster is an oral antiviral agent such as acyclovir, famciclovir, or valacyclovir hydrochloride. The typical dosage for acyclovir is 800 mg taken by mouth five times per day for 7–10 days. This therapy is most effective when initiated within 72 hours of onset of skin eruptions. An antibiotic ointment such as bacitracin–polymyxin B sulfate can be applied to the skin lesions to prevent secondary infection. If the cornea is involved, prescribing cool compresses and preservative-free artificial tears to be used several times per day can provide symptomatic relief. If there is an associated iridocyclitis, a topical steroid such as 1% prednisolone acetate and a cycloplegic such as 2% or 5% homatropine should be prescribed. Topical capsaicin cream and antidepressants can be helpful in managing acute pain and postherpetic neuralgia. Patients who have posterior segment involvement should be comanaged with a retinologist.

It should be noted that herpes zoster is contagious to those that have not had a varicella infection. Pregnant women who have not had chickenpox must be especially careful to avoid contact with someone who has herpes zoster.

ACANTHAMOEBA KERATITIS

Subjective

Acanthamoeba keratitis typically occurs from exposure to contaminated water. For example, contact lens patients who make their own saline solution from tap water or wear their lenses while in a hot tub are at increased risk for acquiring an *Acanthamoeba* infection. Repeated wearing of a contaminated contact lens can cause a chronic keratitis. The patient may present with a history of prior unsuccessful treatment with a topical antiviral or antibacterial medication. Symptoms of *Acanthamoeba* keratitis include irritation, pain, photophobia, and a reduction of vision. The symptoms are often more severe than the clinical presentation would suggest.

Objective

Slit-lamp biomicroscopy reveals lid edema, conjunctival injection, keratitis, and a mild anterior chamber reaction. Early corneal signs include infiltrates in the central or paracentral area and pseudodendrites. Signs of later stages of the disease include radial neuritis, a complete or partial ring of infiltrates in the stroma, and recurrent epithelial defects. Laboratory tests such as Gram's or Giemsa stains are helpful in ruling out other organisms and identifying dormant amoebic cysts. Calcofluor white and immunofluorescent antibody staining of corneal tissues from scrapings or biopsies provide additional diagnostic information. Laboratory analysis of the patient's contact lenses and solutions also may be helpful.

Plan

Acanthamoeba keratitis is difficult to treat; therefore, prompt and aggressive therapy is vital. Medical therapy typically involves prescription of a combination of antibacterial, antifungal, and antiamoebic agents. Agents that have been used include propamidine isethionate, neomycin, paromomycin sulfate, miconazole, clotrimazole, ketoconazole, itraconazole, and polyhexanide biguanide. In some cases, topical corticosteroids have been added to the treatment regimen to control inflammation. Penetrating keratoplasty may be necessary if a corneal scar develops and resultant vision loss occurs. It is important to educate patients about the dangers of improper contact lens cleaning and the wearing of contacts when swimming or soaking in hot tubs in an effort to prevent devastating *Acanthamoeba* infections.

Marginal Limbal Infiltrates

Subjective

Marginal limbal infiltrates are commonly termed *marginal sterile ulcers*. This term is inaccurate because the lesion itself is not infectious, but the result of an antigen-antibody reaction to an infectious organism. It may be secondary to a lid condition such a staphylococcal blepharitis. Typical patient complaints include pain, tearing, photophobia, and foreign body sensation.

Objective

Biomicroscopy reveals one or more circular or oval lesions approximately 0.5–1.5 mm in size in the peripheral cornea. There is typically a clear space between the limbus and the lesion. These lesions most commonly are found in the limbal areas where the lid margins rest on the cornea. In early stages, the infiltrate is slightly raised due to the accumulation of lymphocytes and debris. Later, the overlying epithelium breaks down and becomes ulcerated, staining positively with sodium fluorescein. On some occasions, these defects lead to further ulceration. There is usually minimal anterior chamber reaction associated with marginal corneal infiltrates.

Plan

Topical corticosteroids such as prednisolone acetate may be prescribed to lessen the immune response and resolve the infiltrates. Antibiotic drugs such as gentamicin, tobramycin, polymyxin B sulfate–trimethoprim, or ciprofloxacin may be prescribed in combination with the corticosteroid to reduce or prevent infection. If there are signs of blepharitis, lid scrubs and warm compresses along with topical application of bacitracin or bacitracin–polymyxin B sulfate ointment should be initiated. Corneal cultures may be necessary if there is difficulty in differentiating sterile marginal infiltrates from true infectious ulcers.

SUGGESTED READING

Arffa RC, Grayson M. Grayson's Diseases of the Cornea (4th ed). St. Louis: Mosby–Year Book, 1997.

Bartlett JD, Jaanus SD. Clinical Ocular Pharmacology (3rd ed). Boston: Butterworth–Heinemann, 1995.

Catania LJ. Primary Care of the Anterior Segment (2nd ed). Norwalk, CT: Appleton & Lange, 1995.

Cullom RD, Chang B. The Wills Eye Manual. Office and Emergency Room Diagnosis and Treatment of Eye Disease (2nd ed). Philadelphia: Lippincott, 1994.

Onofrey BE. Clinical Optometric Pharmacology and Therapeutics. Philadelphia: Lippincott, 1994.

Smolin G, Thoft RA. The Cornea: Scientific Foundations and Clinical Practice. Boston: Little, Brown, 1994.

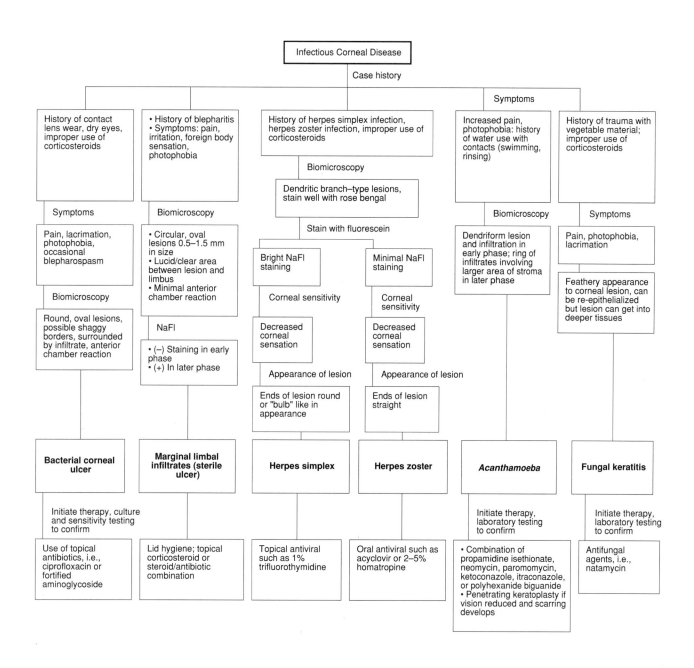

Infectious Corneal Disease

Case history

History of contact lens wear, dry eyes, improper use of corticosteroids

Symptoms

Pain, lacrimation, photophobia, occasional blepharospasm

Biomicroscopy

Round, oval lesions, possible shaggy borders, surrounded by infiltrate, anterior chamber reaction

Bacterial corneal ulcer

Initiate therapy, culture and sensitivity testing to confirm

Use of topical antibiotics, i.e., ciprofloxacin or fortified aminoglycoside

---

• History of blepharitis
• Symptoms: pain, irritation, foreign body sensation, photophobia

Biomicroscopy

• Circular, oval lesions 0.5–1.5 mm in size
• Lucid/clear area between lesion and limbus
• Minimal anterior chamber reaction

NaFl

• (−) Staining in early phase
• (+) In later phase

Marginal limbal infiltrates (sterile ulcer)

Lid hygiene; topical corticosteroid or steroid/antibiotic combination

---

History of herpes simplex infection, herpes zoster infection, improper use of corticosteroids

Biomicroscopy

Dendritic branch–type lesions, stain well with rose bengal

Stain with fluorescein

Bright NaFl staining

Corneal sensitivity

Decreased corneal sensation

Appearance of lesion

Ends of lesion round or "bulb" like in appearance

Herpes simplex

Topical antiviral such as 1% trifluorothymidine

Minimal NaFl staining

Corneal sensitivity

Decreased corneal sensation

Appearance of lesion

Ends of lesion straight

Herpes zoster

Oral antiviral such as acyclovir or 2–5% homatropine

Symptoms

Increased pain, photophobia: history of water use with contacts (swimming, rinsing)

Biomicroscopy

Dendriform lesion and infiltration in early phase; ring of infiltrates involving larger area of stroma in later phase

Acanthamoeba

Initiate therapy, laboratory testing to confirm

• Combination of propamidine isethionate, neomycin, paromomycin, ketoconazole, itraconazole, or polyhexanide biguanide
• Penetrating keratoplasty if vision reduced and scarring develops

---

History of trauma with vegetable material; improper use of corticosteroids

Symptoms

Pain, photophobia, lacrimation

Feathery appearance to corneal lesion, can be re-epithelialized but lesion can get into deeper tissues

Fungal keratitis

Initiate therapy, laboratory testing to confirm

Antifungal agents, i.e., natamycin

21

Corneal Edema

JOHN H. NISHIMOTO

CORNEAL EDEMA AT A GLANCE

Rigid contact lens wear
Soft contact lens wear
Corneal abrasion
Corneal erosion
Corneal ulcer
Medicamentosa
Endothelial dysfunction
   Fuchs' endothelial dystrophy
   Pseudophakic bullous keratopathy
   Congenital hereditary endothelial dystrophy
Angle-closure glaucoma
Congenital glaucoma
Herpes simplex
Herpes zoster
Failed corneal graft
Corneal hydrops from keratoconus
Iridocorneal endothelial syndrome
Trauma

Corneal edema is an excessive hydration of the corneal epithelium, stroma, or both. Corneal hypoxia due to contact lens overwear, infection, medication toxicity, elevated intraocular pressure, or traumatic insult to the epithelium or endothelium also may cause distress to the cornea that results in edema. This chapter discusses some of the conditions that contribute to the development of corneal edema.

EDEMA INDUCED BY RIGID CONTACT LENS WEAR

Subjective

Edema induced by the wearing of polymethylmethacrylate contact lenses was a common occurrence years ago. Today, with the use of rigid gas-permeable (RGP) contact lenses, the frequency of contact lens–induced edema has been reduced. However, the oxygen transmissibility of commonly used extended-wear lenses is still insufficient to eliminate hypoxia. Patients with contact lens–induced edema may be asymptomatic or may note hazy vision, glare, photophobia, and spectacle blur.

Objective

In patients who wear rigid contact lenses, the clinical appearance of edema is an epithelial haze in the area corresponding to the position of the lens (central corneal clouding). This clouding is best observed with the sclerotic-scatter slit-lamp technique. Epithelial microcysts are often associated with RGP lens wear. These appear as small (10–15 μm) circular cysts visible with the biomicroscope. They are first seen in the deeper layers of the epithelium, then migrate anteriorly. Once they erupt to the surface of the epithelium, they cause staining with fluorescein. Keratometry may reveal increased curvature, and the mires often appear distorted. Refraction may reveal a minus shift in correction due to the edema.

Plan

Today the management of rigid-lens edema is quite successful, because a large range of high oxygen permeability RGP lenses are available. The lens material, lens parameters, wearing schedule, or a combination of these may need to be changed to reduce corneal edema. Distorted corneas can be refitted without discontinuing lens wear, and typically the cornea rehabilitates within 3 weeks.

EDEMA INDUCED BY SOFT CONTACT LENS WEAR

Subjective

Patients with corneal edema induced by soft contact lens wear may present with symptoms of glare or colored fringes around lights. The edema is more diffuse and the patient may have fewer symptoms than in RGP lens–induced edema.

Objective

Because the edema associated with soft contact lens wear is diffuse, corneal distortion is less likely to occur than in RGP lens–induced edema. In addition, few if any refractive changes are noted. In soft contact lens wearers, epithelial edema is sometimes associated with superficial punctate keratitis (SPK). These breaks in the epithelial surface allow fluid to move into the epithelium and contribute to light scatter. In addition, stromal edema is found in some soft contact lens wearers. Unlike epithelial edema, stromal swelling must be considerable (> 15%) to produce noticeable light scatter. If the stroma swells at least 6–7%, vertical striae can be observed with slit-lamp biomicroscopy. These folds are most often observed in patients who use extended-wear lenses. Perilimbal stromal edema from thick daily-wear hydrogel lenses may stimulate neovascularization in the limbal region of the cornea.

Plan

Edema induced by soft contact lens wear can be associated with striae, microcysts, neovascularization, and chronic SPK. These signs should prompt discontinuation of lens wear. In less severe cases, enhancing oxygen delivery to the cornea or decreasing wearing time (e.g., changing from extended-wear to daily-wear lenses) may alleviate the problem. Due to the risk of infection from soft contact lens wear, lens wear should be discontinued until persistent epithelial defects are completely healed. At that time, refitting or re-evaluation of wearing schedule can be considered.

CORNEAL ABRASION

Subjective

Patients with a corneal abrasion usually complain of pain, photophobia, excessive lacrimation, and blepharospasm. There may be a history of direct or tangential impact trauma to the cornea from objects such as a fingernail, paper, tree branch, mascara brush, or contact lens.

Objective

The diagnosis of abrasion is usually made on biomicroscopic examination of the cornea. An epithelial defect is best appreciated with the aid of fluorescein or rose bengal stain. There may be edema at the edge of the lesion, which causes negative staining. In addition there may be a minimal anterior chamber reaction. The bulbar and tarsal conjunctiva should be examined carefully with the lid everted to rule out the presence of a foreign body. The cornea should also be thoroughly examined to rule out epithelial basement membrane dystrophy or other conditions that could cause a recurrent corneal erosion.

Plan

Management of a corneal abrasion includes the application of a broad-spectrum antibiotic (e.g., gentamicin) to prevent secondary bacterial keratitis. A cycloplegic agent (e.g., 1% cyclopentolate hydrochloride, 2% or 5% homatropine) is used to minimize the anterior chamber reaction. A pressure patch or bandage contact lens is applied to promote proper re-epithelialization and to prevent shearing forces from the lid's pulling on the new growth of epithelial tissue. The same patch should not be applied to the eye for longer than 24 hours. If the eye must be patched for longer than 24 hours, then application of a new patch and reapplication of an antibiotic is appropriate. When the risk of microbial infection is significant, the eye is not patched and the cornea is treated with antibiotic drops (e.g., ciprofloxacin, tobramycin). Topical steroids should be avoided, especially if inoculation with gram-negative bacteria or fungus is suspected. Topical anesthetics should never be prescribed for extended use, because of the possibility of delayed wound healing and secondary keratitis.

CORNEAL EROSION

Subjective

Corneal erosion is caused by an abnormal adherence of the corneal epithelium to the basement membrane. It is often a recurring condition. The clinician should question the patient about previous similar episodes or previous ocular trauma that caused a corneal abrasion. Other conditions that can predispose a patient to corneal erosions include epithelial basement membrane dystrophy and other corneal dystrophies, herpes simplex keratitis, and ocular surgery. Patients with corneal erosion typically present with severe and acute ocular pain, photophobia, tearing, and blepharospasm. The symptoms often begin when the patient awakens in the morning. The reason is thought to be the adherence of the lid to the loosely attached corneal epithelium, which normally becomes slightly edematous while the eye is closed. When the eye opens, the affected portion of epithelium is pulled away from the basement membrane.

Objective

A corneal erosion is an epithelial defect that stains brightly with fluorescein. The clinician should also look carefully for signs of anterior basement membrane dystrophy (lesions resembling maps, dots, or fingerprints) or stromal dystrophies. There may also be an associated mild anterior chamber reaction with some cells and flare.

Plan

The initial goal in the management of corneal erosion is to promote proper re-epithelialization. This goal can be accomplished by applying a pressure patch or bandage contact lens to the affected eye. A cycloplegic agent and a prophylactic topical antibiotic should be used in conjunction with this therapy. Once healing is complete, nonpreserved artificial tears, 5% sodium chloride drops four times a day, and ointment at night should be used for 2–3 months to prevent further erosions. If proper healing does not occur, the affected area of the cornea can be debrided with a cotton applicator, surgical sponge, or blade. It may be necessary to use bandage lenses for several months. In addition, stromal puncture and excimer laser phototherapeutic keratectomy have been helpful in the treatment of severe, recurrent cases.

BACTERIAL CORNEAL ULCER

Subjective

Trauma, poor hygiene, and contact lens wear (especially extended wear) may introduce bacteria that cause infectious keratitis. Diabetes mellitus is another risk factor. In addition, the clinician should determine whether the patient is using topical corticosteroids. These drugs cause immunosuppression and can contribute to the development or exacerbation of corneal infections. Patients with bacterial corneal ulcers may complain of pain, photophobia, discharge, and decreased vision due to the involvement of the corneal visual axis and the presence of cells

in the anterior chamber. Patients with mild keratitis, however, may have minimal subjective symptoms.

Objective

Signs of bacterial corneal ulcers include not only epithelial and stromal defects but also corneal infiltration and edema. Corneal infiltrates are discrete clusters of inflammatory cells that have migrated throughout the cornea. They originate from the limbal vasculature or from the tears in response to chemotactic factors released from damaged tissues. Conjunctival edema and injection often accompany severe keratitis. An anterior chamber reaction, seen as flare and cells in the aqueous humor, is a common associated finding. Neovascularization, corneal thinning, and scarring may occur after episodes of acute or chronic keratitis. Culturing of corneal samples is helpful in identifying the infectious organism. *Staphylococcus, Streptococcus,* and *Pseudomonas* are some of the more common corneal pathogens.

Plan

Proper initial management of infectious keratitis includes prompt therapeutic intervention and identification of the causative organism. Culturing using blood agar, chocolate and thioglycolate broth, and Gram's staining are useful in identifying most organisms. Bacterial corneal ulcers should be presumed to be caused by *Pseudomonas* until proved otherwise, because of the prevalence of this organism and its potential for rapid sight-threatening damage unless appropriate intervention is instituted. Initial therapy of presumed bacterial keratitis should include broad-spectrum antibiotics with adequate gram-negative coverage. Presumed bacterial corneal ulcers are usually treated with fluoroquinolones such as ciprofloxacin, ofloxacin, and norfloxacin or fortified aminoglycosides such as gentamicin, tobramycin, cefazolin, and vancomycin. Sensitivity testing can help the clinician evaluate and modify the initially selected therapeutic regimen.

MEDICAMENTOSA

Subjective

Medicamentosa is the result of direct chemical irritation of ocular tissues by drugs or preservatives. The toxic effects usually take at least 2 weeks to develop. Patients with this condition often have a history of using a topical ophthalmic medication, either prescription or over the counter. They may report that the condition for which they were taking the medication improved initially, but then seemed to worsen despite proper compliance with the treatment regimen. Symptoms of medicamentosa include irritation, ocular pain, redness, and lid swelling.

Objective

Punctate corneal staining, more prominent with rose bengal than with fluorescein, is the most common finding associated with medicamentosa. Medications that are toxic to the epithelium can inhibit the healing of chronic epithelial defects of the cornea; sometimes pseudodendrites develop. On rare occasions, medicamentosa can produce corneal edema, giving rise to a hazy, ground-glass appearance of the cornea. Other associated findings include disciform stromal infiltrates that resemble Wessely immune rings, and superficial or deep corneal vascularization.

Plan

Treatment for toxic reactions of the ocular surface is quite straightforward. Withdrawal of the offending medication or preservative is the primary and most effective management. Preservative-free artificial lubricants may be prescribed if necessary for symptomatic relief.

FUCHS' ENDOTHELIAL-EPITHELIAL DYSTROPHY

Subjective

Fuchs' dystrophy is a bilateral disease that primarily affects the central cornea. Unlike most other corneal dystrophies, it becomes clinically apparent in the older population. Patients with early Fuchs' dystrophy often present with no symptoms. As the condition progresses, patients experience glare and hazy vision with increased edema. Patients with advanced Fuchs' dystrophy may complain of extreme pain and photophobia as the epithelium becomes involved.

Objective

In the early phases of Fuchs' dystrophy, pigment dusting and guttata in the posterior cornea may be observed with retroillumination or specular reflection. Descemet's membrane becomes opaque and thickened. Stromal edema forms; it is anterior to Bowman's layer at first but can progress to involve the entire stroma. Later in the course of the disease, large epithelial bullae start to appear. When the bullae rupture, the patient often experiences severe pain.

Plan

Corneal hydration control is the objective of effective management of Fuchs' endothelial-epithelial dystrophy. If there is only slight epithelial edema, the use of hypertonic saline drops (5% sodium chloride) by day and hypertonic saline ointment at night is the usual treatment. Blowing warm, dry air at the eye from a hair dryer held at arm's length from the corneal surface may also be of benefit, particularly in the morning when the edema is worst. The application of loosely fitted, thin, high-water-content soft contact lenses may be effective in reducing the pain associated with rupturing of the epithelial bullae. Penetrating keratoplasty is indicated when the pain cannot be controlled and the visual acuity is reduced to an unacceptable level.

ANGLE-CLOSURE GLAUCOMA

Subjective

The most common form of acute angle-closure glaucoma is caused by pupillary blockage of aqueous outflow. Patients with angle-closure glaucoma usually complain of a sudden onset of headache, eye pain, and blurred vision. The patient may note rainbow colors around lights due to corneal edema. The patient may also have associated nausea and vomiting due to the rapid rise in intraocular pressure.

Objective

In angle-closure glaucoma, the intraocular pressure rapidly rises to 40–80 mm Hg. Due to the rise in intraocular pressure, the endothelium becomes distressed, and its pumping action becomes less effective. Edema develops and gives rise to a cloudy cornea. A fixed, mid-dilated pupil is another important clinical sign. The anterior chamber is shallow, and occasionally the iris and cornea touch. This shallowness is best observed with gonioscopy. The conjunctiva is often injected due to ocular congestion. Signs of a mild anterior chamber reaction are usually present. Small, gray-white anterior subcapsular opacities of the lens called *Glaukomflecken* can be observed, especially if previous attacks of angle closure have occurred.

Plan

Angle-closure glaucoma should be considered an ocular emergency. The definitive management of pupillary-block angle-closure glaucoma is surgical; however, medical management should be employed to reduce the intraocular pressure before performing surgery. If the intraocular pressure is greater than 50 mm Hg, the usual treatment is to instill acetazolamide and timolol maleate to initiate pressure reduction. Hyperosmotic agents such as glycerol or mannitol may also be used to help rapidly lower the intraocular pressure. Once the intraocular pressure has decreased below 50 mm Hg, pilocarpine becomes effective in further reducing the intraocular pressure. Topical hyperosmotics such as glycerin may be needed to reduce corneal edema to visualize iris structure. Once the intraocular pressure is lowered, the corneal edema is decreased, and the pupil is miotic from pilocarpine, a peripheral iridotomy should be performed. This procedure creates an opening that allows adequate flow of aqueous humor from the posterior to anterior chamber.

SUGGESTED READING

Arffa RC, Grayson M. Grayson's Diseases of the Cornea (4th ed). St. Louis: Mosby–Year Book, 1997.

Bartlett JD, Jaanus SD. Clinical Ocular Pharmacology (3rd ed). Boston: Butterworth–Heinemann, 1995.

Cullom RD, Chang B. The Wills Eye Manual. Office and Emergency Room Diagnosis and Treatment of Eye Disease (2nd ed). Philadelphia: Lippincott, 1994.

Silbert JA. Anterior Segment Complications of Contact Lens Wear. New York: Churchill Livingstone, 1994.

Smolin G, Thoft RA. The Cornea: Scientific Foundations and Clinical Practice. Boston: Little, Brown, 1994.

Tomlinson A. Complications of Contact Lens Wear. St. Louis: Mosby–Year Book, 1992.

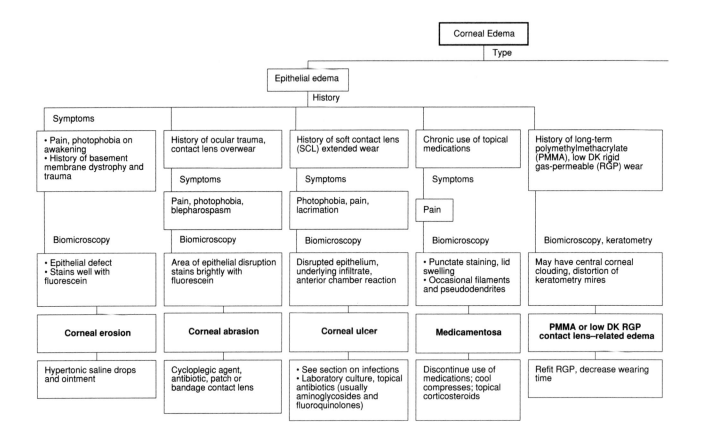

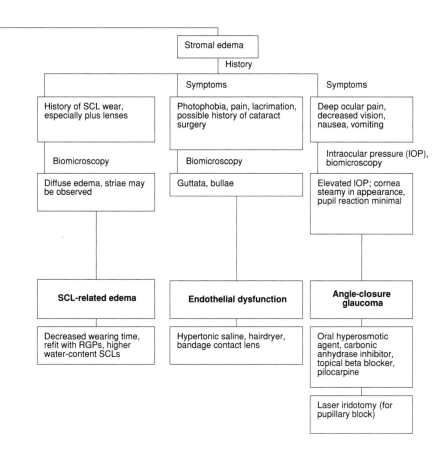

22

Interstitial Keratitis

John H. Nishimoto

INTERSTITIAL KERATITIS AT A GLANCE

Congenital syphilis
Acquired syphilis
Herpes simplex
Herpes zoster
Lyme disease
Tuberculosis
Acanthamoeba
Trachoma
Mumps

Interstitial keratitis (IK) refers to vascularization and infiltration that affect the corneal stroma. Conditions that can cause IK include syphilis, herpes simplex infection, herpes zoster infection, tuberculosis, Lyme disease, mumps, trachoma, and *Acanthamoeba* infection. This chapter discusses several of the ocular and systemic diseases that contribute to IK.

CONGENITAL AND ACQUIRED SYPHILIS

Subjective

Syphilis is caused by the spirochete *Treponema pallidum*. There is evidence that IK is an immune reaction to this organism. There are two basic types of syphilis: congenital and acquired. Congenital syphilis is transmitted from the mother during pregnancy. Both the history and clinical findings are important in the diagnosis of syphilitic IK. The clinician should ask about a history of ocular inflammation in childhood, previous therapy for venereal disease, family history of positive syphilis serology, or family history of stillbirth. IK from congenital syphilis is bilateral approximately 80% of the

time. It is usually diagnosed between the ages of 5 and 20. Patients with acute IK due to congenital syphilis may experience severe eye pain, photophobia, and decreased vision. They may also complain of copious clear discharge and blepharospasm.

Objective

The corneal changes depend on the duration of the disease. The epithelium usually remains intact but may become edematous. In the early phases of this condition, there may be diffuse or sectoral infiltrates in the peripheral stroma. Fine keratic precipitates may or may not be present on the endothelium. As the inflammation increases in intensity, the stroma and epithelium become more edematous and may take on a ground-glass appearance. The stroma typically becomes neovascularized and may exhibit a red hue. There is usually a concurrent anterior chamber reaction and prominent paralimbal injection.

If untreated, the stromal inflammation and vascularization eventually subside. Corneal scarring and impatent "ghost vessels" remain. In congenital syphilitic IK, both eyes are usually affected; involvement of the second eye occurs within 1 year of involvement of the first eye in greater than 75% of cases. Other ocular signs of congenital syphilis include "salt and pepper" chorioretinitis and optic atrophy. Systemic signs include dental and bone malformation (e.g., Hutchinson's teeth, mulberry molars, palatal perforation, frontal bosses, saddle nose, and saber shins), eighth nerve deafness, mental retardation, and behavioral changes.

Acquired syphilis can be subclassified into primary, secondary, and tertiary stages. A chancre at the site of inoculation is the main finding in the primary stage. IK as well as inflammation of numerous other structures of the anterior and posterior segment can be found in the secondary stage. Tertiary syphilis is characterized by tabes dorsalis and other neurologic defects, including those that affect the eye (optic neuritis, optic atrophy, Argyll-Robertson pupils). The pathologic process for the development of IK in acquired syphilis is essentially the same as in congenital syphilis. However, IK due to acquired syphilis tends to be less severe and may remain sectoral. Laboratory testing with a fluorescent treponemal antibody absorption test or microhemagglutination assay for antibody to *T. pallidum* should be performed to help confirm the diagnosis of congenital or acquired syphilis.

Plan

Because syphilitic IK is a manifestation of systemic syphilis, the eye care practitioner should refer the patient for management of the underlying systemic disease. The main medication used to eradicate syphilis is penicillin. It should be noted that antitreponemal therapy is of little help in altering the course or severity of the ocular disease. Topical corticosteroids (e.g., 1% prednisolone acetate) may be prescribed to diminish corneal inflammation and uveitis in an attempt to improve the visual outcome. A topical cycloplegic agent such as 5% homatropine should be added if iritis is present. Patients with significant corneal opacification and visual impairment may require penetrating keratoplasty.

LYME DISEASE

Subjective

Lyme disease is caused by the spirochete *Borrelia burgdorferi*. Cases of Lyme disease most frequently occur in the Northeast, Minnesota, Wisconsin, and along the West Coast; however, cases of the disease have been reported in at least 46 states. It is thought that, in most human cases, the spirochete is transmitted through bites from ticks that fed on infected deer or other animals.

Lyme disease affects almost every organ system and causes a wide array of clinical presentations. Patients with ocular manifestations may complain of decreased vision and show visual acuity ranging from 20/20 to 20/70. Some patients may also complain of pain, photophobia, and epiphora.

Objective

The first dermal sign of the disease is usually a focal, enlarging red rash called *erythema migrans*. The rash may be associated with conjunctivitis and lymphadenopathy.

Other systemic manifestations include arthritis, Bell's palsy, neuritis, meningitis, encephalitis, and heart disease.

In IK secondary to Lyme disease, the patches of infiltration can be found at any depth within the stroma. There is little or no associated anterior chamber reaction. There may be a chorioretinitis with a salt and pepper appearance similar to that seen in congenital syphilis.

Lyme-specific serologic assays such as immunofluorescence, hemagglutination, or enzyme-linked immunosorbent assay (ELISA) should be ordered if Lyme disease is suspected. In addition, Lyme Western blot is a specific test useful when ELISA proves equivocal or falsely negative. It should be noted that the Lyme serology tests may initially show false-negatives due to a long immunologic latency period and that patients with syphilis can produce false-positive results on Lyme titer tests.

Plan

Patients with Lyme disease should be comanaged with an internist. Oral antibiotics such as doxycycline, amoxicillin, tetracycline, or erythromycin are used initially to treat the systemic disease. Intravenous ceftriaxone sodium, cefotaxime sodium, or penicillin may be used in resistant cases. Topical steroids such as 1% prednisolone acetate can help speed the resolution of the IK.

TUBERCULOSIS

Subjective

Tuberculosis is primarily a pulmonary disease but can affect other organ systems, including the eye. It is caused by the bacillus *Mycobacterium tuberculosis*. IK is a rare manifestation of tuberculosis. Those patients who unfortunately develop IK often complain of decreased vision, pain, and photophobia.

Objective

Evidence of tuberculosis includes low-grade fever, weight loss, and a persistent, productive cough. The purified protein derivative (tuberculin) skin test is used to screen for tuberculosis, and chest radiography and sputum culture are used to confirm the diagnosis. IK from tuberculosis tends to be peripheral and sectoral, and is often associated with a focal sclerokeratitis. The inflammation causes dense infiltration involving the anterior and stromal layers. Vascularization is usually confined to the anterior stroma. The resultant scarring is more dense than that found in syphilitic IK due to the more intense inflammation. The clinician should also look for other ocular signs of tuberculosis, including phlyctenular keratoconjunctivitis and anterior and posterior uveitis.

Plan

Referral for systemic treatment of tuberculosis is necessary to eliminate the underlying disease. First-line medications include isoniazid, rifampin, pyrazinamide, ethambutol, and streptomycin. It should be noted that systemic antituberculosis treatment does not affect the corneal inflammation. Corneal inflammation from tuberculosis can be treated with 1% prednisolone sodium phosphate. The steroids are used until symptoms and inflammation are controlled and then slowly decreased. Because tuberculosis is becoming more common in association with acquired immunodeficiency syndrome, screening for infection with human immunodeficiency virus should be considered as well.

HERPES SIMPLEX STROMAL DISEASE

Subjective

Herpes simplex infection is a systemic viral infection that can involve the eye. Stromal involvement usually occurs in recurrent herpes simplex keratitis. Patients with herpes simplex stromal disease may have symptoms of decreased vision, pain, photophobia, and increased lacrimation.

Objective

Slit-lamp examination reveals multiple or diffuse whitish gray stromal infiltrates. The inflammation later leads to thinning and neovascularization. In addition, an anterior chamber reaction commonly occurs, and in severe cases a hypopyon can develop.

It is helpful to note associated signs of herpes simplex to aid in confirming the diagnosis. A history of recurrent vesicular lesions around the mouth or nose (fever blisters) is indicative of herpes simplex infection. Occasionally, the patient may have a history of chronic use of immunosuppressive agents such as topical or systemic steroids, which can exacerbate herpes simplex. Corneal sensitivity testing with a cotton wisp or esthesiometer provides additional information. Decreased corneal sensation at the affected site is commonly found in herpes simplex keratitis. The clinician should also look for a dendritic or geographic staining pattern, which indicates concurrent epithelial herpes simplex keratitis.

Plan

The management goal is to reduce the inflammation that has caused the stromal involvement and to minimize permanent damage. Antiviral treatment should be prescribed along with anti-inflammatories to prevent recurrence of infection. A commonly prescribed initial therapeutic regimen includes 1% prednisolone acetate, 1% trifluorothymidine, and 5% homatropine. If there is dense, nonresolving scarring or perforation is imminent due to necrotizing IK, penetrating keratopathy is indicated.

HERPES ZOSTER STROMAL DISEASE

Subjective

Herpes zoster is caused by reactivation of the latent virus in a person who has previously been infected with varicella. Usually herpes zoster is found in patients over 60 years of age; however, it can affect younger people, particularly if they are immunosuppressed. Unlike herpes simplex, herpes zoster causes burning pain along the distribution of the affected nerves. It can also cause headache, malaise, and depression. If there is corneal involvement, particularly central stromal disease, the patient experiences blurred vision. Pain and photophobia due to secondary uveitis are other symptoms of ocular involvement.

Objective

Classically, there is a history of a vesicular skin rash located along the dermatome of the fifth cranial nerve. The lesions usually appear on the forehead and upper eyelid and may extend to the tip of the nose (Hutchinson's sign). They do not cross the vertical midline. These lesions can leave permanent scars.

Ocular signs of herpes zoster include the presence of pseudodendrites (mucous plaques on the corneal epithelium), uveitis, scleritis, and iritic atrophy. Subepithelial and peripheral anterior stromal infiltrates are signs of deeper corneal involvement. Disciform keratitis may develop later. A dilated fundus examination should be performed to rule out optic neuritis and optic atrophy, and the patient should be monitored for the development of secondary glaucoma.

Plan

Early treatment of herpes zoster with oral antiviral agents such as acyclovir or famciclovir is desirable to prevent or reduce complications. This therapy is most effective when initiated within 72 hours of the onset of the skin lesions. To treat stromal keratitis, topical steroids such as 1% prednisolone acetate and cycloplegic agents such as 5% homatropine are useful in reducing the inflammation. The use of prophylactic antibiotic ointment such as bacitracin can reduce the occurrence of secondary infection.

SUGGESTED READING

Arffa RC, Grayson M. Grayson's Diseases of the Cornea (4th ed). St. Louis: Mosby–Year Book, 1997.

Bartlett JD, Jaanus SD. Clinical Ocular Pharmacology (3rd ed). Boston: Butterworth–Heinemann, 1995.

Chandler JW, Sugar JS, Edelhauser HF. External Diseases: Cornea, Conjunctiva, Sclera, Eyelids, Lacrimal System. In Textbook of Ophthalmology, Vol 8. New York: Gower Medical, 1993.

Cullom RD, Chang B. The Wills Eye Manual: Office and Emergency Room Diagnosis and Treatment of Eye Disease (2nd ed). Philadelphia: Lippincott, 1994.

Onofrey BE. Clinical Optometric Pharmacology and Therapeutics. Philadelphia: Lippincott, 1994.

Smolin G, Thoft RA. The Cornea: Scientific Foundations and Clinical Practice. Boston: Little, Brown, 1994.

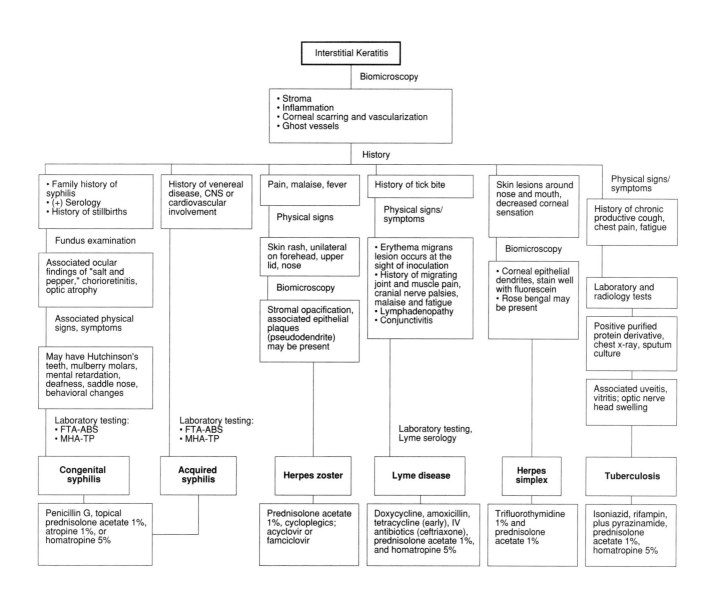

Interstitial Keratitis

Biomicroscopy

- Stroma
- Inflammation
- Corneal scarring and vascularization
- Ghost vessels

History

Congenital syphilis path:
- Family history of syphilis
- (+) Serology
- History of stillbirths

Fundus examination

Associated ocular findings of "salt and pepper," chorioretinitis, optic atrophy

Associated physical signs, symptoms

May have Hutchinson's teeth, mulberry molars, mental retardation, deafness, saddle nose, behavioral changes

Laboratory testing:
- FTA-ABS
- MHA-TP

Congenital syphilis

Penicillin G, topical prednisolone acetate 1%, atropine 1%, or homatropine 5%

Acquired syphilis path:
History of venereal disease, CNS or cardiovascular involvement

Laboratory testing:
- FTA-ABS
- MHA-TP

Acquired syphilis

Herpes zoster path:
Pain, malaise, fever

Physical signs

Skin rash, unilateral on forehead, upper lid, nose

Biomicroscopy

Stromal opacification, associated epithelial plaques (pseudodendrite) may be present

Herpes zoster

Prednisolone acetate 1%, cycloplegics; acyclovir or famciclovir

Lyme disease path:
History of tick bite

Physical signs/ symptoms

- Erythema migrans lesion occurs at the sight of inoculation
- History of migrating joint and muscle pain, cranial nerve palsies, malaise and fatigue
- Lymphadenopathy
- Conjunctivitis

Laboratory testing, Lyme serology

Lyme disease

Doxycycline, amoxicillin, tetracycline (early), IV antibiotics (ceftriaxone), prednisolone acetate 1%, and homatropine 5%

Herpes simplex path:
Skin lesions around nose and mouth, decreased corneal sensation

Biomicroscopy

- Corneal epithelial dendrites, stain well with fluorescein
- Rose bengal may be present

Herpes simplex

Trifluorothymidine 1% and prednisolone acetate 1%

Tuberculosis path:
Physical signs/ symptoms

History of chronic productive cough, chest pain, fatigue

Laboratory and radiology tests

Positive purified protein derivative, chest x-ray, sputum culture

Associated uveitis, vitritis; optic nerve head swelling

Tuberculosis

Isoniazid, rifampin, plus pyrazinamide, prednisolone acetate 1%, homatropine 5%

23

Corneal Neovascularization

John H. Nishimoto

CORNEAL NEOVASCULARIZATION AT A GLANCE

Soft contact lens wear
Rosacea (acne rosacea)
Superior limbic keratoconjunctivitis
Phlyctenular keratoconjunctivitis
Ocular pemphigoid
Peripheral corneal degeneration (Terrien's marginal degeneration, Mooren's ulcer)
Graft rejection
Interstitial keratitis
Infectious corneal disease (bacterial, viral, fungal, chlamydial)
Bullous keratopathy
Disciform keratitis
Chronic irritation (e.g., trichiasis, exposure keratoconjunctivitis)
Thermal or chemical burn
Atopic keratoconjunctivitis

Beyond the limbus, the cornea is avascular tissue. Abnormal blood vessel growth (neovascularization) of the cornea is usually secondary to hypoxia, inflammation, or infection. This chapter discusses the major conditions that may lead to corneal neovascularization.

SOFT CONTACT LENS WEAR

Subjective

Corneal neovascularization secondary to contact lens wear is an indication of poor lens tolerance. Patients with contact lens–related neovascularization are often asymp-

tomatic, especially if the condition is caused by low-grade chronic hypoxia. Some patients complain of mild irritation with prolonged lens wear. If neovascularization encroaches on the central cornea, the patient may complain of decreased vision.

Objective

Contact lens–related neovascularization can result from hypoxia, lens decentration causing peripheral edema or restriction of venous drainage, epithelial disturbances, limbal hyperemia, and overwear. Some of these problems are more prevalent with extended-wear than with daily-wear soft contact lenses. Hydrogel lens wear can be associated with corneal softening, which can promote the development of tortuous epithelial or stromal vessels that arise from the limbal region. Vessels that loop back toward the limbus are of less significance than those that have small projections spiking toward the central cornea.

Plan

When contact lens–induced corneal vascularization is managed successfully, the new vessels empty and become ghost vessels. Reduction in wearing time is a key factor in the management of all cases of corneal vascularization. Extended-wear lenses should be changed to daily-wear lenses as a first step. Daily-wear hours should be reduced to allow the cornea periods of greater oxygenation during waking hours. Poorly centered or tight lenses may impinge on the limbus and cause localized irritation or interference with limbal circulation. Remedial steps include refitting to improve lens centration, reducing edge clearance and thickness, using a more oxygen-permeable or more wettable material, alleviating tear deficiencies, and promoting proper blinking habits. Promoting better lens care can also be helpful. In extreme cases, contact lens wear may need to be discontinued.

ROSACEA (ACNE ROSACEA)

Subjective

Rosacea is a dermal disease that can affect the eyes. It is most common in middle-aged adults. The condition may be aggravated by the ingestion of certain substances, including tea, coffee, other hot drinks, alcoholic beverages, and spicy foods, and by tobacco use. Focal infections, vitamin deficiencies, diseases of the gastrointestinal tract, endocrine abnormalities, menopause, psychosocial problems, and allergies are other aggravating factors. Symptoms of rosacea involving the cornea include pain, photophobia, and foreign body sensation.

Objective

Telangiectasia, erythema, papules, and papulomacular skin lesions, especially at the flush areas of the face, are characteristic cutaneous signs of rosacea. Rhinophyma is a sign of more advanced disease and is usually more pronounced in males than in females. Hyperemic, thickened eyelids with telangiectasia of the eyelid margins is a common ocular sign. Blepharoconjunctivitis, hordeola, chalazia, and episcleritis may also be observed. The keratitis of rosacea initially manifests as a marginal infiltrate that typically involves the lower two-thirds of the cornea. Vessels from the limbus then advance into the zone of infiltration. Other corneal manifestations include superficial punctate keratopathy and subepithelial infiltrates. In some cases ulcers may develop in those areas with pannus and cause subsequent scarring.

Plan

Oral tetracycline, doxycycline, minocycline, and other related drugs are commonly used to treat both ocular and cutaneous rosacea. If tetracycline is not tolerated by the patient, erythromycin can be used. Some patients are maintained on a low dosage of tetracycline (250 mg qd) indefinitely. Topical corticosteroids such as 1% prednisolone acetate or steroid-antibiotic combinations may be useful in managing the blepharoconjunctivitis and corneal infiltrates. Other associated conditions such as hordeola, chalazia, and dry eyes should be treated as well.

SUPERIOR LIMBIC KERATOCONJUNCTIVITIS

Subjective

Superior limbic keratoconjunctivitis (SLK) is a chronic inflammatory condition that occasionally is associated with soft contact lens wear or thyroid disease. Symptoms of SLK include pain, photophobia, and blepharospasm. In some instances, patients squint and create a bandage effect in an attempt to keep the lesion covered.

Objective

SLK is usually bilateral but may be asymmetric. In chronic cases pannus develops, especially in the superior region of the cornea. Corneal filaments are commonly found in this condition. Conjunctival findings include papillary hypertrophy, chemosis, and hyperemia of the bulbar conjunctiva, particularly in the limbal region.

Plan

If SLK is associated with soft contact lens use, discontinuance of lens wear is the most effective therapy. In all forms of SLK, ocular lubricants and topical corticosteroids can be used to provide symptomatic relief. Topical acetylcysteine and cromolyn sodium have been effective in some cases. Silver nitrate followed by irrigation has been used to debride degenerating epithelial cells. In addition, pressure patching may be used to promote proper re-epithelialization. If the cause of the SLK is not evident, a thyroid profile should be ordered to rule out associated thyrotoxicosis.

PHLYCTENULAR KERATOCONJUNCTIVITIS

Subjective

Phlyctenules represent a hypersensitivity reaction to microbial antigens such as those produced by *Staphylococcus* and *Mycobacterium tuberculosis*. The clinician should question the patient about prior tubercular infection or exposure and note coughing or other symptoms that may indicate current tubercular infection. Symptoms of phlyctenular keratoconjunctivitis include foreign body sensation, discomfort, pain, and photophobia. Occasionally the patient may complain of itching and mucoid discharge.

Objective

There are generally two types of phlyctenular presentation: conjunctival and corneal. Conjunctival phlyctenules are usually located in the bulbar conjunctiva. They appear as small, whitish yellow, lymphocytic nodules surrounded by hyperemic vessels. Corneal phlyctenules are usually located at the limbus but may migrate toward the center of the cornea. There may be a linear area of neovascularization extending from the limbus to the lesion. Associated signs include blepharitis and conjunctivitis if the condition is caused by hypersensitivity to staphylococcal exotoxins. Patients at risk for tuberculosis should be screened with a purified protein derivative (tuberculin) skin test. Chest radiography and sputum culture may be used to confirm the diagnosis.

Plan

Because phlyctenulosis is a hypersensitivity reaction, topical corticosteroids such as 1% prednisolone acetate or rimexolone have proved effective in reducing signs and symptoms. In addition, it is important to eliminate the underlying cause. If the condition is associated with blepharitis, proper lid hygiene and an antibiotic ointment such as bacitracin or bacitracin–polymyxin B sulfate can be prescribed to decrease the population of *Staphylococcus* organisms. Patients with suspected or confirmed tuberculosis should be referred to an internist for further evaluation and treatment.

OCULAR PEMPHIGOID

Subjective

Cicatricial pemphigoid is an autoimmune disorder that affects the skin and mucous membranes. It is most commonly found in patients aged 55 and older. Some cases are triggered by the use of topical drugs such as epinephrine, pilocarpine, trifluorothymidine, or aminoglycosides, or are secondary to Stevens-Johnson syndrome. Patients with ocular pemphigoid present with dry-eye symptoms, tearing, and photophobia. There may be a history of similar episodes.

Objective

In pemphigoid, bullous vesicles form in the mucous membranes of the nose, mouth, pharynx, and other sites. Scarring of the affected tissues often results. Ocular pemphigoid typically is bilateral. Symblepharon formation involving the inferior conjunctiva is a common sign. The lower fornix may be shortened, and this shortening induces entropion and trichiasis. Due to goblet cell abnormalities, this condition results in severe dry eye. Initially this causes superficial punctate keratopathy. Severe, chronic dry eye

can lead to corneal opacification, pannus formation, ulceration, and keratinization.

Plan

Severe dry eye can be treated initially with frequent instillation of preservative-free ocular lubricants. Topical tretinoin, punctal occlusion, and bandage contact lenses have also been used to provide relief. In addition, the use of goggles and spectacles with shields can help provide a moist environment.

Pemphigoid should be comanaged with an internist and dermatologist. Systemic steroids such as prednisone can decrease symptoms during acute episodes. Immunosuppressives and dapsone have been used in more severe cases. Cryotherapy or electrolysis can be used to eliminate trichiasis. In cases with severe scarring, it may be necessary to refer the patient to an oculoplastic specialist for surgical reconstruction of the fornices by mucous membrane grafting.

GRAFT REJECTION

Subjective

Corneal graft rejection can occur several weeks to years after a penetrating keratoplasty procedure. The predominant symptoms are decreased vision, mild pain, tearing, and photophobia.

Objective

On slit-lamp examination, the clinician may note keratic precipitates or a line of white blood cells on the corneal endothelium called an endothelial rejection line. Stromal and epithelial edema are common findings. Subepithelial infiltrates and a demarcated line of elevated epithelium termed an *epithelial rejection line* are other important corneal signs. In some cases, neovascularization forms adjacent to or extends into the grafted corneal button. Other ocular findings include anterior chamber reaction and circumlimbal injection. It is important to note that an anterior chamber reaction may be from recent graft surgery and not from true graft rejection.

Plan

Topical steroid therapy should be initiated or increased immediately to suppress the immune response. Prednisolone acetate 1% or rimexolone can be used for both epithelial and endothelial rejection. Dexamethasone ointment should be added at night to manage endothelial rejection. Topical steroids must be tapered very slowly once improvement is observed. If the graft fails to respond to topical steroids, then oral, subconjunctival, or intravenous administration of steroids should be considered.

SUGGESTED READING

Bartlett JD, Jaanus SD. Clinical Ocular Pharmacology (3rd ed). Boston: Butterworth–Heinemann, 1995.

Catania LJ. Primary Care of the Anterior Segment (2nd ed). Norwalk, CT: Appleton & Lange, 1995.

Kaufman HE. The Cornea (2nd ed). Boston: Butterworth–Heinemann, 1997.

Silbert JA. Anterior Segment Complications of Contact Lens Wear. New York: Churchill Livingstone, 1994.

Smolin G, Thoft RA. The Cornea: Scientific Foundations and Clinical Practice. Boston: Little, Brown, 1994.

Tomlinson A. Complications of Contact Lens Wear. St. Louis: Mosby–Year Book, 1992.

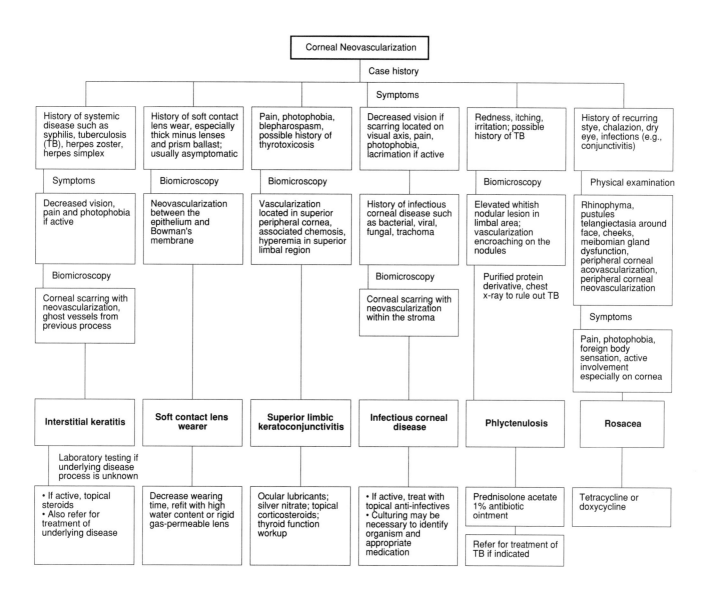

24

Corneal Pigmentation

John H. Nishimoto

CORNEAL PIGMENTATION AT A GLANCE

Keratic precipitates
Corneal guttata
Krukenberg's spindle
Hudson-Stähli line
Systemic medications (e.g., phenothiazines, amiodarone, chloroquine, indomethacin)
Fleischer's ring
Kayser-Fleischer ring
Stocker's line
Melanosis
Corneal blood staining from hyphema
Rust ring
Ferry's line
Band keratopathy
Fabry's disease
Alkaptonuria

Pigmented discoloration of the cornea may be caused by degenerative changes, medications, iron deposition, pigment cell deposition, or inflammation. This chapter reviews some of the more common corneal pigmentations, their etiologies, and associated conditions.

KERATIC PRECIPITATES

Subjective

Keratic precipitates (KPs) are deposits of white blood cells on the endothelium that indicate prior or concurrent anterior uveitis. The patient may have a history of a systemic disease that causes the inflammation, such as ankylosing spondylitis, sarcoidosis, syphilis, tuberculosis, or Reiter's disease. If the uveitis is active, the patient may complain of pain, photophobia, and tearing. In chronic low-grade uveitis or resolved uveitis, the patient may be asymptomatic.

Objective

Recently deposited KPs are light colored, whereas long-standing KPs often become pigmented. Pigmented KPs may be confused with corneal guttata or liberated iris pigment cells. Keratic precipitates are classified into two categories based on their biomicroscopic appearance: granulomatous and nongranulomatous. Granulomatous precipitates are large and yellowish white, often have a greasy appearance, and are termed *mutton-fat* KPs. Other signs that may accompany granulomatous KPs are Koeppe and Busacca iris nodules, vitreous "snowballs," chorioretinal granulomas, and retinal vascular "candle-wax drippings." Diseases that may cause some or all of these presentations include sarcoidosis, toxoplasmosis, tuberculosis, syphilis, Vogt-Koyanagi-Harada syndrome, and sympathetic ophthalmia.

Nongranulomatous precipitates are small, fine, and initially white or yellow. Conditions such as ankylosing spondylitis, Fuchs' heterochromic iridocyclitis, juvenile rheumatoid arthritis, and Reiter's disease may cause KPs that have a nongranulomatous appearance on biomicroscopic examination.

The workup of uveitis should include a thorough ocular and systemic history and a complete examination. In addition, laboratory and radiologic testing are useful in identifying any underlying systemic cause. Laboratory testing is particularly useful in bilateral and chronic or recurrent conditions. Relevant tests include HLA level and fluorescent treponemal antibody absorption testing. Radiography of the chest and sacroiliac joint is also useful. Other tests may be indicated based on the clinical presentation.

Plan

If the patient presents with an active inflammation, topical corticosteroids such as 1% prednisolone acetate and cycloplegic agents such as 2–5% homatropine can help reduce the inflammatory response, prevent synechiae, and improve comfort. Any underlying ocular or systemic cause of the inflammation should be treated as well. Systemic therapy includes antibiotics if the underlying condition is infectious as well as corticosteroids or nonsteroidal anti-inflammatory agents.

CORNEAL GUTTATA

Subjective

Guttata are focal excrescences of Descemet's membrane often observed in patients of middle-age and older. Occasionally the patient with guttata may have a history of previous cataract surgery or other trauma causing endothelial damage. Patients with corneal guttata are often asymptomatic. However, if the guttata are more prominent and the endothelial pump becomes compromised, corneal edema results. This outcome can occur in Fuchs' endothelial-epithelial dystrophy. In this condition, the patient may complain of decreased vision, photophobia, and, in advanced cases, pain.

Objective

Guttata on Descemet's membrane may be observed through a slit-lamp biomicroscope. They are usually bilateral, symmetric, and more prominent in the central cornea. When specular reflection is used, the endothelial cells demonstrate a loss of size uniformity, and the excrescences appear as small focal dark areas. Some clinicians have described the appearance as similar to that of an orange peel or beaten metal. The clinician should also look for signs of endothelial dysfunction associated with guttata, such as corneal thickening, stromal edema, and epithelial bullae.

Plan

If there is no corneal edema present, management consists of monitoring the patient annually. If there is a slight epithelial edema, instillation of hypertonic 5% sodium chloride drops during the day and hypertonic sodium chloride ointment at night is the usual treatment. Holding a hair dryer at arm's length and gently blowing air toward the eye for 5–10 minutes every morning is beneficial in some cases. If intraocular pressure is elevated (22 mm Hg or more), a topical beta blocker such as 0.25–0.50% timolol

maleate can be used to reduce stress on the endothelium. In severe cases of Fuchs' dystrophy in which vision is significantly compromised or the patient's pain cannot be controlled, a penetrating keratoplasty may be indicated.

KRUKENBERG'S SPINDLE

Subjective

Pigment from the iris travels with aqueous humor, eventually flowing to the trabecular meshwork. Because of the current of the aqueous, the pigment usually travels vertically along the posterior surface of the corneal endothelium. Excessive pigment is deposited in a vertical pattern on the central endothelium; this pattern is termed *Krukenberg's spindle*. In addition, pigment may deposit in the limbal area of the posterior surface of the corneal endothelium. Krukenberg's spindle is often associated with pigment dispersion syndrome. Occasionally a Krukenberg's spindle pigment pattern is associated with cocaine abuse. As the pupil becomes dilated, the iris rubs against the ciliary zonules, liberating pigment. Unless the intraocular pressure is greatly elevated (>40 mm Hg), patients with Krukenberg's spindle are usually asymptomatic. If the pressure becomes quite elevated, the patient may complain of eye pain, photophobia, and hazy vision.

Objective

When the conical-beam slit-lamp technique is used, the clinician may observe pigment cells floating in the anterior chamber in addition to the characteristic pattern of pigment deposition on the corneal endothelium. Defects in the iris representing areas of pigment sloughing are best viewed with a transillumination technique. Gonioscopy should be performed to look for excessive pigment in the anterior chamber angle, especially in the trabecular meshwork and adjacent to Schwalbe's line. Tonometry should be used to detect fluctuations in intraocular pressure. During intraocular pressure spikes associated with pigmentary glaucoma, pigment cells may be seen floating within the anterior chamber. Corneal edema may be present if the intraocular pressure becomes markedly elevated. Threshold visual fields should also be assessed to determine whether significant damage to the retinal nerve fibers has occurred.

Plan

If the patient has pigmentary glaucoma, topical medications such as 0.5% timolol maleate or 1–4% pilocarpine is prescribed to lower the intraocular pressure. Miotics are the medical treatment of choice, because they minimize contact between the iris and the ciliary zonules; however, they may not be tolerated by younger patients. The use of beta blockers is especially indicated for prepresbyopic patients, whereas the miotics are a more appropriate choice for presbyopes. In pigmentary glaucoma patients with reverse pupillary block, laser peripheral iridotomy has been shown to be effective because it allows the iris to move away from the zonules.

SYSTEMIC MEDICATIONS

Phenothiazines

Subjective

Phenothiazines are a group of medications used primarily in the treatment of psychoses. If the patient is taking thioridazine hydrochloride (Mellaril) in doses of greater than 2,000 mg per day, or if the patient has been taking 800 mg per day for several years, a toxic level may be reached that produces corneal pigmentation and other ocular signs. In general, the deposits on the cornea have no adverse effects and do not cause decreased vision.

Objective

On slit-lamp examination, pigmented deposits appearing near Descemet's membrane can be seen in the interpalpebral cornea. These are accompanied by similar granules in the interpalpebral conjunctiva. The distribution of the deposits suggests that exposure to light contributes to the formation of the pigment granules.

Associated findings include yellow-brown deposits on the lens arranged in a stellate pattern. Vision is rarely affected unless there is associated retinal involvement. Chlorpromazine hydrochloride (Thorazine) taken at 1,200–2,400 mg per day for longer than 12 months can cause toxic retinopathy. This condition manifests as pigment clumps between the posterior pole and the equator, areas of retinal depigmentation, and retinal edema. The toxic effect of the medication can also cause visual field abnormalities (central scotoma and generalized constriction), and an extinguished or diminished response on electroretinogram.

Plan

The deposits of the lens, cornea, and conjunctiva tend to subside slowly with cessation of drug administration. Patients with these changes require no treatment other than regular monitoring. If drug levels are high enough to cause toxic changes in the retina, however, then a reevaluation of medication or dosage is necessary.

Aminoquinolines (Chloroquine, Hydroxychloroquine Sulfate, and Amiodarone Hydrochloride)

Subjective

Chloroquine (Aralen) and hydroxychloroquine sulfate (Plaquenil) are aminoquinolines used to treat malaria as well as rheumatoid arthritis, systemic lupus erythematosus, and other inflammatory diseases. Typically, patients taking these medications are visually asymptomatic. However, if the dosage is high enough (hydroxychloroquine, >300 g total cumulative dose or >750 mg per day taken over months to years), decreased vision may occur due to retinal changes.

Objective

Chronic ingestion of or environmental exposure to chloroquine can produce deposits on the cornea that are visible with the biomicroscope. They are seen as many fine yellowish deposits or white dots in the epithelium. At first they may have a linear appearance resembling a Hudson-Stähli line, but the most common appearance is that of an epithelial vortex. This pattern is very much like the pattern seen in Fabry's disease. Associated retinal changes include a "bull's-eye" macula (ring of increased pigmentation) and loss of the foveal reflex. Color vision and the central visual field may also be affected.

Plan

The corneal deposits do no harm and usually disappear after the medication is discontinued or the dosage is decreased. The major ocular consequence is retinopathy, which can result in permanent vision loss. Patients on these medications should be examined every 6 months to monitor for the development of retinopathy.

HUDSON-STÄHLI LINE

Subjective

Histologically, a Hudson-Stähli line is a band of iron deposition in the basal corneal epithelial cells. Such an iron deposit can be found in patients of any age and is sometimes associated with tear disturbances. The Hudson-Stähli line itself causes no symptoms; however, the patient may report irritation or other symptoms associated with dry eyes.

Objective

A Hudson-Stähli line typically is found in the interpalpebral zone of the cornea. It appears as a brown, green, yellow, or white irregular horizontal line in the central deep epithelium.

Plan

Hudson-Stähli lines require no treatment and should merely be noted during routine examinations. If the patient has dry-eye syndrome, then lubricating drops and ointments or punctal occlusion can be beneficial.

FLEISCHER'S KERATOCONUS RING

Subjective

Fleischer's keratoconus ring is an area of iron deposition along the base of the cone in keratoconus. Patients with keratoconus may complain of decreased vision and, on occasion, slight pain and photophobia. The symptoms are due almost entirely to the distortion and thinning of the cornea or corneal hydrops.

Objective

With slit-lamp biomicroscopy, Fleischer's keratoconus ring appears as a ring of brown pigment around the base of the cone. There can be associated signs of increased visibility of corneal nerves and vertical striae. Reflexes as measured by retinoscopy and ophthalmoscopy are distorted. Keratometry or corneal topographical analysis reveal steepening, usually in the inferior nasal region of the cornea. In later stages, Munson's sign may be noted. This sign is a deviation of the lower lid during downward gaze that is caused by the protruding apex of the cone.

Plan

There is no treatment for Fleischer's ring itself. However, the underlying condition, keratoconus, usually requires management. Keratoconus management includes the use of spectacles to correct the decreased vision as long as possible. More advanced cases may be managed with contact lenses, especially rigid gas-permeable lenses. Penetrating keratoplasty can be performed when vision can no longer be corrected by either spectacles or contact lenses.

KAYSER-FLEISCHER RING

Subjective

A Kayser-Fleischer ring is associated with Wilson's disease, a congenital error of copper metabolism that results in chronic liver disease. The disorder has an autosomal recessive mode of inheritance. Wilson's disease has been found to be such a common cause of hepatic dysfunction in children that it should be suspected in any child with cirrhosis until evidence proves otherwise. In addition to liver dysfunction, patients with this disease may develop personality changes or behavioral abnormalities. The Kayser-Fleischer ring itself causes no ocular symptoms.

Objective

A Kayser-Fleischer ring may be seen grossly as a golden brown, green, or ruby red band over the peripheral cornea. It is better viewed with the use of slit-lamp biomicroscopy. The ring typically appears first superiorly between the 10- and 2-o'clock positions, then medially, and finally laterally. A pigment deposition band develops in Descemet's membrane beginning at the limbus and gradually extending centrally and circumferentially. Gonioscopy may be used to visualize pigment in the peripheral region of Descemet's membrane. Associated signs include anterior and posterior subcapsular copper deposition in the crystalline lens, which produces a "sunflower" cataract.

Laboratory tests to measure ceruloplasmin and serum and urinary copper levels are used to confirm the diagnosis of Wilson's disease.

Plan

A referral is necessary for any patient suspected of having Wilson's disease. Without proper treatment, Wilson's disease can be fatal. The cause of death may be dysfunction of the hepatic, renal, or central nervous system. Treatment involves the reduction of copper through oral medications such as penicillamine, trientine hydrochloride, or zinc acetate, as well as dietary control. The efficacy of the therapy is monitored by observing the disappearance of the Kayser-Fleischer ring; therefore, the eye care practitioner can play an important role in the management of this systemic disease.

STOCKER'S LINE

Subjective

Stocker's line is a brownish deposit of hemosiderin observed in the corneal epithelium adjacent to the leading apical edge of a pterygium. Patients with this condition may have a history of chronic exposure to sunlight. Although Stocker's line itself does not produce symptoms, the associated pterygium may cause the patient to complain of irritation, redness, or decreased vision.

Objective

A pterygium is a triangular growth of fibrovascular conjunctival tissue that extends onto the cornea. The apex of the triangle points to the center of the cornea. Stocker's line is a thin brownish line that is just anterior to the leading edge of a pterygium and follows its contour.

Plan

There is no treatment for Stocker's line itself. However, the associated pterygium should be closely monitored and excised when indicated. Protection from UV radiation and topical lubricants may be of some benefit in impeding progress of the pterygium. Because postoperative recurrence is a problem, surgery is often delayed until the pterygium has become large enough to pose a threat to vision.

EPITHELIAL MELANOSIS

Subjective

Corneal melanosis is usually an extension of conjunctival melanosis. It occurs most commonly in persons with dark complexions. Patients with corneal melanosis are typically asymptomatic but may express concern about the cosmetic appearance of the melanosis.

Objective

Melanosis usually appears in the peripheral region of the corneal epithelium. The most common associated finding is conjunctival melanosis, in which patches of pigmentation occur in various areas throughout the conjunctiva.

Plan

No treatment is necessary for epithelial melanosis other than routine observation. If the area of pigmentation enlarges significantly or other changes occur, a melanoma should be ruled out.

RUST RING

Subjective

A rust ring results when a metallic foreign body, usually iron or steel, has become embedded in the cornea. In many cases the patient is aware of the event that caused the foreign body insult. For example, metallic foreign bodies many be produced during hammering or use of a grinding wheel. Most patients with a corneal rust ring experience excessive lacrimation, photophobia, and irritation, especially upon blinking or moving the eye.

Objective

After removal of the metallic foreign body, a rust deposit may remain. This deposit has a characteristic circular or ringlike appearance. Associated signs may include an infiltrate or edema surrounding the lesion and an anterior chamber reaction, indicated by the appearance of cells, flare, and circumlimbal injection. The practitioner should perform a Seidel test, assess chamber angle depth, and perform a dilated fundus examination to rule out a perforating injury. These steps are particularly important if the trauma was due to a small, high-velocity projectile.

Plan

The rust should be removed, because it is toxic to the corneal epithelium and could result in secondary infection and impairment of healing. The use of a spinning burr (Alger brush or Orthobur) is effective in removing the rust. When the area is touched gently with the brush, the rust easily spins off. After rust removal, application of a topical broad-spectrum antibiotic (e.g., gentamicin, bacitracin–polymyxin B sulfate) can prevent secondary infection. A cycloplegic agent such as 1% cyclopentolate hydrochloride or 2% or 5% homatropine can be used to prevent or reduce secondary iritis. Pressure patching or application of a bandage contact lens can promote proper re-epithelialization and improve comfort.

CORNEAL BLOOD STAINING FROM HYPHEMA

Subjective

A hyphema is blood in the anterior chamber and often occurs as a result of trauma. Corneal blood staining is more likely to occur in patients with hyphema who have an elevated intraocular pressure. The rise in pressure causes malfunction of the endothelial pump and forces the hemoglobin into the cornea. Corneal staining also is more likely to occur in patients with corneal dystrophies. Patients with hyphema may complain of gradual or sudden blurred vision resulting either from blood's filling the anterior chamber and interfering with the visual axis, or from blood's staining the cornea.

Objective

Slit-lamp examination reveals blood that has mostly or completely filled the anterior chamber. The staining of the cornea is distributed diffusely in the endothelium and posterior stroma. Tonometry often reveals an elevated intraocular pressure. If it is not treated, the corneal staining may remain for several months to years.

Plan

Because corneal blood staining threatens vision, it is recommended that a patient with hyphema who shows any sign of corneal staining be referred for surgical intervention to remove the blood from the anterior chamber. In addition, the elevated intraocular pressure should be managed with topical or oral antiglaucoma agents.

SUGGESTED READING

Arffa RC, Grayson M. Grayson's Diseases of the Cornea (4th ed). St. Louis: Mosby–Year Book, 1997.

Bartlett JD, Jaanus SD. Clinical Ocular Pharmacology (3rd ed). Boston: Butterworth–Heinemann, 1995.

Fingeret M, Lewis T. Primary Care of the Glaucomas. Norwalk, CT: Appleton & Lange, 1992.

Kanski JJ. Clinical Ophthalmology (3rd ed). Oxford, UK: Butterworth–Heinemann, 1994.

Nussenblatt RB, Whitcup SM, Palestine AG. Uveitis: Fundamentals and Clinical Practice (2nd ed). St. Louis: Mosby–Year Book, 1996.

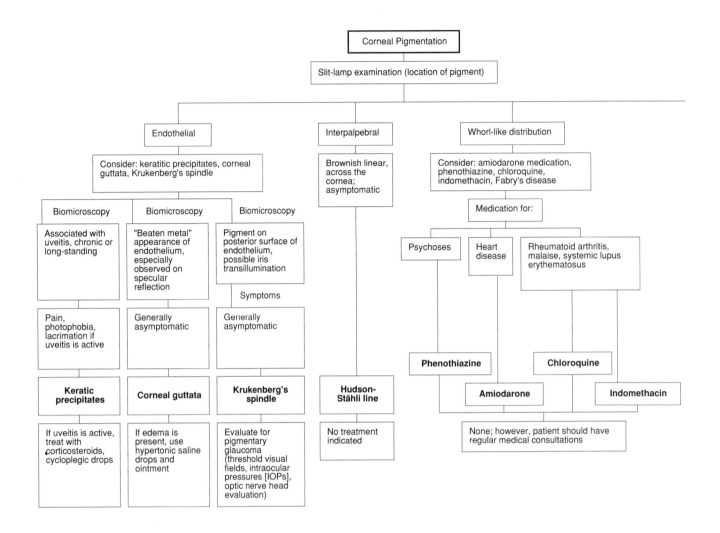

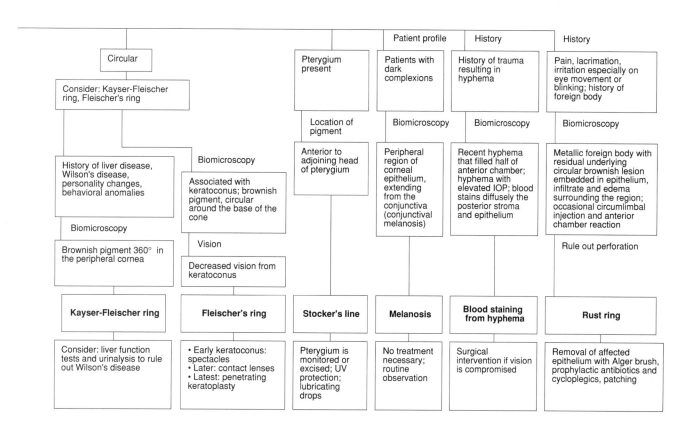

Circular

Consider: Kayser-Fleischer ring, Fleischer's ring

History of liver disease, Wilson's disease, personality changes, behavioral anomalies

Biomicroscopy

Brownish pigment 360° in the peripheral cornea

Biomicroscopy

Associated with keratoconus; brownish pigment, circular around the base of the cone

Vision

Decreased vision from keratoconus

Patient profile

History

History

Pterygium present

Patients with dark complexions

History of trauma resulting in hyphema

Pain, lacrimation, irritation especially on eye movement or blinking; history of foreign body

Location of pigment

Biomicroscopy

Biomicroscopy

Biomicroscopy

Anterior to adjoining head of pterygium

Peripheral region of corneal epithelium, extending from the conjunctiva (conjunctival melanosis)

Recent hyphema that filled half of anterior chamber; hyphema with elevated IOP; blood stains diffusely the posterior stroma and epithelium

Metallic foreign body with residual underlying circular brownish lesion embedded in epithelium, infiltrate and edema surrounding the region; occasional circumlimbal injection and anterior chamber reaction

Rule out perforation

Kayser-Fleischer ring

Fleischer's ring

Stocker's line

Melanosis

Blood staining from hyphema

Rust ring

Consider: liver function tests and urinalysis to rule out Wilson's disease

• Early keratoconus: spectacles
• Later: contact lenses
• Latest: penetrating keratoplasty

Pterygium is monitored or excised; UV protection; lubricating drops

No treatment necessary; routine observation

Surgical intervention if vision is compromised

Removal of affected epithelium with Alger brush, prophylactic antibiotics and cycloplegics, patching

25

Corneal Opacification

John H. Nishimoto

CORNEAL OPACIFICATION AT A GLANCE

Foreign body trauma (Coats' white ring)
Corneal ulcer
Interstitial keratitis
Corneal dystrophies
   Epithelial basement membrane dystrophy
   Macular dystrophy
   Lattice dystrophy
   Granular dystrophy
   Fuchs' endothelial dystrophy
   Congenital hereditary epithelial dystrophy
   Reis-Bücklers dystrophy
   Gelatinous drop–like dystrophy
   Central crystalline dystrophy
   Flecked dystrophy
   Central cloudy dystrophy
   Pre-Descemet's dystrophy
   Posterior amorphous corneal dystrophy
   Congenital hereditary stromal dystrophy
   Posterior polymorphous dystrophy
   Congenital hereditary endothelial dystrophy
Corneal degenerations
   Corneal arcus
   Band keratopathy
   Limbal girdle of Vogt
   Corneal farinata
   Crocodile shagreen of Vogt
   Corneal amyloidosis
   Salzmann's nodular degeneration
   Hyaline degeneration
   Lipid degeneration
   Pigmentary degeneration
   Pellucid marginal degeneration

   Terrien's marginal degeneration
   Climatic droplet degeneration
Rosacea
Superior limbic keratoconjunctivitis
Trachoma
Vernal keratoconjunctivitis
Herpes simplex
Epidemic keratoconjunctivitis
Phlyctenulosis
Toxic keratopathy
Pterygium
Hydrops secondary to keratoconus
Peter's anomaly
Mucopolysaccharidoses
Carcinoma in situ

Corneal opacification results from a variety of conditions, including traumatic insult, infection, inflammation, and congenital abnormalities. This chapter discusses some of the more common conditions that cause decreased corneal transparency.

COATS' WHITE RING

Subjective

Coats' white ring is a small corneal opacity that is the residue of previous injury by a metallic foreign body; therefore, it is important to take a careful history of previous ocular injuries. Patients with Coats' white ring complain of decreased vision if the lesion is located on the visual axis. At the time of diagnosis there are usually no complaints of pain or photophobia.

Objective

On slit-lamp examination, the ring is seen as a small, granular, white, oval ring. It is caused by an inflammatory response to iron deposition in Bowman's layer or the anterior stroma. Coats' white ring is an indication that the lesion is inactive.

Plan

Because at this time the lesion has healed and there is no indication of activity, the patient is usually instructed to return for examinations on a routine basis.

CORNEAL ULCER

Subjective

Infectious corneal ulcers can be caused by bacteria, viruses, fungi, or amoebae. Sterile corneal ulcers are the result of inflammation. The clinician should question the patient carefully about contact lens wear, especially extended wear; recent ocular trauma; and topical steroid use. Patients with corneal ulcer usually complain of pain, photophobia, lacrimation, and, on occasion, blepharospasm. The symptoms usually get progressively worse with each passing day.

Objective

An ulcer exists if there is a focal white opacity in the corneal stroma (infiltrate), an overlying epithelial defect that stains with fluorescein, and stromal loss. Typically, an ulcer or infiltrate is opaque, whereas stromal edema is more transparent. Associated signs are conjunctival injection, corneal thinning, stromal edema and inflammation surrounding the infiltrate, folds in Descemet's membrane, anterior chamber reaction (cells and flare), hypopyon, mucopurulent discharge, and upper eyelid edema. Corneal ulcers are described in greater detail in Chapter 20.

Plan

Ulcers and infiltrates are generally treated initially as bacterial unless there is a high suspicion of another form of infection (fungus, *Acanthamoeba*, herpes simplex). The initial management consists of prescribing a topical fluoroquinolone such as ciprofloxacin, ofloxacin, or norfloxacin and a cycloplegic such as 5% homatropine or 0.25% scopolamine. Stained corneal scrapings, cultures, and sensitivity testing are needed to determine the causative agent and the most appropriate course of ther-

apy. If the ulcer does not respond to the initial treatment, fortified antibiotics such as tobramycin, gentamicin and cefazolin, or vancomycin may be substituted based on the results of sensitivity testing.

INTERSTITIAL KERATITIS

Subjective

A number of diseases can cause interstitial keratitis. Syphilis, herpes simplex, herpes zoster, and tuberculosis are among the more common causes. In the acute phase of interstitial keratitis, patients may complain of pain, photophobia, tearing, and red eye. The clinician should try to determine whether the patient has a positive history of viral eye disease or whether the patient's mother has a history of venereal disease during pregnancy.

Objective

In the acute phase of interstitial keratitis, there are patent corneal stromal blood vessels and edema. Other signs of the acute phase of interstitial keratitis include conjunctival injection, fine keratic precipitates on the corneal endothelium, and anterior chamber cells and flare.

Signs of inactive interstitial keratitis include deep corneal haze or scarring, stromal blood vessels containing no blood ("ghost vessels"), and stromal thinning. There may be an associated finding of corneal nerves that are segmentally thickened like beads on a string. The clinician should also note whether iris nodules are present (found in tuberculosis or leprosy) and look for patchy hyperemia of the iris with fleshy pink nodules (found in syphilis). In addition, the fundus may have an associated "salt and pepper" appearance, which is commonly noted in syphilis.

Plan

Acute interstitial keratitis is treated with a topical cycloplegic agent such as 5% homatropine or 1% atropine, and a topical steroid such as 1% prednisolone acetate. Laboratory testing should be performed to rule out syphilis (VDRL test or rapid plasma reagin test, *Treponema pallidum* microhemagglutination assay, or fluorescent treponemal antibody absorption test) and tuberculosis (purified protein derivative test and chest radiography), and to try to determine the underlying cause of the interstitial keratitis. Once the cause is determined, it may be concurrently treated if indicated. For inactive interstitial keratitis, penetrating keratoplasty may improve vision when vision has been impaired by central corneal scarring.

EPITHELIAL BASEMENT MEMBRANE DYSTROPHY

Subjective

Epithelial basement membrane dystrophy (EBMD) is one of the most commonly diagnosed corneal dystrophies. Patients with this condition may be asymptomatic or may complain of irritation, pain, excessive lacrimation, or photophobia, especially on awakening. In some instances, the symptoms abate later in the day.

Objective

Slit-lamp examination may reveal diffuse gray patches (termed *maps*), large or tiny cysts (termed *dots*), or fine refractile lines (termed *fingerprints*) in the corneal epithelium. They are most easily viewed with retroillumination or indirect illumination from the side. EBMD can be a precursor to corneal erosion, in which large amounts of epithelium are roughened or sloughed. Spontaneous corneal epithelial erosions often arise after sleep due to the development of increased corneal edema behind the closed lid. The use of sodium fluorescein is very helpful in the diagnosis of EBMD. Areas of negative staining are seen that indicate poor adhesion, edema, and thickened basement membrane. There also may be areas of positive staining that indicate disrupted or poorly adhering epithelium.

Plan

If the patient is asymptomatic, usually there is no treatment. If the patient is experiencing pain and lacrimation, hypertonic saline drops and ointments are helpful to promote better adhesion and reduce edema. The management of corneal erosions is discussed in Chapter 21.

STROMAL DYSTROPHIES

Subjective

The three most common types of stromal dystrophy are macular (Groenouw's type II), lattice (Biber-Haab-Dimmer), and granular (Groenouw's type I). It is helpful to determine if there is a significant family history of corneal disease, because there is a genetic predisposition for the stromal dystrophies. Granular and lattice dystrophies have an autosomal dominant mode of inheritance, whereas macular dystrophy has an autosomal recessive mode. The most common patient complaint associated with stromal dystrophies is decreased vision. The onset of reduced vision occurs in the first decade of life for macular dys-

trophy, in the 20s or 30s for lattice dystrophy, and in the 40s or 50s for granular dystrophy. In addition, the patient may experience bouts of pain and lacrimation due to recurrent erosions.

Objective

Of the discussed stromal dystrophies, macular dystrophy is considered to have the most severe presentation. The earliest change is a diffuse clouding of the central superficial stroma, first noted between 3 and 9 years of age. With time, indistinct gray spots develop; there is clouding in between the spots that extends peripherally and into the deeper stroma. By adolescence the opacification involves the entire thickness of the cornea and may ultimately extend to the limbus, giving the cornea a ground-glass appearance.

In granular dystrophy, the corneal opacities appear in the first decade as small, discrete, sharply demarcated, grayish white opacities in the anterior axial stroma. These lesions have a bread-crumb appearance and are separated by areas of clear stroma. As the condition advances, the lesions become larger, increase in number, coalesce, and extend into the deeper stroma. As with most other corneal dystrophies, the changes are bilateral and fairly symmetric.

In lattice dystrophy, the shape of the lesions is quite different from that found in granular dystrophy. Early in the disease, the lesions typically appear as fine, translucent, irregular lines and dots. They are located mainly in the axial cornea and involve anterior stroma and Bowman's layer. With progression, the lattice of linear lesions becomes thicker and more opaque. The stroma between the lines progresses from clear to hazy. Eventually a central disciform opacity develops, impairing vision.

Plan

The treatment of stromal dystrophies consists of penetrating keratoplasty or excimer laser phototherapeutic keratectomy. However, the procedures are usually delayed until significant reduction in acuity is measured, because the dystrophy can reappear in as little as 3 years.

FUCHS' ENDOTHELIAL DYSTROPHY

Subjective

Fuchs' endothelial dystrophy is different from most other corneal dystrophies in that patients with this condition rarely become symptomatic before the age of 50. Although often classified as an endothelial dystrophy, it may affect the entire thickness of the cornea. The major complaints associated with Fuchs' dystrophy include glare and blurred vision, especially on awakening. In cases with significant epithelial involvement, the patient may experience severe pain. A careful history should be taken to determine whether the patient has had cataract surgery, especially surgery in which an intraocular lens has been implanted in the anterior chamber, because this procedure can lead to bullous keratopathy.

Objective

Fuchs' dystrophy is usually bilateral but may be asymmetric. Corneal guttata, best seen by specular reflection, and fine pigment dusting on the endothelium are early signs of Fuchs' dystrophy. With increasing edema due to malfunction of the endothelial pump, the cornea may develop a hazy, ground-glass appearance. Folds in Descemet's membrane and cystic epithelial edema develop. In the more severe cases, bullous keratopathy develops. Ruptured bullae cause epithelial disruption that is visible with sodium fluorescein stain and can be quite painful. Tonometry can provide additional information useful in both the diagnosis and management of Fuchs' dystrophy. Increased intraocular pressure may cause the endothelium to be further distressed and malfunction, with a resulting increase in corneal edema.

Plan

Sodium chloride 5% drops during the day and ointment at night is the standard initial treatment. In addition, it may be helpful to hold a hair dryer at arm's length and gently blow warm air toward the eyes for 5–10 minutes every morning to dehydrate the cornea. If the intraocular pressure is greater than 20 mm Hg, a reduction of pressure with antiglaucoma medications such as timolol maleate or levobunolol hydrochloride can assist in decreasing stress on the endothelium. When epithelial bullae are present, bandage contact lenses are helpful in providing symptomatic relief. Penetrating keratoplasty is usually indicated when visual acuity becomes significantly decreased or the disease becomes advanced and painful.

CORNEAL ARCUS

Subjective

Corneal arcus is an opacification of the peripheral cornea caused by deposition of cholesterol, phospholipids, and triglycerides. Often it is an age-related corneal degener-

ation, but in some cases there is concurrent hyperlipidemia. Patients with corneal arcus, especially those less than 50 years old, should be questioned about familial hyperlipidemia and cardiac disease. Corneal arcus is an asymptomatic condition because the affected area is located away from the visual axis.

Objective

Corneal arcus is located in the periphery of the cornea along the region of Descemet's membrane and stroma. The opacification varies in appearance from a faint haze that slightly obscures the underlying iris to a dense opacity through which the iris cannot be observed. Corneal arcus usually begins inferiorly and superiorly, then moves circumferentially to encompass the entire periphery. There is a small interval of clear cornea separating the arcus from the limbus.

Plan

If the patient is unaware of his or her serum cholesterol level, then an evaluation to determine the lipid profile is indicated. This evaluation is particularly important for younger patients. The majority of these patients have an abnormal lipid profile, and there is a strong correlation between corneal arcus and a high ratio of total cholesterol to high-density lipoprotein.

BAND KERATOPATHY

Subjective

Band keratopathy is a lateral corneal opacification. It may be caused by a number of factors, including chronic uveitis (especially in juvenile rheumatoid arthritis), interstitial keratitis, hypercalcemia, chronic corneal edema, glaucoma, phthisis bulbi, renal failure, and exposure to chemicals. Patients with band keratopathy may be asymptomatic or may complain of foreign body sensation. They also may be concerned about the cosmetic appearance of the cornea. Band keratopathy can lead to decreased vision, because the lesion can cover the interpalpebral zone of the cornea.

Objective

Band keratopathy is a plaque of calcium at the level of Bowman's membrane. The plaque extends laterally across the cornea in the interpalpebral zone and is separated from the limbus by clear cornea at the 3- and 9-o'clock positions. Holes are often present in the plaque, giving it a Swiss cheese appearance. Band keratopathy can cause decreased acuity ranging from 20/25 to 20/200. Intraocular pressure may vary from abnormally low if there is associated uveitis or phthisis bulbi to abnormally high if there is associated long-standing glaucoma.

Plan

Treatment depends on the severity of the condition. If the band keratopathy is mild, vision is not reduced, and there is only mild foreign body sensation, then artificial tears may be the only treatment necessary. For more severe manifestations, the calcium must be removed to decrease irritation and improve vision and cosmetic appearance. The traditional treatment consists of debriding the epithelium and then swabbing the area of band keratopathy with 3% ethylenediaminetetraacetic acid until the calcified area clears. After the treatment, application of a cycloplegic agent such as 5% homatropine and a prophylactic antibiotic ointment such as bacitracin–polymyxin B sulfate, followed by pressure patching for 24 hours, is necessary for proper re-epithelialization. An oral analgesic agent may be helpful for relief of symptoms. Surgical removal can be repeated if the band keratopathy recurs. More recently, excimer laser phototherapeutic keratectomy has proved effective in removing band keratopathy.

LIMBAL GIRDLE OF VOGT

Subjective

Limbal girdle of Vogt is a common age-related degeneration that may be caused by chronic exposure to sunlight.

Patients with this condition are usually asymptomatic. In rare cases, however, patients may complain of irritation and foreign body sensation. Generally, there is no history of ocular or systemic disease associated with this condition.

Objective

Limbal girdle of Vogt is a subepithelial lesion located in the interpalpebral zone adjacent to the limbus. This thin, crescent-shaped lesion has a whitish, chalky appearance. Occasionally, the lesion may be elevated and thus cause irritation when the lids move over the lesion. Because the lesion involves only the peripheral cornea, there is no interference with vision.

Plan

No treatment is necessary for limbal girdle of Vogt. If irritation exists, artificial lubricants can be recommended for symptomatic relief. In rare severe cases of irritation or cosmetic concern, surgical removal can be considered.

SUGGESTED READING

Arffa RC, Grayson M. Grayson's Diseases of the Cornea (4th ed). St. Louis: Mosby–Year Book, 1997.

Classé JG (ed). Corneal Disease Update. Norwalk, CT: Appleton & Lange, 1995.

Duane TD, Jaeger EA. Clinical Ophthalmology. Philadelphia: Lippincott, 1996.

Silbert JA. Anterior Segment Complications of Contact Lens Wear. New York: Churchill Livingstone, 1994.

Smolin G, Thoft RA. The Cornea: Scientific Foundations and Clinical Practice. Boston: Little, Brown, 1994.

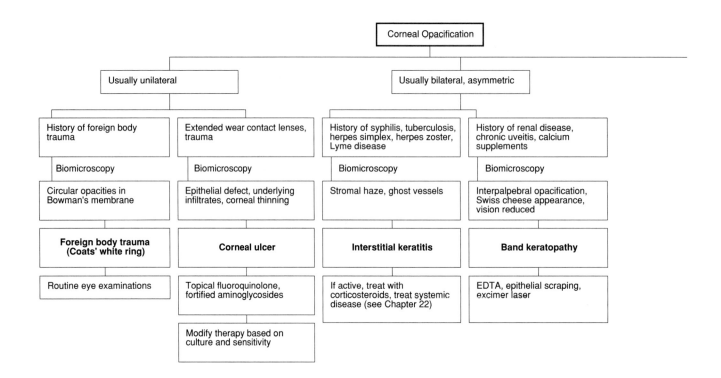

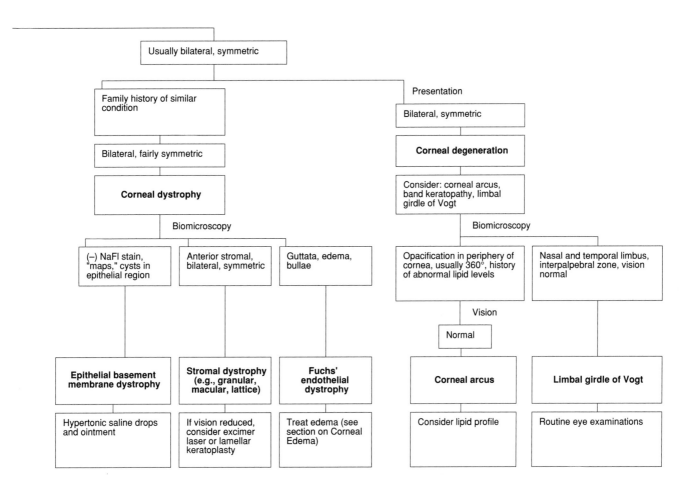

26

Corneal Thinning

JOHN H. NISHIMOTO

CORNEAL THINNING AT A GLANCE

Keratoconus
Terrien's marginal degeneration
Mooren's ulcer
Pellucid marginal degeneration
Dellen
Keratoglobus
Corneal ulcer
Senile furrows
Traumatic injury
Congenital glaucoma
Staphylococcal hypersensitivity
Collagen-vascular disease
    Rheumatoid arthritis
    Systemic lupus erythematosus
    Scleroderma
    Polyarteritis nodosa
    Relapsing polychondritis
    Wegener's granuloma
Neurotrophic keratopathy
Vernal keratoconjunctivitis
Rosacea
Inflammatory bowel disease
Idiopathic

This chapter reviews some of the disorders that cause the cornea to be of less than average thickness. Thinning may be due to degenerative conditions, inflammatory disease, or desiccation, or may be idiopathic.

KERATOCONUS

Subjective

Keratoconus is a progressive steepening of the curvature of areas of the cornea. The condition usually becomes apparent around puberty. In some cases, keratoconus is associated with Down syndrome, contact lens wear, chronic allergies, or hard eye rubbing. Patients with keratoconus usually experience a gradual decrease in vision that may not be correctable with spectacles. In advanced cases, ruptures in Descemet's membrane can occur suddenly, and an acute decrease in vision is caused by the ensuing edema.

Objective

Keratoconus is usually bilateral but may be asymmetric. Early keratoconus can be difficult to diagnose; however, corneal topographic analysis is useful in the detection of corneal irregularity in the early stages of keratoconus before slit-lamp findings are evident.

Slit-lamp findings include reduced corneal thickness at the apex of the lesion. Viewed with an optic section, the cone appears to be approximately one-half normal corneal thickness. Vertical Vogt's striae may be noted in the posterior cornea, and the visibility of corneal nerves also may be increased. At the base of the cone, there may be a ring of iron pigment (Fleischer's ring). Another useful procedure is to have the patient look down as the upper lids are raised. The lower lid conforms to the cone and is displaced in a distinctive cone shape (Munson's sign). In later stages the cone can become scarred, and corneal sensation is sometimes reduced.

Due to the corneal steepening and irregularity, keratometry mires may be distorted. An increase in myopia and irregular astigmatism frequently are noted. Examination using Placido's disk and computerized corneal topographic analysis typically shows increased inferior or central steepening and irregular rings. In addition, a "scissors" reflex on retinoscopy and distorted reflex on ophthalmoscopy may be observed.

Plan

Patients with keratoconus should wear corrective spectacles as long as these are helpful. However, in many cases rigid contact lenses are used, especially when vision can no longer be corrected adequately with spectacles. There is evidence that the condition may be aggravated when contact lenses are fitted.

If the patient cannot tolerate contact lens wear or if vision cannot be adequately corrected by refractive means, penetrating keratoplasty is recommended. The visual prognosis after this procedure is generally quite favorable.

TERRIEN'S MARGINAL DEGENERATION

Subjective

Terrien's marginal degeneration is more common in males than in females and can occur at any age. It is often bilateral but may be asymmetric. In many cases of Terrien's marginal degeneration, the patient has decreased vision. This decrease in vision is due to thinning of the superior or inferior cornea, which causes corneal steepening 90 degrees away from the midpoint of the thinned area. Some patients with this condition experience episodic inflammation that can be quite painful.

Objective

Corneal topographic analysis is very helpful in diagnosing Terrien's marginal degeneration. Topographic analysis reveals flattening over the areas of thinning. Refraction typically reveals against-the-rule astigmatism or oblique astigmatism. When the cornea is viewed with a biomicroscope in the early stages of the disease, fine, white, peripheral subepithelial opacities are present; the limbus appears normal and intact. The opacities eventually coalesce, and this coalescence leads to corneal guttering that progresses circumferentially. There is a thin lucid zone adjacent to the limbus. In most cases, the overlying epithelium remains intact, but it is susceptible to perforation, even from mild trauma. Often the eye remains white and quiet. In some young patients, however, inflammation can cause necrosis and neovascularization of the peripheral cornea with associated episcleritis or scleritis.

Plan

Because slight trauma can lead to perforation of the thinned cornea, protective eyewear should be prescribed. Routine observation may be the only management. If thinning becomes extreme, a full-thickness or lamellar corneoscleral graft may be necessary to reinforce this area.

MOOREN'S ULCER

Subjective

Mooren's ulcer is a progressive serpiginous ulceration of the peripheral cornea. It is unilateral approximately 70% of the time. Generally the condition is found in older adults and affects both sexes equally; however, one form of this condition is more common among young African-American males. Patients with Mooren's ulcer often experience severe pain, photophobia, and excessive lacrimation. There can be vision loss due to corneal scarring or irregular astigmatism induced by peripheral corneal thinning.

Objective

Mooren's ulcer usually begins in the periphery of the cornea. In most cases this process begins as a narrow gray zone of infiltration near the limbus, which breaks down to form the marginal ulceration within a few weeks. Unlike in Terrien's degeneration, the involvement extends to the limbus. Conjunctival and episcleral tissue adjacent to the ulcer are edematous and hyperemic. The degeneration may progress circumferentially or centrally and eventually may involve the entire cornea. The thinned area may have associated vascularization and opacification. Complications include anterior uveitis, glaucoma, and cataract formation.

Plan

The initial treatment of Mooren's ulcer typically is the application of a topical cycloplegic agent and therapeutic soft contact lens for symptomatic relief. Topical corticosteroids such as 1% prednisolone acetate can be used to suppress secondary uveitis. In severe cases, immunosuppressants such as cyclophosphamide and methotrexate can be of benefit. If topical therapeutic management cannot control the progression of the lesion, surgical excision or cryotherapy of the perilimbal conjunctiva may be necessary. Lamellar keratoplasty and conjunctival flap surgery are other forms of treatment that have been beneficial in some cases.

PELLUCID MARGINAL DEGENERATION

Subjective

Pellucid marginal degeneration is a bilateral, slowly progressive condition that causes thinning of the inferior peripheral cornea. It occurs most commonly in young and middle-aged adults. Typically, patients with this condition do not experience pain but notice a slow, progressive decrease in vision.

Objective

On slit-lamp examination, the inferior peripheral cornea shows thinning between the 4- and 8-o'clock positions, and there is an area of corneal protrusion above the thinned area. The result is inferior corneal steepening and an increase in against-the-rule astigmatism. There is no inflammation, infection, or anterior chamber reaction, and the corneal epithelium remains intact. Unlike in keratoconus, there is no Fleischer's ring or cone formation.

Plan

Because the cornea has thinned, the risk of perforation secondary to trauma is increased. Thus, the patient should use protective eyewear, especially during vigorous physical activity. The treatment for pellucid marginal degeneration is similar to that for keratoconus. Spectacles are prescribed initially in mild cases, and rigid gas-permeable contact lenses are prescribed in more advanced cases. Lamellar keratoplasty may be indicated in severe cases; however, the prognosis is not as favorable as it is in keratoconus.

DELLEN

Subjective

Dellen are small depressions in the peripheral cornea caused by desiccation. The desiccation leads to a shrinkage of the stroma. Patients with dellen may complain of dry eye, irritation, photophobia, or foreign body sensation. Because the lesion is located in the peripheral cornea, vision is usually not affected.

Objective

In many cases, the dellen are produced by an adjacent elevated structure that causes lid vaulting and reduced tear distribution over that area of the cornea. This tear reduction results in a focal area of desiccation. Common causes include pinguecula, pterygium, edematous limbal tissue (such as after muscle, glaucoma, or cataract surgery), and lagophthalmos. Sodium fluorescein staining may show pooling if only the stroma is affected, but positive staining may occur if the epithelial cells become disrupted. Dellen are usually transient and typically last only 24–48 hours; however, if they are chronic, they can lead to scarring.

Plan

The goal for therapy is to lubricate the desiccated areas. This lubrication can help hydrate the cornea and subsequently allow the area to return to its original thickness. Artificial tears are helpful in providing lubrication during the daytime. Patching with an application of bland ointment for 24 hours and then every night has also been successful. Removing the adjacent elevation that is causing the dellen (e.g., pinguecula, pterygium) is probably the most effective way to eliminate the area of dryness. The cornea usually returns to its normal size within 1 week after the elevation is removed.

SUGGESTED READING

Arffa RC, Grayson M. Grayson's Diseases of the Cornea (4th ed). St. Louis: Mosby–Year Book, 1997.

Bartlett JD, Jaanus SD. Clinical Ocular Pharmacology (3rd ed). Boston: Butterworth–Heinemann, 1995.

Catania LJ. Primary Care of the Anterior Segment (2nd ed). Norwalk, CT: Appleton & Lange, 1995.

Cullom RD, Chang B. The Wills Eye Manual. Office and Emergency Room Diagnosis and Treatment of Eye Disease (2nd ed). Philadelphia: Lippincott, 1994.

Gills JP, Sanders DR, Thornton SP, et al. Corneal Topography: The State of the Art. New York: Slack Inc., 1995.

Smolin G, Thoft RA. The Cornea: Scientific Foundations and Clinical Practice. Boston: Little, Brown, 1994.

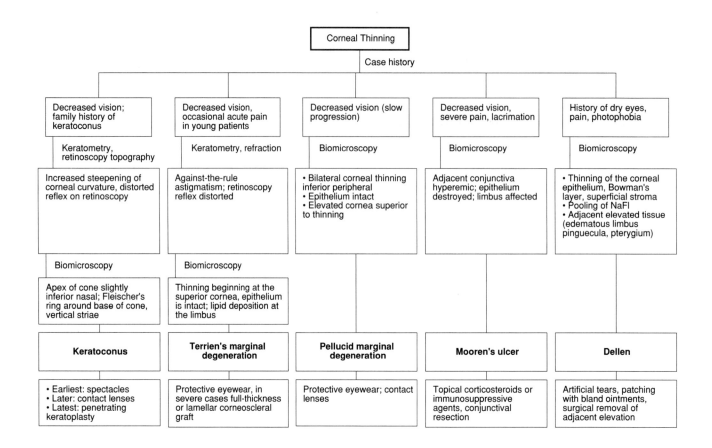

27

Anomalies of Corneal Size and Curvature

JOHN H. NISHIMOTO

ANOMALIES OF CORNEAL SIZE AND CURVATURE AT A GLANCE

Congenital glaucoma
Keratoconus
Megalocornea
Microcornea
Microphthalmos
Nanophthalmos
Keratoglobus
Pellucid marginal degeneration

Anomalies of corneal size and curvature may suggest the presence of associated ocular and systemic conditions. This section discusses some of the more common causes of anomalies of corneal size and shape. Because many of these conditions have a hereditary component, pedigree analysis can provide useful information, and genetic counseling may be indicated.

CONGENITAL GLAUCOMA

Subjective

Patients with congenital glaucoma usually present to the eye care practitioner at a young age. Symptoms include light sensitivity, blepharospasm, excessive lacrimation, and eye rubbing. The parent also may express concern over the cosmetic appearance of the eye. If congenital glaucoma is suspected, it is important to ask the parents about a history of conditions such as aniridia, Rieger's anomaly, and Marfan syndrome.

Objective

The enlargement of the cornea associated with congenital glaucoma is termed *buphthalmos*. The clinician should measure the diameter of the cornea, especially in the horizontal meridian. The average diameter for a normal infant is 10 mm. A diameter of greater than 12 mm in an infant or an asymmetry between the eyes exceeding 1.5 mm is suggestive of congenital glaucoma. The anterior segment examination may have to be performed with a penlight, loupe, or handheld slit lamp rather than by standard means. The affected cornea typically appears hazy, and ruptures in Descemet's membrane may be visible. If possible, the anterior chamber angle should be evaluated with gonioscopy to look for membranes and structural abnormalities that inhibit aqueous outflow. Tonometry provides additional useful information. Intraocular pressures greater than 18 mm Hg suggest glaucoma in an infant. The elevated intraocular pressure can cause an increase in axial length measurable with A-scan ultrasonography. On ophthalmoscopy, a cup-to-disc ratio of greater than 0.3 or cupping asymmetry also is suggestive of congenital glaucoma.

Plan

Due to the delay in diagnosis and initiation of medical therapy that frequently occurs in congenital glaucoma as well as the poor response to medical therapy, surgical management is often necessary. Goniotomy and trabeculotomy procedures can provide adequate control of intraocular pressure; in most instances, however, the most effective treatment is a combination of surgery and antiglaucoma medications. Even with aggressive treatment, some cases of congenital glaucoma continue to progress. If intraocular pressure is not controlled, damage to the cornea results in irregular astigmatism, and damage to the nerve fiber layer results in visual field loss.

MICROCORNEA

Subjective

Microcornea can be one manifestation of a number of syndromes, including Ehlers-Danlos, Rieger's, Axenfeld's, Weill-Marchesani, and Laurence-Moon-Biedl. Ocular symptoms vary, but if angle-closure (narrow-angle) glaucoma is present, the patient may experience pain, photophobia, headache, and reduced vision. Associated systemic symptoms may include deafness and mental retardation.

Objective

In cases of microcornea, the corneal diameter is typically less than 10 mm. Other commonly associated anterior segment findings include cataract and posterior embryotoxon (a prominent Schwalbe's line). Prominent iris processes and narrowed chamber angle are best viewed with gonioscopy. Other ocular findings such as sclerocornea, coloboma, aniridia, lenticonus, lens subluxation, or macular hypoplasia may be present when other hereditary anomalies are found in association with microcornea.

Plan

If glaucoma is present, the intraocular pressure must be lowered. Beta blockers and carbonic anhydrase inhibitors are the most effective medical agents. The lens should be monitored for subluxation, and, if lens opacification causes decreased vision, cataract extraction should be considered. Genetic counseling is important because conditions associated with microcornea often show an autosomal dominant mode of inheritance. In cases with an associated aniridia, a complete physical examination should be performed by a pediatrician or family practitioner to assess blood pressure and rule out Wilms' tumor.

MEGALOCORNEA

Subjective

Megalocornea is more common in males than in females. Approximately 90% of cases are bilateral. Megalocornea may be an isolated finding or one component of a disorder such as Down, Marfan, or Rieger's syndrome. Most patients

with isolated megalocornea are asymptomatic; however, if the condition is associated with congenital glaucoma or a systemic syndrome, related symptoms may be present.

Objective

To be diagnosed as megalocornea, the cornea should be greater than 14 mm in diameter in an infant. The cornea may be clear, or it may be hazy due to epithelial and stromal edema. As in microcornea, cataract is frequently an associated finding. The cataracts may be located throughout the lens and can be quite variable in density. Ectopia lentis may occur later in life. Other associated anterior segment findings include aniridia, anisocoria, and an anteriorly displaced Schwalbe's line. Refraction often reveals a high refractive error, particularly myopia or astigmatism. Tonometry should be performed to rule out elevated intraocular pressure.

Plan

The patient with megalocornea should be referred to a pediatrician to rule out associated systemic syndromes. Genetic counseling also may be in order. Significant cataracts should be removed, and refractive errors should be corrected as soon as possible to prevent amblyopia. Because the intraocular pressure can become elevated at any time, it should be monitored closely (every 3–6 months when patients are under the age of 6, then annually thereafter). If glaucoma develops, beta blockers and carbonic anhydrase inhibitors are more effective than miotics in maintaining pressure control. In addition, the patient should be monitored for the development of ectopia lentis.

CORNEA PLANA

Subjective

Cornea plana is an abnormal flattening of the corneal curvature caused by a reduction in development of ocular tissues during the fourth month of gestation. Associated systemic conditions include osteogenesis imperfecta and Hurler's syndrome. Patients with cornea plana often have reduced vision. Because the anterior chamber is shallow in this condition, the patient is at risk for developing angle-closure glaucoma. If this condition occurs, the patient may experience pain, photophobia, steamy vision, headache, or nausea.

Objective

The corneal curvature in cornea plana is usually 30–35 D. If the curvature of the cornea appears to be the same as that of the sclera, cornea plana is suggested. The limbus appears indistinct, and the sclera seems to protrude from the cornea. There may be central corneal opacities in the recessive form of this disorder. Other ocular conditions that may be associated with cornea plana include hyperopia, cataract, and aniridia.

Plan

The management of cornea plana is similar to that of megalocornea and microcornea. Correcting the refractive error is important to improve vision and prevent amblyopia. Cataract extraction or penetrating keratoplasty may be indicated if significant media opacification reduces vision. If glaucoma is present, medical therapy including beta blockers and carbonic anhydrase inhibitors should be used initially to reduce intraocular pressure; surgical intervention should follow. Referral for evaluation for associated systemic syndromes and for genetic counseling also may be indicated.

KERATOCONUS

Subjective

Keratoconus is a focal steepening of the cornea that usually manifests around adolescence. The patient may have a history of contact lens wear, chronic allergies, or frequent eye rubbing. Keratoconus can also be found in Down syndrome. Patients with keratoconus usually experience a progressive decrease in vision that eventually cannot be corrected with spectacles. In some cases, corneal sensation is reduced. In advanced cases, Descemet's membrane can rupture; such rupturing causes acute corneal edema, termed *hydrops*. The patient with hydrops may experience irritation, pain, photophobia, increased lacrimation, and a sudden decrease in vision.

Objective

Keratoconus is usually bilateral but may be asymmetric. Early keratoconus can be difficult to diagnose; however, corneal topographic analysis is useful for detecting corneal irregularity in the early stages of keratoconus before slit-lamp findings are evident.

Slit-lamp findings include reduced corneal thickness at the apex of the lesion. Viewed with an optic section, the cone appears to be approximately one-half normal corneal thickness. Vertical Vogt's striae may be noted in the posterior cornea, and the visibility of corneal nerves also may be increased. At the base of the cone, there may be a ring of iron pigment (Fleischer's ring). Another useful procedure is to have the patient look down as the upper lids are raised. The lower lid conforms to the cone and is displaced in a distinctive cone shape (Munson's sign). In later stages, the cone can become scarred, and corneal sensation is sometimes reduced.

Due to the corneal steepening and irregularity, keratometry mires may be distorted. An increase in myopia and irregular astigmatism frequently are noted. Examination using Placido's disk and computerized corneal topographic analysis typically shows increased inferior or central steepening and irregular rings. In addition, a "scissors" reflex on retinoscopy and distorted reflex on ophthalmoscopy may be observed.

Plan

Patients with keratoconus should wear corrective spectacles as long as these are helpful. However, in many cases rigid contact lenses are used, especially when vision can no longer be corrected adequately with spectacles. There is evidence that the condition may be aggravated when contact lenses are fitted.

If the patient cannot tolerate contact lens wear or if vision cannot be adequately corrected by refractive means, penetrating keratoplasty is recommended. The visual prognosis after this procedure is generally quite favorable.

SUGGESTED READING

Arffa RC, Grayson M. Grayson's Diseases of the Cornea (3rd ed). St. Louis: Mosby–Year Book, 1991.

Bartlett JD, Jaanus SD. Clinical Ocular Pharmacology (3rd ed). Boston: Butterworth–Heinemann, 1995.

Cullom RD, Chang B. The Wills Eye Manual: Office and Emergency Room Diagnosis and Treatment of Eye Disease (2nd ed). Philadelphia: Lippincott, 1994.

Roy FH. Ocular Differential Diagnosis (5th ed). Philadelphia: Lea & Febiger, 1993.

Roy FH, Fraunfelder FI. Current Ocular Therapy 4. Philadelphia: Saunders, 1995.

Smolin G, Thoft RA. The Cornea: Scientific Foundations and Clinical Practice. Boston: Little, Brown, 1994.

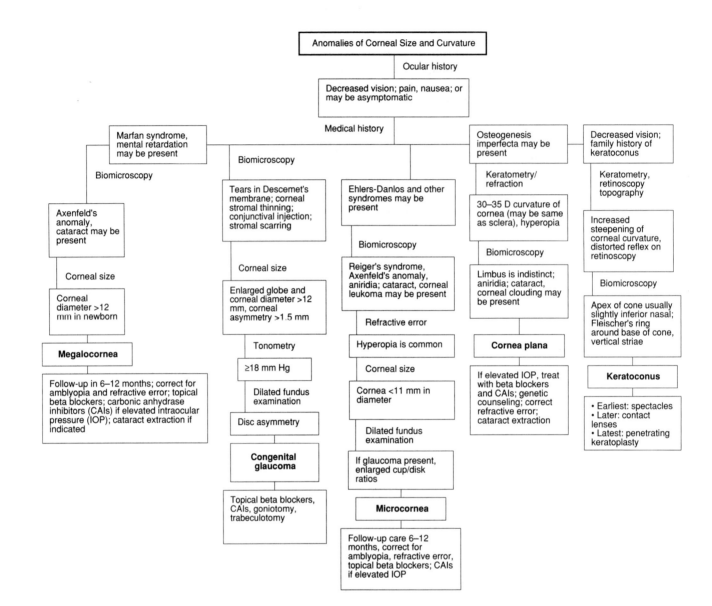

28

Lacrimal System Disorders

CARL H. SPEAR AND DAVID K. TALLEY

LACRIMAL SYSTEM DISORDERS AT A GLANCE

Dry eye
  Collagen vascular disease
  Sjögren's syndrome
  Medication-induced desiccation
  Filamentary keratitis
  Lid abnormalities
    Ectropion
    Entropion
    Lagophthalmos
  Corneal or conjunctival disorders
    Dellen
    Poor surface for tear layer
  Environmental desiccation
  Vitamin A deficiency
  Pemphigoid
  Chemical and thermal burns
Wet eye
  Punctal stenosis
  Nasolacrimal duct obstruction
    Congenital
    Acquired
  Lid abnormalities
    Ectropion
    Entropion
  Allergies
  Viral conjunctivitis
  Trauma
  Corneal defects of any etiology
  Reflex tearing due to dry eye (from any cause)

Patients with dry eye often have vague complaints that may be overlooked. They usually present complaining of a foreign body sensation and burning eyes. However, other complaints such as itching or irritated eyes and even blurred vision may also be due to ocular surface disease. The astute clinician should also keep in mind that patients with dry eye may complain of watery eyes due to reflex tearing that occurs when the corneal epithelium becomes disrupted. Many of these patients have an associated systemic disorder such as a collagen vascular disease or Sjögren's syndrome. A careful case history should also be taken to discover whether the patient is using medications that may exacerbate dry eye. Objective findings include a decreased tear meniscus (< 1 mm), superficial punctate keratitis, staining with rose bengal, and a decreased Schirmer's or phenol red thread tear test. Treatment is based on the severity of the disorder and may range from application of artificial tears to punctal occlusion to tarsorrhaphy. Whatever the treatment modality, it is essential to educate the patient that dry eye is a chronic condition that requires judicious treatment to alleviate the symptoms.

DRY-EYE SYNDROME

Subjective

Patients with dry-eye syndrome present complaining of burning, foreign body sensation, and possibly excess tearing (pseudoepiphora). They are generally elderly or have a history of collagen vascular disease, Sjögren's syndrome, or use of medications known to inhibit tear production.

Objective

A tear meniscus of less than 1 mm and a tear break-up time of less than 10 seconds are essential criteria for the diagnosis of dry-eye syndrome. Superficial punctate keratitis is often present, typically in the interpalpebral region. Staining with rose bengal is also a common finding.

Decreased tear production can be confirmed by Schirmer's test or phenol red thread test.

Plan

Treatment of dry-eye syndrome depends on severity. In mild cases, the patient's symptoms may be relieved with artificial tears alone. In moderate to severe cases, more frequent use of artificial tears, addition of lubricating ointments, or punctal occlusion may be required to provide satisfactory patient comfort. In extreme cases, tarsorrhaphy may be necessary. Environmental and geographic factors should also be taken into consideration. Concomitant ocular disorders such as blepharitis or lid abnormalities should be treated as indicated. Underlying systemic disorders should be comanaged with the patient's primary care physician.

NOCTURNAL LAGOPHTHALMOS

Subjective

Patients with lagophthalmos may present complaining of burning and foreign body sensation that is more severe on awakening in the morning.

Objective

Superficial punctate keratitis is present in the lower one-third of the cornea. Incomplete closure of eyelids can be noted as well.

Plan

Lid taping in conjunction with application of lubricating ointments and artificial tears is very effective at treating this condition.

FILAMENTARY KERATITIS

Subjective

Patients with filamentary keratitis may report moderate pain, foreign body sensation, and photophobia. They often have a history of dry-eye syndrome.

Objective

Slit-lamp examination reveals small mucous strands attached to the cornea that stain with fluorescein.

Plan

Debridement of the filaments and instillation of artificial tears should be the first line of treatment. Alternative treatments include use of acetylcysteine, hypertonic solutions, and bandage contact lenses.

ECTROPION

Subjective

Patients with ectropion may present with tearing or eyelid irritation, or they may be asymptomatic.

Objective

The critical finding is an eyelid that is not in direct contact with the globe. Superficial punctate keratitis, keratinization of the lid margin, and conjunctival injection may also be present.

Plan

Use of artificial tears or lid taping may be sufficient to treat the associated keratopathy. However, surgical repair is the definitive treatment for ectropion regardless of the cause.

ENTROPION

Subjective

Patients with entropion present complaining of foreign body sensation, tearing, and eye redness.

Objective

The salient feature of entropion is an inward turning of the eyelid margin. Superficial punctate keratitis or more coalesced areas of staining and conjunctival injection may also be noted. Corneal abrasions secondary to lash contact may also be observed.

Plan

Immediate temporary treatment includes epilation of eyelashes in direct contact with the cornea, lid taping, and application of bandage contact lenses. Surgical management is the definitive therapy for entropion.

PUNCTAL STENOSIS

Subjective

Patients with punctal stenosis present complaining of excessive tearing and irritated ocular adnexa.

Objective

Slit-lamp examination reveals an occluded punctum. A Jones' No. 2 test can be used to diagnose this condition.

Plan

A Bowman's probe may be used to open the punctum. In some cases, more extensive surgical intervention may be required.

NASOLACRIMAL DUCT OBSTRUCTION (CONGENITAL)

Subjective

Newborns or infants with nasolacrimal duct obstruction present with excessive tearing, mattering, and a chronic low-grade discharge.

Objective

Watery eyes are a typical finding in these patients, and reflux of a mucopurulent discharge from the punctum is also frequently observed. The patient may also have a concomitant dacryocystitis or bacterial conjunctivitis.

Plan

For patients younger than 1 year, conservative therapy with digital massage and application of erythromycin ointment is the treatment of choice. Surgical probing may be performed after age 1 if the obstruction does not resolve spontaneously.

SUGGESTED READING

Bartlett JD, Jaanus SD. Clinical Ocular Pharmacology (3rd ed). Boston: Butterworth–Heinemann, 1995.

Catania LJ. Primary Care of the Anterior Segment (2nd ed). Norwalk, CT: Appleton & Lange, 1995.

Fraunfelder FT, Roy FH. Current Ocular Therapy 4. Philadelphia: Saunders, 1995.

Kanski JJ. Clinical Ophthalmology (3rd ed). Oxford, UK: Butterworth–Heinemann, 1994.

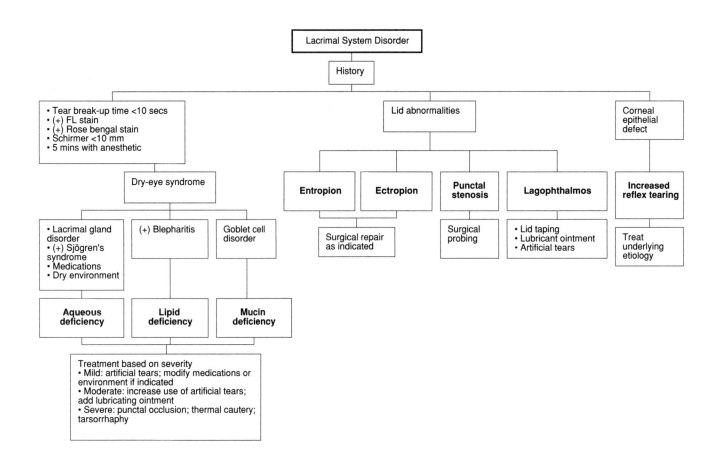

29

Lid Inflammation

DEBRA J. BEZAN

LID INFLAMMATION AT A GLANCE

Angular blepharitis
Staphylococcal marginal blepharitis
   Acute
   Chronic
Seborrheic blepharitis
Mixed staphylococcal/seborrheic blepharitis
Meibomian gland dysfunction
   Primary
   Secondary to rosacea
   Associated with seborrhea
Allergic blepharitis
   Type I
   Type IV
   Mixed hypersensitivity
Viral blepharitis
   Herpes simplex
   Herpes zoster
   Adenovirus
Hordeolum
Chalazion
Preseptal cellulitis
Canaliculitis
Orbital cellulitis
Endophthalmitis

When a patient presents complaining of swollen eyelids, the clinician should gather some pertinent information about the onset and duration of the condition, history of ocular trauma, and associated ocular symptoms such as pain, itching, or double vision. In addition, a careful history of systemic diseases, allergies, and medications should be obtained.

Gross observation and slit-lamp examination with attention to the laterality of the condition, the location and nature of the inflammation, and associated signs are other important aspects of the initial evaluation.

ANGULAR BLEPHARITIS

Subjective

Angular blepharitis is most commonly caused by *Staphylococcus* and *Moraxella* species. The patient with this condition may complain of tenderness near the lateral canthus.

Objective

Hyperemia, maceration, excoriation, and occasionally ulceration of the lateral canthus region are signs of angular blepharitis. The patient may also have an associated conjunctivitis.

Plan

Bacitracin or erythromycin ointment is usually effective for angular blepharitis caused by *Staphylococcus*. Zinc sulfate ointment is generally effective if *Moraxella* is the causative organism.

STAPHYLOCOCCAL MARGINAL BLEPHARITIS

Subjective

Staphylococcal marginal blepharitis is usually caused by *Staphylococcus aureus*, although *Staphylococcus epidermidis* is also commonly found in cultures from these patients. This condition is more common in women than in men. Patients may be asymptomatic or may complain of irritation of the lids or cornea. Staphylococcal marginal blepharitis is often a chronic condition with exacerbations and remissions.

Objective

Inflammation of the lid margins with collarette formation on the lashes is characteristic of staphylococcal marginal blepharitis. There is often an associated mild conjunctivitis and keratitis, usually involving the lower third of the cornea. Marginal corneal infiltration, phlyctenules, or hordeola are occasionally seen in association with this condition. In chronic cases tylosis (lid thickening) and madarosis (loss of cilia) may be observed.

Plan

Good lid hygiene, including application of warm compresses and lid scrubs, is the first step in managing marginal blepharitis. Applying an antibiotic ointment such as bacitracin or erythromycin or drops such as polymyxin B sulfate–trimethoprim to the lid margins is helpful in controlling the underlying staphylococcal infection.

SEBORRHEIC BLEPHARITIS

Subjective

Seborrheic blepharitis can be a separate entity or can be found in conjunction with staphylococcal blepharitis or meibomitis. It tends to affect older people and is often chronic. Patients with this condition are often asymptomatic.

Objective

Greasy scales or scurf on the lids and lashes is characteristic of seborrheic blepharitis. The patient often has associated dandruff of the brows and scalp. The lids tend to be less red and inflamed with this form of blepharitis than with staphylococcal or mixed staphylococcal/seborrheic blepharitis.

Plan

Application of warm compresses and lid scrubs are usually effective in managing seborrheic blepharitis. A selenium sulfide–based dandruff shampoo is also helpful in managing an associated seborrheic scalp condition. If the blepharitis is thought to have an infectious component, addition of an antibiotic ointment effective against *Staphylococcus* is recommended.

MEIBOMIAN GLAND DYSFUNCTION

Subjective

Inflammation associated with meibomian gland dysfunction (meibomitis) can be a primary condition or it can be secondary to rosacea. It can also be found in association with seborrheic blepharitis. Patients with this condition may complain of dry eyes or a foreign body sensation.

Objective

Domes of lipid material or "pouting" of the meibomian orifices on the lid margins is a sign of meibomitis. The lids may be slightly thickened but have minimal inflammation. The tear film is usually foamy, and patients with this condition often demonstrate a superficial punctate keratopathy secondary to the tear film abnormality.

Plan

The initial management of meibomitis consists of application of warm compresses, meibomian gland expression, and lid scrubs. Oral tetracycline or doxycycline therapy is also helpful, particularly in those patients with rosacea. It should be avoided, however, in pregnant or lactating women.

ALLERGIC BLEPHARITIS

Type I hypersensitivity reactions (anaphylactic, immediate, IgE-mediated reactions) of the eyelids include hay fever blepharitis and angioneurotic edema. Pollens, molds, and animal dander are common causes of hay fever blepharoconjunctivitis, whereas reactions to foods, ingested medications, or insect stings can cause angioneurotic edema.

Type IV hypersensitivity reactions (delayed, cell-mediated reactions) require a previous sensitizing exposure to the offending agent. Common allergens that cause contact blepharitis include poison ivy, nail polish, dyes, nickel, preservatives, and topical medications.

Mixed reactions have some characteristics of both type I and type IV reactions. Vernal and atopic conditions are examples of this type of reaction.

Subjective

Itching is the classic symptom of allergic blepharitis.

Objective

Type I hypersensitivity blepharitis is characterized by significant lid edema. The lid is more erythremic in hay fever blepharitis than in angioneurotic edema. In type IV reactions, the lid is mildly edematous and often develops scaly eruptions. In mixed reactions, the lid often has a corrugated appearance. All of these conditions are usually found in association with conjunctivitis, and the eyes often have a serous or mucoid discharge.

Plan

Type I lid reactions are initially managed with the use of cool compresses and oral antihistamines. Type IV and mixed reactions are managed with the use of cool compresses and topical corticosteroid ointments or creams for symptomatic relief. Mast cell stabilizers are helpful in preventing subsequent histamine release in type I and mixed reactions. Avoidance of the offending allergen whenever possible is the best way to prevent recurrence of any type of allergic reaction.

VIRAL BLEPHARITIS

Subjective

Viral blepharitis is usually found in association with viral keratoconjunctivitis. The most common forms of viral blepharokeratoconjunctivitis are herpes simplex, herpes zoster, and adenoviral infections. Patients with these conditions often complain of burning, tearing, and blurred vision. Patients with herpes zoster may also experience considerable pain.

Objective

Viral blepharitis causes mild lid edema and erythema. In the case of primary herpes simplex and herpes zoster, vesicular lid lesions are also present. Associated signs include conjunctivitis, punctate or dendriform epithelial keratopathy, subepithelial infiltrates, stromal keratitis, or uveitis.

Plan

Application of cool compresses helps provide symptomatic relief in viral blepharitis. Topical steroids can also be used to provide symptomatic relief in adenoviral infections. The lid lesions of herpes simplex are self-limiting and usually require no treatment. Topical antiviral agents are used to manage the epithelial keratopathy associated with herpes simplex. The lid lesions of herpes zoster are also self-limiting but may be severe enough to cause permanent scarring. The oral antivirals acyclovir, famciclovir, or valacyclovir are used to reduce the severity of herpes zoster infections, and topical capsaicin cream is occasionally used to reduce discomfort. Topical antibiotics can be used to prevent secondary infection of vesicular lesions.

ORBITAL CELLULITIS

Subjective

Orbital cellulitis is an inflammatory response that is associated with infections of the sinus, orbit, or teeth, or with orbital trauma, including surgery. Symptoms include headache, blurred vision, diplopia, fever, and pain, especially on eye movement.

Objective

Orbital cellulitis is typically a unilateral condition that is characterized by diffuse hyperemic edema of the lid. Conjunctival hyperemia and chemosis are usually present. Proptosis and restricted extraocular muscle motility are common accompanying signs.

Plan

Patients presenting with orbital cellulitis should be carefully evaluated for an underlying cause. Diagnostic tests include computed tomographic scan of the orbit and sinuses, complete blood count and differential, blood cultures, culture and Gram's staining of any discharge, and lumbar puncture if meningitis is suspected.

Initial treatment consists of broad-spectrum antibiotics such as ceftriaxone sodium plus vancomycin or nafcillin administered intravenously. After improvement is demonstrated, the patient may be switched to oral antibiotics such as amoxicillin or cefaclor until the condition resolves.

PRESEPTAL CELLULITIS

Subjective

Preseptal cellulitis is a generalized inflammatory condition involving the lid structures anterior to the orbital septum. It may be caused by traumatic injuries or infections such as nonresolving hordeola, dacryocystitis, or sinusitis. In preseptal cellulitis the lid is warm and tender to the touch, and the patient may have fever and malaise.

Objective

This unilateral condition is characterized by generalized erythema and edema of the lid, which often cause marked ptosis. The patient does not have proptosis, significant pain on eye movement, or restriction of gaze, findings that help differentiate this condition from orbital cellulitis.

Plan

Preseptal cellulitis is treated with oral antibiotics such as amoxicillin or cefaclor that are effective against *Streptococcus* and some of the common anaerobic species. In children, *Haemophilus influenzae* should always be suspected. Pediatric patients should be treated more aggressively with intravenous antibiotics such as ceftriaxone sodium and vancomycin followed by oral therapy to prevent meningitis.

HORDEOLUM

Subjective

Hordeola are acute infections involving the glands of the eyelids. Internal hordeola involve glands of Zeis and Moll, whereas external hordeola involve the meibomian glands. These lesions tend to be quite tender or painful to the touch.

Objective

Hordeola present as a focal areas of redness and swelling on the lid. They often develop a yellow point and drain spontaneously within a few days of the onset of the condition.

Plan

Application of warm compresses is often the first line of therapy for hordeola. Topical antibiotic ointments are sometimes used to prevent draining lesions from infecting surrounding tissues. Stab incision and drainage may help reduce pain and inflammation and promote the resolution of the lesion. Oral antibiotics such as doxycycline, minocycline, erythromycin, or dicloxacillin may be used to treat resistant cases.

CHALAZION

Subjective

A chalazion is a focal granuloma of a meibomian gland. It may be a sequela of chronic blepharitis or hordeolum. In contrast to an acute hordeolum, a chalazion is relatively asymptomatic.

Objective

A chalazion appears as a firm, nontender, flesh-colored lump of variable size on the lid.

Plan

Small chalazia may be treated conservatively with warm compresses. Recalcitrant small lesions (< 6 mm in diameter) may respond to intralesional injections of triamcinolone. Larger lesions often require surgical incision and curettage.

SUGGESTED READING

Bartlett JD, Jaanus SD. Clinical Ocular Pharmacology (3rd ed). Boston: Butterworth–Heinemann, 1995.

Cullom RD, Chang B. The Wills Eye Manual: Office and Emergency Room Diagnosis and Treatment of Eye Disease (2nd ed). Philadelphia: Lippincott, 1994.

Fitzpatrick TB, Johnson RA, Polano MK, et al. Color Atlas and Synopsis of Clinical Dermatology (2nd ed). New York: McGraw-Hill, 1992.

Fraunfelder FT, Roy FH. Current Ocular Therapy 4. Philadelphia: Saunders, 1995.

Roberts DK, Terry JE. Ocular Disease: Diagnosis and Treatment (2nd ed). Boston: Butterworth–Heinemann, 1996.

van Heuven WAJ, Zwaan JT. Decision Making in Ophthalmology. St. Louis: Mosby–Year Book, 1992.

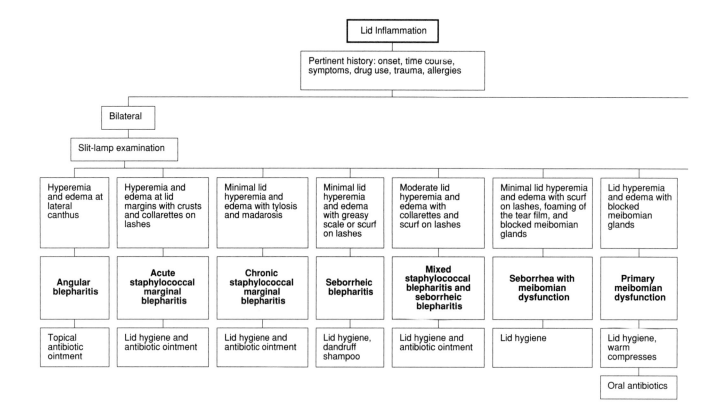

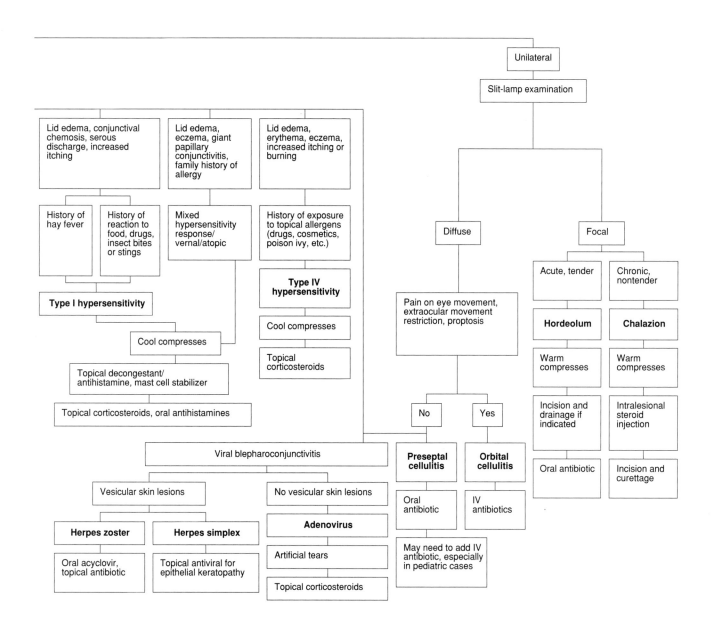

Unilateral

Slit-lamp examination

Lid edema, conjunctival chemosis, serous discharge, increased itching

Lid edema, eczema, giant papillary conjunctivitis, family history of allergy

Lid edema, erythema, eczema, increased itching or burning

History of hay fever

History of reaction to food, drugs, insect bites or stings

Mixed hypersensitivity response/ vernal/atopic

History of exposure to topical allergens (drugs, cosmetics, poison ivy, etc.)

Type I hypersensitivity

Type IV hypersensitivity

Cool compresses

Cool compresses

Topical decongestant/ antihistamine, mast cell stabilizer

Topical corticosteroids

Topical corticosteroids, oral antihistamines

Diffuse

Focal

Acute, tender

Chronic, nontender

Pain on eye movement, extraocular movement restriction, proptosis

Hordeolum

Chalazion

Warm compresses

Warm compresses

No

Yes

Incision and drainage if indicated

Intralesional steroid injection

Viral blepharoconjunctivitis

Preseptal cellulitis

Orbital cellulitis

Oral antibiotic

Incision and curettage

Vesicular skin lesions

No vesicular skin lesions

Oral antibiotic

IV antibiotics

Herpes zoster

Herpes simplex

Adenovirus

Oral acyclovir, topical antibiotic

Topical antiviral for epithelial keratopathy

Artificial tears

May need to add IV antibiotic, especially in pediatric cases

Topical corticosteroids

30

Diffuse Eyelid Swelling

Debra J. Bezan

DIFFUSE EYELID SWELLING AT A GLANCE

Preseptal cellulitis
Dacryoadenitis
Canaliculitis
Insect bite or bee sting
Bacterial blepharitis
Viral blepharitis
Allergic blepharitis
Orbital cellulitis
Traumatic lid edema
Infectious endophthalmitis
Cavernous sinus fistula
Blepharochalasis
Orbital fat herniation
Neoplasm
   Hemangioma
   Neurofibroma
   Dermoid
   Lymphoma
   Leukemia
   Rhabdomyosarcoma
Orbital pseudotumor
Cardiac disease
Renal disease
Hypothyroidism
Pregnancy

When a patient presents with eyelid swelling, the clinician is usually able to note immediately with gross observation whether the condition is unilateral or bilateral. Pertinent history questions include the following: When did the condition begin? Was the onset gradual or sudden? Is it associated with any symptoms such as itching or pain? Have you had any recent ocular injuries or surgery? Do you have any systemic illnesses? Do you have any allergies? Are you taking any medications? Slit-lamp examination can also reveal signs associated with eyelid edema to aid in the differential diagnosis.

ORBITAL CELLULITIS

Subjective

Orbital cellulitis is an inflammatory response that is associated with infections of the sinus, orbit, or teeth, or with orbital trauma, including surgery. Symptoms include headache, blurred vision, diplopia, fever, and pain, especially on eye movement.

Objective

Orbital cellulitis is characterized by diffuse hyperemic edema of the lid. Conjunctival hyperemia and chemosis are usually present. Proptosis and restricted extraocular muscle motility are common accompanying signs.

Plan

Patients presenting with orbital cellulitis should be carefully evaluated for an underlying cause. Diagnostic tests include computed tomographic (CT) scan of the orbit and sinuses, complete blood count and differential, blood cultures, culture and Gram's stain of any discharge, and lumbar puncture if meningitis is suspected.

Initial treatment consists of broad-spectrum antibiotics such as ceftriaxone sodium, vancomycin, or nafcillin administered intravenously. After improvement is demonstrated, the therapy may be switched to oral antibiotics such as amoxicillin or cefaclor until the condition resolves.

PRESEPTAL CELLULITIS

Subjective

Preseptal cellulitis is a generalized inflammatory condition involving the lid structures anterior to the orbital septum. It may be caused by traumatic injuries or infections such as nonresolving hordeola, dacryocystitis, or sinusitis. In preseptal cellulitis the lid is warm and tender to the touch. The patient also may complain of fever and malaise.

Objective

This unilateral condition is characterized by generalized erythema and edema of the lid, which often cause marked ptosis. The patient does not have proptosis, significant pain on eye movement, or restriction of gaze, findings that help differentiate this condition from orbital cellulitis.

Plan

Preseptal cellulitis is treated with oral antibiotics such as amoxicillin or cefaclor that are effective against *Streptococcus* and some of the common anaerobic species. In young children, *Haemophilus influenzae* should always be suspected. Pediatric patients should be treated more aggressively with intravenous antibiotics such as ceftriaxone sodium and vancomycin followed by oral therapy to prevent meningitis.

DACRYOADENITIS

Subjective

Dacryoadenitis is an inflammation of the lacrimal gland secondary to bacterial or viral infection. It is most commonly found in children and young adults. Symptoms include fever and tenderness or pain on the affected side.

Objective

Dacryoadenitis is characterized by hyperemia and edema of the lateral third of the superior lid. Other signs include tearing, conjunctival chemosis, and preauricular lymphadenopathy.

Plan

Patients with dacryoadenitis should be evaluated thoroughly to determine the underlying cause. The treatment for bacterial dacryoadenitis usually consists of administering an oral broad-spectrum antibiotic such as amoxicillin or cephalexin. Intravenous antibiotics may be indicated in severe cases. Use of cool compresses and analgesics is helpful supportive therapy for patients with dacryoadenitis secondary to viral infections such as mumps, influenza, or infectious mononucleosis.

CANALICULITIS

Subjective

Canaliculitis is an inflammatory condition of the canaliculus most often caused by bacterial, fungal, or viral infection. It is occasionally associated with allergy. Patients with this condition usually complain of tenderness or pain in the nasal portion of the lid.

Objective

Hyperemia and edema of the nasal lid and a "pouting" punctum are characteristic signs of canaliculitis. Finger pressure can be applied beneath the punctum to express mucopurulent discharge or concretions. Chronic conjunctivitis is a common associated condition.

Plan

Any material expressed from the punctum should be prepared for smears and cultures. Treatment consists of removing any obstructing concretions and irrigating with antibiotic solution. Oral antibiotics are needed in some cases. Application of warm compresses also helps the condition resolve. In severe cases surgery may be indicated.

INSECT BITE OR BEE STING

Subjective

Insect bites or bee stings can cause an acute unilateral inflammatory reaction of the lid. Symptoms include itching, burning, or pain.

Objective

In these cases the lid appears edematous and hyperemic.

Plan

Treatment of bee sting consists of gently scraping off the stinger, if present. Use of cool compresses, oral antihistamines, and analgesics can provide symptomatic relief.

Susceptible patients should be monitored closely for anaphylactic reactions.

BACTERIAL BLEPHARITIS

Subjective

Bacterial blepharitis can be either unilateral or bilateral, acute or chronic. It is most commonly caused by *Staphylococcus aureus* or *Staphylococcus epidermidis*. Symptoms of this condition include burning, foreign body sensation, itching, and sticky mattering of the lids, particularly in the morning.

Objective

Acute staphylococcal blepharitis is characterized by mild edema and hyperemia of the lid margins, crusty scales on the lids and lashes, and minimal mucopurulent discharge. The inferior cornea often shows superficial punctate keratopathy from the release of bacterial exotoxins. Lost of cilia (madarosis) and thickening of the lid margins (tylosis) are more commonly associated with chronic staphylococcal blepharitis.

Plan

The management of staphylococcal blepharitis includes lid scrubs and application of topical antibiotic ointments. A steroid-antibiotic combination may be helpful if there is a significant inflammatory component. It can also facilitate effective lid hygiene by reducing tenderness.

VIRAL BLEPHARITIS

Subjective

Viral blepharitis is usually found in association with viral keratoconjunctivitis. The most common forms of viral blepharokeratoconjunctivitis are herpes simplex, herpes zoster, and adenoviral infections. Patients with this condition often complain of burning, tearing, and blurred vision.

Objective

Viral blepharitis causes mild lid edema and erythema. In the case of primary herpes simplex and herpes zoster, vesicular lid lesions are also present. Associated symptoms include conjunctivitis, punctate or dendriform epithelial keratopathy, subepithelial infiltrates, or stromal keratitis, depending on the infectious agent.

Plan

Application of cool compresses helps provide symptomatic relief in viral blepharitis. Topical antiviral agents are most commonly used to manage the epithelial keratopathy associated with herpes simplex, whereas oral antivirals are used more commonly to manage herpes zoster. Topical lubricants or steroids can provide symptomatic relief in adenoviral infections.

ALLERGIC BLEPHARITIS

Type I hypersensitivity reactions (anaphylactic, immediate, IgE-mediated reactions) of the eyelid include hay fever blepharitis and angioneurotic edema. Pollens, molds, and animal dander are common causes of hay fever blepharoconjunctivitis, while reactions to foods, ingested medications, or insect stings can cause angioneurotic edema.

Type IV hypersensitivity reactions (delayed, cell-mediated reactions) require a previous sensitizing exposure to the offending agent. Common allergens that cause contact blepharitis include poison ivy, nail polish, dyes, nickel, preservatives, and topical medications.

Mixed reactions have some characteristics of both type I and type IV reactions. Vernal and atopic conditions are examples of this type of reaction.

Subjective

Itching is the classic symptom of allergic blepharitis. Some patients may experience a burning sensation.

Objective

Type I hypersensitivity blepharitis is usually bilateral and characterized by significant lid edema. The lid is more erythremic in hay fever blepharitis than in angioneurotic edema. In type IV reactions, the lid is mildly edematous and often develops scaly eruptions. In mixed reactions, the lid often has a corrugated appearance. All of these conditions are often found in association with conjunctivitis, and the eyes frequently exhibit a serous or mucoid discharge.

Plan

Type I lid reactions are initially managed with the use of cool compresses and oral antihistamines. Type IV and mixed reactions are initially managed with the use of cool compresses and topical corticosteroid ointments or creams for symptomatic relief. Mast cell stabilizers are helpful in preventing subsequent histamine release in type I and mixed reactions. Avoidance of the offending allergen whenever possible is the best therapy to prevent recurrence of any type of allergic reaction.

TRAUMATIC BLEPHARITIS

Subjective

Lid edema can be caused by many forms of trauma, including blunt and sharp trauma. UV radiation and chemical and thermal burns can also cause lid edema. The symptoms associated with traumatic lid injuries range from mild discomfort to severe pain.

Objective

Blunt trauma causes lid edema, hyperemia, and often ecchymosis. Depending on the nature of the injury, radiologic evaluation may be indicated to rule out orbital fracture, and the chamber angle and posterior segment should be examined for evidence of damage. The edema associated with sharp trauma is usually centered around a puncture or laceration site. Overexposure to UV radiation causes diffuse edema and hyperemia. Chemical and thermal burns, in contrast, usually have focal areas of tissue damage that later necrose and may lead to scar formation.

Plan

Application of cool compresses provides some symptomatic relief in cases of traumatic injury to the lid. Antibiotic therapy is indicated any time the epithelium is disrupted. Lacerations usually need surgical repair. Lids with chemical injuries should be thoroughly irrigated before initiating other forms of therapy.

INFECTIOUS ENDOPHTHALMITIS

Subjective

Infectious endophthalmitis may be induced by trauma and is one of the most serious complications of intraocular surgery. Symptoms range from mild to severe eye pain and blurred vision.

Objective

The presence of lid edema is one sign used to help differentiate infectious endophthalmitis from other forms of postoperative uveitis. Infectious endophthalmitis is usually found in association with corneal edema, conjunctival chemosis, and the presence of inflammatory debris in the anterior chamber and vitreous. Culture of vitreous aspirate can be used to confirm the diagnosis.

Plan

Aggressive therapy with antibiotics administered topically, subconjunctivally, orally, intravenously, or intravitreously is used to treat the underlying infection in this type of endophthalmitis. Agents used include gentamicin, tobramycin, clindamycin, vancomycin, cefazolin sodium, and ceftriaxone sodium. In addition, cycloplegic agents and corticosteroids are used to manage the inflammatory component.

CAVERNOUS SINUS FISTULA

Subjective

Carotid cavernous fistulas or cavernous sinus arteriovenous malformations can form spontaneously or can be the result of trauma. Patients may complain of audible bruits or diplopia. They may report vision loss if the optic nerve is involved.

Objective

In addition to edema and hyperemia of the lid, common anterior segment manifestations include proptosis, arterialized conjunctival vessels, extraocular muscle palsies, iritis, iris atrophy, and ischemia. Posterior segment signs include retinal hemorrhages, macular edema, and papilledema. Secondary glaucoma may also occur.

Plan

Management includes monitoring or radiation treatment performed with low-flow shunts. Surgical embolization or radiation treatment with high-flow shunts is used if the condition is sight threatening.

BLEPHAROCHALASIS

Subjective

Blepharochalasis is a rare condition with an onset that typically occurs between the ages of 7 and 20. Patients with this condition are usually asymptomatic but may complain of the cosmetic appearance of the lids.

Objective

Blepharochalasis is characterized by recurrent episodes of bilateral lid and periorbital edema. The condition results in progressive damage to the lid tissues, which causes fat prolapse and ptosis. In some cases exacerbations are triggered by fever or sun exposure. The episodes tend to diminish with age.

Plan

Surgical repair of the damaged lids may be attempted after the attacks diminish in frequency.

ORBITAL FAT HERNIATION

Subjective

This condition occurs when orbital fat herniates around the rim of the orbital septum. It is more common in older persons. The condition is asymptomatic, but the appearance of the lids is often cosmetically unacceptable to the patient.

Objective

Orbital fat herniation presents as bilateral baggy lids. It can affect both the superior and inferior lids.

Plan

Surgical repair of this condition may be indicated for cosmetic reasons.

EYELID EDEMA SECONDARY TO SYSTEMIC DISEASE

Subjective

Lid edema is occasionally associated with systemic conditions, including cardiac disease, renal disease, and hypothyroidism, as well as with pregnancy. The ocular condition is asymptomatic; however, the patient may experience symptoms characteristic of the underlying systemic disease.

Objective

This condition manifests as bilateral nonerythematous baggy lids. Laboratory evaluation and a cardiovascular workup are helpful in the differential diagnosis of the underlying disease.

Plan

Referral for management of the underlying systemic condition is the treatment of choice for this type of lid edema.

TUMORS

Subjective

A number of different types of tumor of the lids and orbit can cause the lids to have an edematous appearance. These include lymphoma, hemangioma, dermoid, leukemia, neurofibroma, rhabdomyosarcoma, and orbital pseudotumor. The lid lesions are usually asymptomatic; however, a lesion that causes significant ptosis in a young child can lead to amblyopia.

Objective

These lesions vary in their shape and appearance. Most are flesh-colored; however, hemangiomas tend to be red or purple. Associated proptosis or globe displacement suggests an orbital lesion. CT scan or magnetic resonance imaging is helpful in the differential diagnosis of these lesions.

Plan

Most benign tumors can be monitored routinely; however, any tumor that obstructs vision and has the potential to cause amblyopia in a young child requires removal. Patients with suspected malignancies should be referred to an oncologist for further evaluation and management.

SUGGESTED READING

Bartlett JD, Jaanus SD. Clinical Ocular Pharmacology (3rd ed). Boston: Butterworth–Heinemann, 1995.

Berkow R, Fletcher AJ. The Merck Manual of Diagnosis and Therapy. Rahway, NJ: Merck, 1992.

Cullom RD, Chang B. The Wills Eye Manual: Office and Emergency Room Diagnosis and Treatment of Eye Disease (2nd ed). Philadelphia: Lippincott, 1994.

Fitzpatrick TB, Johnson RA, Polano MK, et al. Color Atlas and Synopsis of Clinical Dermatology (2nd ed). New York: McGraw-Hill, 1992.

Fraunfelder FT, Roy FH. Current Ocular Therapy 4. Philadelphia: Saunders, 1995.

Margo CE, Hamed LM, Mames RN. Diagnostic Problems in Clinical Ophthalmology. Philadelphia: Saunders, 1994.

Roberts DK, Terry JE. Ocular Disease: Diagnosis and Treatment (2nd ed). Boston: Butterworth–Heinemann, 1996.

Roy FH. Ocular Differential Diagnosis (5th ed). Philadelphia: Lea & Febiger, 1993.

van Heuven WAJ, Zwaan JT. Decision Making in Ophthalmology. St. Louis: Mosby–Year Book, 1992.

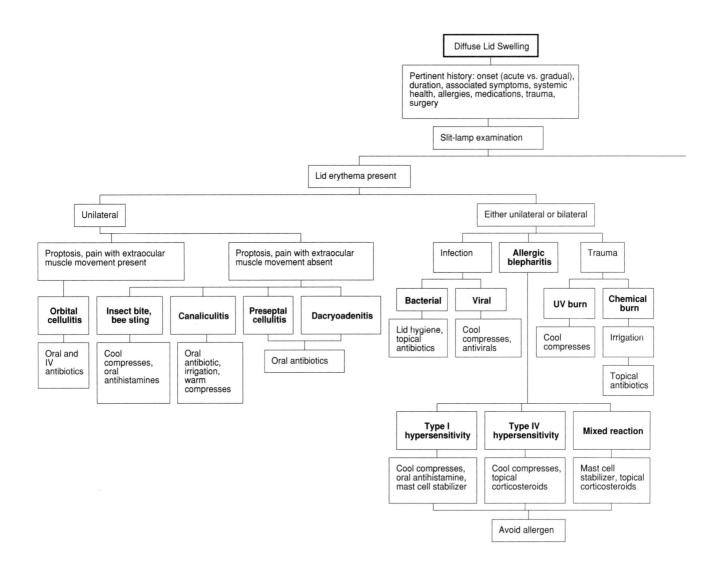

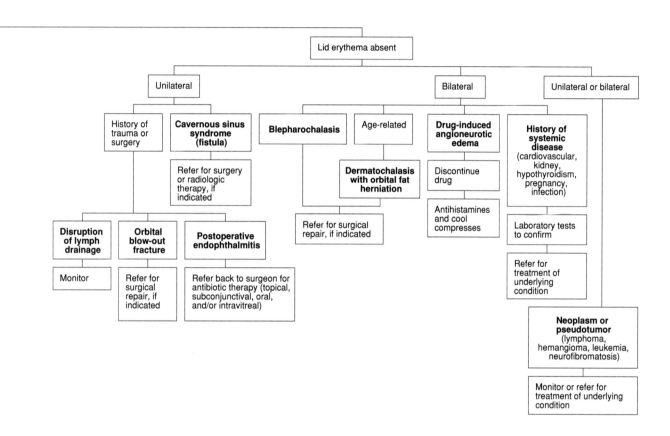

31

Lid Lesions

Debra J. Bezan

LID LESIONS AT A GLANCE

Black or brown
  Lentigines
  Ephelis
  Comedones
  Seborrheic keratosis
  Melanotic nevus
  Lentigo (senilis or maligna)
  Melanoma
  Pigmented basal cell carcinoma
  Allergic shiner
  Café-au-lait spot
  Melasma
  Radiation
  Drug deposition
  Xeroderma pigmentosum
Red
  Hordeolum
  Preseptal cellulitis
  Chickenpox
  Herpes zoster
  Hemangioma
  Rubella
  Rubeola
  Impetigo
  Contact dermatitis
  Urticaria
  Basal cell carcinoma
  Squamous cell carcinoma
  Keratoacanthoma
Blue
  Blue nevus
  Nevus of Ota
Purple
  Ecchymosis

Kaposi's sarcoma
Port-wine stain
Dermatomyositis (heliotrope)
White or yellow
  Sebaceous cyst
  Sudoriferous cyst
  Epidermal inclusion cyst
  Xanthelasma
  Actinic keratosis
  Primary herpes simplex
  Vitiligo
  Psoriasis
  Albinism
  Tuberous sclerosis
  Trauma
  Drug-induced depigmentation
Flesh-colored
  Chalazion
  Verruca
  Squamous papilloma
  Cutaneous horn
  Nevus
  Molluscum contagiosum
  Basal cell carcinoma
  Sebaceous carcinoma
  Sebaceous adenoma
  Neurofibroma

When a patient presents with a lesion of the eyelid and adnexa, pertinent questions to ask include the following: When was the lesion first noted? Did it appear suddenly or gradually? Has it changed in appearance over time? Is it symptomatic? Lid lesions should be examined grossly and microscopically. Manual palpation of the lesion often reveals additional important diagnostic information.

LENTIGO

Subjective

Lentigo is most commonly seen in elderly patients and is typically asymptomatic. Lentigo senilis is benign, whereas lentigo maligna (melanotic freckle of Hutchinson) is a precursor to malignant melanoma.

Objective

Lentigo appears as a flat, darkly pigmented lesion of irregular size and shape.

Plan

Lentigo lesions should be monitored closely for change. A lesion that is suspected to be premalignant or is undergoing malignant transformation should be excised.

MALIGNANT MELANOMA

Subjective

Melanomas are relatively uncommon malignancies of the eyelids that are usually asymptomatic. They may appear spontaneously or may develop from a lentigo maligna (melanotic freckle of Hutchinson) or a dysplastic nevus.

Objective

Melanomas tend to be asymmetric lesions with irregular borders. Although most are darkly pigmented, the color often varies within a single lesion, ranging from black to blue, red, or even white. Melanomas also vary in size, but most are greater than 6 mm in diameter.

Plan

Patients with suspected melanomas should be referred immediately for excisional biopsy and subsequent systemic evaluation by an oncologist. It is important to remember that malignant melanomas account for approximately 65% of skin cancer–related deaths. The prognosis is much better when lesions are detected while they are still shallow than when the lesions are deep and have already metastasized.

PIGMENTED BASAL CELL CARCINOMA

Subjective

Basal cell carcinoma is the most common form of skin cancer and usually occurs in areas of the skin that have received long-term sun exposure. Although most basal cell lesions are flesh colored, some may be darkly pigmented. They are usually asymptomatic.

Objective

Basal cell carcinomas are nodular lesions with rolled borders. They often have telangiectatic vessels coursing over the borders and an umbilicated center. This center may erode, so that the lesion has a rodent-ulcer appearance.

Plan

Basal cell carcinomas should be removed. They rarely metastasize but can be locally invasive. Lesions in the nasal canthus area may be lethal if they invade beyond the orbit.

COMEDONES

Subjective

Comedones (commonly known as *blackheads*) are often associated with sebaceous cysts. These asymptomatic lesions are most commonly found in older adults in areas of the skin that have received long-term sun exposure.

Objective

Comedones appear as pinpoint black dots filling a pore of the skin.

Plan

These lesions are benign and need no treatment. They may be expressed for cosmetic reasons but have a tendency to recur.

LENTIGINES

Subjective

Lentigines or ephelis (commonly known as *freckles*) are benign skin lesions found in sun-exposed areas, including the lids.

Objective

These lesions are small, flat, and uniformly pigmented. They usually occur in multiples.

Plan

Lentigines are benign and should merely be noted during routine examination. However, it is important to remember that fair-skinned people who develop lentigines have an increased likelihood of developing malignant skin lesions.

ALLERGIC SHINER

Subjective

An allergic shiner is an uncommon manifestation of allergic blepharitis. It is usually accompanied by symptoms of itching.

Objective

An allergic shiner appears as a darkening of the periorbital skin that somewhat resembles traumatic ecchymosis. It is often found in association with other signs of allergy, including edema and erythema of the lids and conjunctiva, watery or mucoid ocular discharge, and allergic rhinitis.

Plan

Treatment with cool compresses and oral antihistamines may give some symptomatic relief. The most definitive cure, however, is to eliminate the allergen.

CAFÉ-AU-LAIT SPOTS

Subjective

Café-au-lait spots are dermal signs associated with neurofibromatosis (Recklinghausen's disease) and occasionally with tuberous sclerosis (Bourneville's disease). They may be found anywhere on the skin, including the lids, and are asymptomatic.

Objective

Café-au-lait spots present as flat lesions with the characteristic coffee-with-cream brown color. When there are six or more of these lesions and the largest is greater than 5 mm in diameter in a preadolescent or greater than 15 mm in diameter in a postadolescent, then neurofibromatosis is suggested. Other ocular signs of neurofibromatosis include lid neurofibromas, ptosis, proptosis, Lisch nodules of the iris, early-onset posterior subcapsular cataract, choroidal nevi, astrocytic hamartoma, and optic nerve glioma.

Plan

No treatment is indicated for café-au-lait spots, but suspected cases should be further evaluated to rule out neurofibromatosis.

NEVUS

Subjective

Nevi (moles) are found on the skin of most white adults; they occur less commonly among more pigmented races. Nevi are classified as junctional, dermal, or compound according to their location. They may be found on the eyelids and are usually asymptomatic.

Objective

Nevi are quite variable in their appearance. They can be nearly flat, dome shaped, or pedunculated. They can range in color from dark brown to nearly flesh colored. Dysplastic nevi often have variegated coloration and slightly irregular borders. These may be a precursor to malignant melanoma.

Plan

Most nevi can be monitored routinely. Nevi may be removed surgically if they are dysplastic, exposed to constant irritation, or are cosmetically unacceptable to the patient.

SEBORRHEIC KERATOSIS

Subjective

The two forms of keratosis that involve the lids are seborrheic keratosis and actinic keratosis. Seborrheic keratoses are benign asymptomatic lesions most commonly found in older adults.

Objective

These lesions are usually dark brown or brownish gray and have a waxy or slightly scaly surface. They are elevated, with well-defined borders, and have a characteristic "stuck-on" appearance.

Plan

Seborrheic keratoses should be noted and monitored during routine examinations.

DRUG DEPOSITION

Subjective

Many drugs and chemicals can cause asymptomatic discoloration of the lids, including sulfacetamide, sulfisoxazole, testosterone, thimerosal, mercuric oxide, fluorouracil, silver, gold, iron, and vitamins A and D.

Objective

Discoloration due to drugs usually presents as a darkening or hyperpigmentation involving both of the lids symmetrically.

Plan

Patients with drug-induced hyperpigmentation should be monitored, and the drug therapy should be modified if appropriate.

HERPES ZOSTER

Subjective

The varicella virus causes both chickenpox and herpes zoster. Chickenpox, the primary infection, is a highly contagious disease found mainly in children. It causes fever, malaise, and itchy vesicular lesions of the skin, including the lids. Herpes zoster, the secondary infection, is primarily found in relatively immunosuppressed adults. It is often accompanied by a painful neuralgia.

Objective

The skin lesions of herpes zoster usually begin as a cluster of slightly reddish vesicular lesions located over a sensory dermatome. The lesions do not cross the vertical midline. Lesions on the tip of the nose (Hutchinson's sign) suggest ocular involvement. As they resolve, the lesions form yellowish brown crusts and may ultimately leave scars. Other ocular signs of herpes zoster include keratitis, conjunctivitis, scleritis, iridocyclitis, cataracts, chorioretinitis, optic neuritis, and secondary glaucoma.

Plan

The lid lesions may be treated prophylactically with a topical broad-spectrum antibiotic to prevent secondary bacterial infection. Corticosteroid or combination ointments are helpful with particularly symptomatic lid lesions. If initiated early in the course of the disease, oral acyclovir, famciclovir, or valacyclovir is helpful in reducing the duration and severity of ocular manifestations. Topical capsaicin is helpful in treating specific areas of neuralgia. Oral corticosteroids, analgesics, sedatives, and antidepressants are also used to treat postherpetic neuralgia and associated depression.

It is important to remember that herpes zoster is usually triggered by immune suppression. In young adults with herpes zoster, acquired immunodeficiency syndrome (AIDS) should be ruled out.

HORDEOLUM

Subjective

Hordeola are acute infections involving the glands of the eyelids. Internal hordeola involve glands of Zeis and Moll, whereas external hordeola involve the meibomian glands. These lesions tend to be quite tender or painful to the touch.

Objective

A hordeolum presents as a focal area of redness and swelling on the lid. It often develops a yellow point and drains spontaneously within a few days of the onset of the condition.

Plan

Application of warm compresses is often the first line of therapy for hordeola. Topical antibiotic ointments are sometimes used to prevent draining lesions from infecting surrounding tissues. Stab incision and drainage may help reduce pain and inflammation and promote resolution of the lesion. Oral antibiotics such as doxycycline, erythromycin, or dicloxacillin may be used to treat resistant cases.

PRESEPTAL CELLULITIS

Subjective

Preseptal cellulitis is a generalized inflammatory condition involving the lid structures anterior to the orbital septum. It may be caused by traumatic injuries or infections such as nonresolving hordeola, dacryocystitis, or sinusitis. In preseptal cellulitis the lid is warm and tender to the touch, and the patient may have fever and malaise.

Objective

This unilateral condition is characterized by generalized erythema and edema of the lid, which often cause marked ptosis. The patient does not have proptosis, significant pain on eye movement, or restriction of gaze, findings that help differentiate this condition from orbital cellulitis.

Plan

Preseptal cellulitis is treated with oral antibiotics such as amoxicillin or cefaclor that are effective against *Streptococcus* and some of the common anaerobic species. In children, *Haemophilus influenzae* should always be suspected. Children with moderate to severe preseptal cellulitis should be treated more aggressively with intravenous antibiotics, such as ceftriaxone and vancomycin, followed by oral therapy to prevent meningitis.

HEMANGIOMA

Subjective

Hemangiomas are benign blood vessel tumors. When they involve the lid, they are usually asymptomatic unless they cause significant ptosis. Large, long-standing lid hemangiomas in young children may result in amblyopia ex anopsia. Sturge-Weber syndrome should also be considered if lid hemangiomas are associated with a facial port-wine stain.

Objective

Hemangiomas are reddish lesions of variable size and shape. A helpful test is to apply pressure to the lesion, causing it to blanch, and then to watch for refilling of the vessels when the pressure is removed. Other ocular signs of Sturge-Weber syndrome include choroidal hemangiomas and secondary glaucoma.

Plan

Most hemangiomas should be monitored during routine examinations. Large lid lesions that cause reduced vision or are cosmetically unacceptable may be treated with a laser procedure. Sturge-Weber syndrome should also be ruled out in suspicious cases.

KERATOACANTHOMA

Subjective

Keratoacanthomas are benign skin lesions typically found in middle-aged and elderly individuals. They are usually asymptomatic.

Objective

Keratoacanthoma manifests as an elevated red lesion with a central crater filled with yellowish keratin debris. These lesions are characterized by rapid growth and thus are often mistaken for malignancies.

Plan

Keratoacanthomas can be conservatively managed by close monitoring, and most resolve spontaneously. They may also be removed via surgical excision, curettage, or electrocautery.

SQUAMOUS CELL CARCINOMA

Subjective

Squamous cell carcinomas are most commonly found in fair-skinned older adults in sun-exposed areas of the skin. They are found on the lids far less frequently than basal cell carcinomas and are usually asymptomatic.

Objective

These lesions present as reddish, elevated, scaly plaques. They tend to bleed easily and often have central ulceration with an overlying serosanguineous crust.

Plan

Squamous cell carcinomas should be surgically excised. Unlike basal cell carcinomas, they have a tendency to metastasize to regional lymphatics. A referral for oncologic evaluation is indicated in most cases.

KAPOSI'S SARCOMA

Subjective

Kaposi's sarcoma is a malignant skin tumor associated with immunosuppression. It is found in approximately one-third of AIDS patients. These lesions are usually asymptomatic.

Objective

The tumors present as nodular or plaquelike skin lesions that range in color from pink to dark purple. They may become ulcerated. These sarcomas most often occur on the extremities but occasionally may be found on the eyelids.

Plan

Kaposi's sarcoma is slowly progressive and may be monitored or treated more aggressively with radiation, surgical excision, electrosurgery, topical immunotherapy, or systemic chemotherapy. All patients with Kaposi's sarcoma should be evaluated for an underlying systemic condition such as AIDS.

ECCHYMOSIS

Subjective

Lid ecchymosis, or bruising, is usually caused by trauma, including surgery, although it is occasionally drug induced. It is usually asymptomatic unless accompanied by inflammation and edema.

Objective

Lid ecchymosis initially presents as a diffuse reddish purple area. After a few days, as the blood resorbs, it takes on a green then yellow hue.

Plan

Lid ecchymosis tends to resolve spontaneously.

BLUE NEVUS AND NEVUS OF OTA

Subjective

Nevi of the lids can occasionally take on a blue hue. In oculodermal disease, or nevus of Ota, both the episclera and lid are involved. These lesions are asymptomatic.

Objective

Lid nevi tend to be elevated lesions with well-defined borders. In nevus of Ota, both the episclera and ipsilateral periocular skin have a blue-gray pigmentation. The iris and choroid may also be more darkly pigmented on that side than on the unaffected side.

Plan

Blue nevi should be monitored on routine examination. Patients with nevus of Ota are predisposed to developing malignancies of the uvea, orbit, and brain, and thus should be monitored with increased vigilance.

VITILIGO

Subjective

Vitiligo is an asymptomatic patchy depigmentation of the skin. The lids are occasionally involved. It may appear as an isolated finding or be associated with other conditions such as Vogt-Koyanagi-Harada syndrome or scleroderma.

Objective

In Vogt-Koyanagi-Harada syndrome, the dermal depigmentation or vitiligo is usually accompanied by poliosis (whitening of the cilia) and alopecia (baldness). Other ocular signs include Dalen-Fuchs nodules and exudative detachment of the retina.

In scleroderma the skin, including the eyelids, is tight and thickened. The patient may also suffer from arthralgia, Raynaud's phenomenon, and various visceral disorders. Other ocular signs include lagophthalmos, dry eye, and uveitis.

Plan

Patients with vitiligo should be monitored, and underlying systemic conditions should be ruled out.

DRUG-INDUCED LID DEPIGMENTATION

Subjective

A number of drugs can cause depigmentation of the lid. Among these are chloramphenicol, hydroxychloroquine sulfate, thiotepa, and corticosteroids. These lesions are asymptomatic but may be cosmetically unacceptable to the patient.

Objective

The induced depigmentation may be focal or diffuse, unilateral or bilateral, depending on the drug dosage and route of administration.

Plan

These lesions should be noted on routine examination, and the drug therapy should be modified if appropriate.

PRIMARY HERPES SIMPLEX

Subjective

Primary herpes simplex usually occurs in childhood. Many cases are subclinical; overt cases are usually accompanied by fever and malaise.

Objective

If primary herpes simplex involves the lid, the lesions occur as clusters of yellowish white vesicles. Other signs include follicular conjunctivitis, keratitis, gingivosto-matitis, and lymphadenopathy.

Plan

The lid lesions of primary herpes simplex are self-limiting and generally need no treatment. It is important to remember that patients who have had primary herpes simplex are at risk for developing recurrent herpes simplex.

XANTHELASMA

Subjective

Xanthelasma (xanthoma) is a benign, asymptomatic lesion of the lids composed of cells containing cholesterol and other lipids. It is most commonly found in adults with hyperlipidemia or diabetes.

Objective

Xanthelasma presents as a yellow, plaquelike lesion found near the nasal canthus. It can occur on either the superior or inferior lid.

Plan

These lesions may be routinely monitored or removed surgically if they are cosmetically unacceptable. A lipid profile and fasting blood glucose level or similar test should also be ordered for these patients to rule out hyperlipidemia and diabetes.

SEBACEOUS CYST

Subjective

Sebaceous cysts are asymptomatic lesions formed from hyperplastic sebaceous glands. These are often found in older adults in areas of the skin that have received long-term sun exposure.

Objective

Sebaceous cysts present as yellow, slightly elevated, donut-shaped lesions. They often have associated comedones (blackheads).

Plan

These cysts are benign and should simply be noted during routine examination. However, they may be expressed or excised for cosmetic reasons.

SUDORIFEROUS CYST

Subjective

Sudoriferous cysts are asymptomatic inclusion cysts involving sweat glands.

Objective

These cysts appear as elevated, pinkish white lesions filled with clear fluid. They can be transilluminated.

Plan

Sudoriferous cysts should simply be monitored routinely, but they may be incised or excised for improved cosmetic appearance. They have a tendency to recur unless the inner wall of the cyst is removed.

ACTINIC KERATOSIS

Subjective

Actinic keratoses are asymptomatic premalignant lesions. They occur most frequently in older adults in sun-exposed areas of the skin.

Objective

Actinic keratoses typically present as yellowish, rough lesions with a crust that can be easily scraped off, leaving a pink patch. The lesions tend to bleed easily. They may also take the form of a cutaneous horn.

Plan

Because of their tendency to transform into squamous cell carcinomas, actinic keratoses should be monitored closely or removed using cryotherapy, electrocautery, or surgical excision.

NEUROFIBROMA

Subjective

Neurofibromas are asymptomatic benign peripheral neuromas. They are associated with neurofibromatosis (Recklinghausen's disease) and may be found in children or adults.

Objective

Neurofibromas present as multiple elevated, flesh-colored lesions. Other ocular signs of neurofibromatosis include dermal café-au-lait spots, ptosis, proptosis, Lisch nodules of the iris, early-onset posterior subcapsular cataract, choroidal nevi, astrocytic hamartoma, and optic nerve glioma.

Plan

No treatment is indicated for neurofibromas, but their presence indicates that the patient should be evaluated further for the presence of other manifestations of neurofibromatosis.

SEBACEOUS ADENOMA

Subjective

Sebaceous adenomas are asymptomatic facial angiofibromas that may be associated with tuberous sclerosis (Bourneville's disease).

Objective

Sebaceous adenomas present as elevated, reddish yellow or flesh-colored papules distributed in a butterfly pattern on the cheeks. They are often first noted in childhood. Other dermal manifestations of tuberous sclerosis include shagreen patches, ash-leaf sign, and occasionally café-au-lait spots. Other signs that may be found as part of this syndrome include astrocytic hamartoma, seizures, and mental retardation.

Plan

Patients with sebaceous adenomas require no treatment but should be thoroughly evaluated for the presence of tuberous sclerosis.

MOLLUSCUM CONTAGIOSUM

Subjective

Molluscum contagiosum is a dermal infection caused by a poxvirus. Contrary to what its name implies, it is only mildly contagious. It is most commonly found in children or immunosuppressed adults.

Objective

These lesions are dome-shaped, umbilicated, flesh-colored nodules that are usually found in clusters. Lesions located on the lid margins may shed viral toxins that can cause follicular conjunctivitis and pannus.

Plan

Molluscum contagiosum is usually self-limiting; however, the lesions may be removed surgically or with cryother-

apy or chemical cautery. Evaluation for an underlying immunosuppressive condition such as AIDS should be considered for adults with this condition.

SQUAMOUS PAPILLOMA

Subjective

Squamous papillomas are asymptomatic benign epithelial tumors most commonly found on the lids of older adults.

Objective

A squamous papilloma appears as a flesh-colored, cauliflower-like lesion with a central vascular core in each lobe. It is similar in appearance to verruca.

Plan

Squamous papillomas require only routine monitoring; however, they may be removed surgically or by cryoablation or chemical cauterization for cosmetic reasons.

VERRUCA

Subjective

Verrucae are asymptomatic skin lesions caused by papillomavirus. They are found most frequently among children and young adults.

Objective

Verrucae present as multilobed, flesh-colored lesions that may have a pedunculated stalk (verruca vulgaris) or may be rounded and cauliflower-like (verruca plana). Lesions on the lid margins may shed viral toxins that cause a chronic follicular conjunctivitis.

Plan

Verrucae usually resolve spontaneously but often recur. They may be removed by surgical excision, cryoablation, electrocautery, or chemical cautery if desired.

CHALAZION

Subjective

A chalazion is a focal granuloma of a meibomian gland. It may be a sequela of chronic blepharitis or hordeolum. In contrast to an acute hordeolum, a chalazion is nontender and relatively asymptomatic.

Objective

A chalazion appears as a flesh-colored lump of variable size on the lid.

Plan

Small chalazia may be treated conservatively with the application of warm compresses. Recalcitrant small lesions (<6 mm in diameter) may respond to intralesional injections of triamcinolone. Larger lesions often require surgical incision and curettage.

SKIN TAG AND CUTANEOUS HORN

Subjective

Skin tags and cutaneous horns are asymptomatic lesions that may be found on the lids. Cutaneous horns are sometimes associated with actinic keratosis.

Objective

These lesions appear as flesh-colored projections. Cutaneous horns are often slightly scaly.

Plan

The lesions should be routinely monitored or may be removed by surgical excision, cryoablation, electrocautery, or chemical cautery.

SEBACEOUS GLAND CARCINOMA

Subjective

Sebaceous gland carcinomas are malignant tumors that may involve the meibomian glands on the lids. They are most often found in middle-aged or older adults and are typically asymptomatic.

Objective

Sebaceous gland carcinomas are elevated lesions on the lids that resemble recurrent chalazia or intractable blepharitis. Loss of cilia and changes in meibomian orifice morphology in the region of these lesions suggest a malignant, rather than benign, process.

Plan

Excisional biopsy is indicated in cases of suspected sebaceous gland carcinoma. Systemic oncologic evaluation may also be indicated, because orbital extension and metastasis can occur with these tumors.

NONPIGMENTED BASAL CELL CARCINOMA

Subjective

Basal cell carcinoma is the most common form of skin cancer and usually occurs in older adults on areas of the skin that have received long-term sun exposure. It is usually asymptomatic.

Objective

Basal cell carcinomas are nodular lesions with rolled borders. Although most basal cell lesions are flesh colored, some may be darkly pigmented. They often have telangiectatic vessels coursing over the borders and an umbilicated center. This center may erode, so that the lesion has a rodent-ulcer appearance.

Plan

Basal cell carcinomas should be removed. They rarely metastasize but can be locally invasive. Lesions in the nasal canthus area may be lethal if they invade beyond the orbit.

SUGGESTED READING

Bartlett JD, Jaanus SD. Clinical Ocular Pharmacology (3rd ed). Boston: Butterworth–Heinemann, 1995.

Bezan DJ. An overview of dermatology for primary care providers. J Am Optom Assoc 1991;62:138–145.

Fitzpatrick TB, Johnson RA, Polano MK, et al. Color Atlas and Synopsis of Clinical Dermatology (2nd ed). New York: McGraw-Hill, 1992.

Marks ES, Adamczyk DT, Thomann KH. Primary Eyecare in Systemic Disease. Norwalk, CT: Appleton & Lange, 1995.

Roy FH. Ocular Differential Diagnosis (5th ed). Philadelphia: Lea & Febiger, 1993.

van Heuven WAJ, Zwaan JT. Decision Making in Ophthalmology. St. Louis: Mosby–Year Book, 1992.

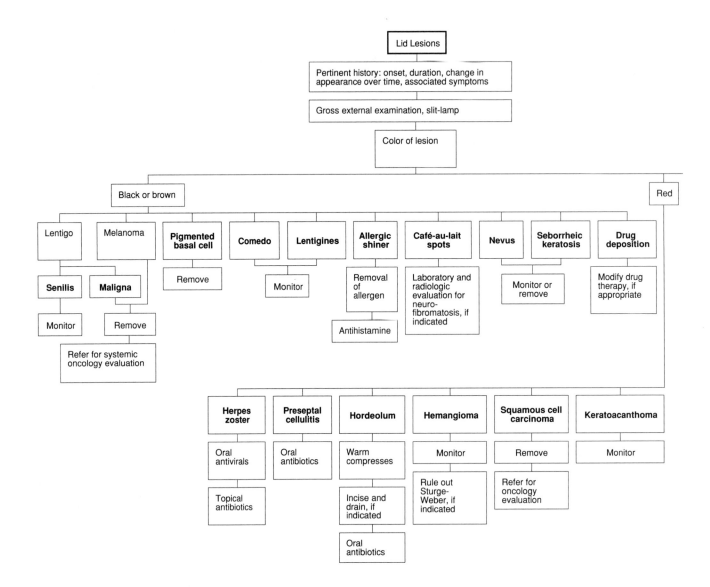

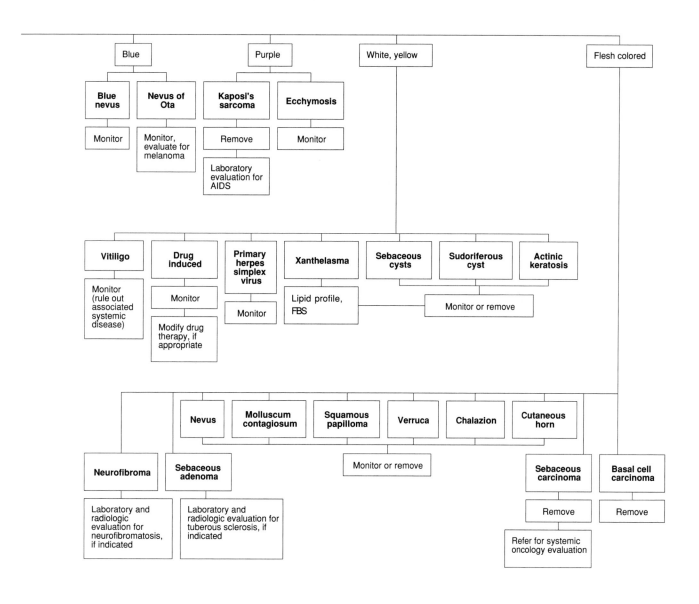

32

Anomalies of Lid Position

DEBRA J. BEZAN

**ANOMALIES OF LID POSITION
AT A GLANCE**

Lagophthalmos
  Physiologic (nocturnal)
  Orbital (proptotic)
  Mechanical (cicatricial)
  Paralytic (seventh nerve palsy)
Congenital ptosis
  With normal superior rectus function (simple)
  With diminished superior rectus function
  With blepharophimosis
  Synkinetic
    Marcus Gunn syndrome (jaw-winking)
    Misdirected third nerve
Acquired ptosis
  Neurogenic
    Horner's syndrome
    Third nerve palsy
    Cerebral palsy
    Multiple sclerosis
    Syphilis
    Riley-Day syndrome
  Myogenic
    Muscular dystrophy (myotonic dystrophy)
      or atrophy
    Myasthenia gravis
    Progressive external ophthalmoplegia
    Involutional
    Pharmacologic
  Traumatic
    Damage to muscles or nerves
    Post–anterior segment surgery
    Post–botulinum toxin injection
  Mechanical
    Tumor

    Blepharochalasis
    Vernal conjunctivitis
    Cicatrization
Pseudoptosis
  Lid edema
    Inflammatory
    Noninflammatory
  Dermatochalasis
  Blepharospasm
  Microphthalmos
  Enopthalmos
Phthisis bulbi
Lid retraction
  Associated only with ocular conditions
    Compensatory
    Brown's syndrome
    Aberrant third nerve regeneration
    Duane's syndrome
  Associated with systemic conditions
    Graves' disease
    Encephalitis
    Midbrain tumor
    Syphilis
Entropion
  Congenital
  Acquired
    Inflammatory
    Mechanical
    Involutional
    Cicatricial
Ectropion
  Congenital
  Acquired
    Spastic
    Involutional
    Cicatricial

Atonic seventh nerve palsy
Allergic
Tumor
Floppy eyelid syndrome

Anomalies of lid position are often visible with gross observation. They may be mentioned as one of the patient's chief concerns or may initially be noted by the clinician in the course of routine examination. When anomalies of lid position are identified, the clinician should take a careful history of the onset and duration of the condition; aggravating or relieving factors; associated ocular or systemic signs and symptoms; and ocular disease or trauma including surgery, systemic disease, and medication use. Careful evaluation of the lids and other ocular structures with the biomicroscope as well as evaluation of the pupillary responses and extraocular motilities are also part of the initial workup.

LAGOPHTHALMOS

Subjective

Lagophthalmos is subclassified according to its underlying cause as nocturnal (physiologic), orbital (usually associated with thyroid eye disease), mechanical (cicatricial), and paralytic (usually associated with seventh nerve palsy). Symptoms of lagophthalmos are irritation, dryness, or foreign body sensation due to desiccation of the inferior conjunctiva and cornea.

Objective

In lagophthalmos, the lids cannot close completely. This condition can usually be assessed with gross observation. Placing the patient in a supine position and evaluating the closed lids can be helpful in diagnosing nocturnal lagophthalmos. Other useful diagnostic tests include exophthalmometry, assessment of the seventh cranial nerve, and slit-lamp examination for evidence of lid scarring and drying of the inferior conjunctiva and cornea.

Plan

Initial treatment for patients with lagophthalmos is the application of lubricant drops or ointments to provide symptomatic relief. Lid taping at night can be particularly helpful for patients with nocturnal lagophthalmos. More severe cases can be treated with bandage contact lenses, moisture chambers, or lid surgery. Patients with suspected thyroid disease should be referred to an endocrinologist.

DERMATOCHALASIS

Subjective

Dermatochalasis is found primarily in elderly patients. It is usually asymptomatic unless the excess skin blocks the visual axis. Patients may also complain about the cosmetic appearance.

Objective

Dermatochalasis presents as a wrinkled, drooping eyelid caused by age-related loss of skin elasticity.

Plan

If dermatochalasis affects vision or is a cosmetic concern, blepharoplasty is indicated.

BLEPHAROSPASM

Blepharospasm may have no other associated conditions (benign essential blepharospasm), or it may be secondary to ocular irritation. See Chapter 9 for more information.

LID EDEMA

Lid edema can cause a relative ptosis. A number of inflammatory conditions, vascular diseases, and other disorders can cause swollen eyelids. See Chapter 30 for more information.

CONGENITAL PTOSIS

Subjective

Congenital ptosis is due to an incomplete development of the levator muscle or its innervation. The condition usually has an autosomal dominant mode of inheritance. The ptosis is unilateral in approximately 75% of cases. The condition may be symptomatic if the lid droop is pronounced enough to block the visual axis.

Objective

Congenital ptosis is classified according to the presence or absence of other associated findings, including diminished superior rectus function, blepharophimosis, Marcus Gunn syndrome (jaw-winking), or misdirected third nerve. Clinical evaluation of suspected congenital ptosis includes gross observation and measurement of the palpebral fissures, evaluation of levator function while the frontal muscle is stabilized, evaluation for the presence of lid lag on downgaze, and evaluation of lid position while chewing. Slit-lamp examination of the lids should also be performed, and the clinician should note whether the lid fold is less distinct on the side with the ptosis. Tear function, corneal sensitivity, and refractive error should also be assessed.

Plan

Mild cases of congenital ptosis can be monitored routinely. If the ptosis is severe enough to block the visual axis, surgical intervention is required to prevent amblyopia.

HORNER'S SYNDROME

Subjective

Horner's syndrome is an oculosympathetic palsy or paresis. It can be congenital or acquired. Acquired forms can be secondary to trauma, ischemia, inflammation, or compression from a space-occupying lesion. The condition is further classified as central, preganglionic, or postganglionic depending on the location of the lesion. Patients with Horner's syndrome are generally asymptomatic; however, if they also have Raeder's syndrome, they may experience headache or facial pain. Associated arm pain is suggestive of Pancoast's tumor.

Objective

Signs of Horner's syndrome include unilateral ptosis, elevation of the lower lid (upside-down ptosis), miosis on the affected side, greater anisocoria in dim illumination than in bright, pupil dilation lag, and ipsilateral lack of facial sweating (anhydrosis). Heterochromia iridis, in which the iris on the affected side is less pigmented, is associated with congenital or neonatal Horner's syndrome.

Pharmacologic evaluation is indicated to confirm the diagnosis of Horner's syndrome and to differentiate postganglionic from preganglionic or central lesions. If the affected pupil fails to dilate within 30 minutes after one to two drops of 10% cocaine solution has been bilaterally instilled, the diagnosis of Horner's syndrome is confirmed. If the affected pupil fails to dilate within 30 minutes after bilateral instillation of one to two drops of 1% hydroxyamphetamine, the lesion is considered postganglionic. Instil-

lation of 2.5% phenylephrine hydrochloride causes a temporary reduction of the ptosis in Horner's syndrome.

Plan

Patients with postganglionic Horner's syndrome can be monitored routinely. Those with persistent associated symptoms such as headache or signs of other cranial-nerve involvement should be referred for a neurologic evaluation. Patients with preganglionic Horner's syndrome should be referred to a family practitioner or internist to rule out Pancoast's tumor of the lung as well as other causes. Patients with suspected central lesions require referral to a neurologist.

THIRD NERVE PALSY

Subjective

Acquired, isolated third nerve palsies may be aneurysmal, ischemic, traumatic, neoplastic, or of undetermined origin. The chief complaint associated with third nerve palsy is diplopia. The patient may or may not experience pain.

Objective

The hallmarks of isolated third nerve palsy are ptosis and restriction of extraocular motility in all but the inferotemporal field of gaze. It is important to assess whether the pupil is involved (fixed and dilated) or spared. Pupil involvement is suggestive of an aneurysmal origin, whereas pupil sparing is more suggestive of an ischemic origin.

All patients with third nerve palsies should be evaluated for aberrant regeneration and screened for evidence of involvement of other cranial nerves. Patients with pupil sparing should have a laboratory workup including complete blood count, fasting blood sugar level, erythrocyte sedimentation rate, syphilis screening, antinuclear antibody test, and blood pressure assessment. A radiographic skull series is also indicated. All patients with pupil involvement should immediately have a magnetic resonance imaging (MRI), magnetic resonance angiography, or four-vessel cerebral angiography to rule out an aneurysm. Patients who have no evidence of ischemic disease, have aberrant regeneration, have involvement of other cranial nerves, or do not show improvement in 3 months should also have these radiologic tests performed.

Plan

Patients with confirmed ischemic third nerve palsy can be monitored carefully. Most show recovery within 3 months. All other patients should be referred for further neurologic assessment and treatment.

MYASTHENIA GRAVIS

Subjective

Myasthenia gravis (MG) is an autoimmune neuromuscular disorder involving the acetylcholine receptor. It is found in all age groups and among males and females. It can be either congenital or acquired. Certain drugs, including beta blockers, steroids, and antibiotics, can also cause MG. The primary symptom of MG is weakness and fatigability of the muscles of the extremities, neck, or face. The patient may also complain of difficulty in speaking, swallowing, or breathing. Ocular symptoms include lid twitch or droop, blurred vision, and diplopia. The symptoms vary depending on the time of day and on the patient's physical activity level, stress, and general health.

Objective

Unilateral or bilateral ptosis that worsens with fatigue or in bright illumination is often the initial manifestation of MG. Extraocular motility and convergence may be reduced due to MG-induced ophthalmoplegia. The patient may also have incomplete lid closure with secondary keratitis.

Several tests may be performed to aid in the diagnosis of MG. In the lid twitch test, the clinician looks for a twitching of the lid when the patient is instructed to blink. In the sustained upgaze test, the palpebral apertures are measured before and after approximately 1 minute of sustained upgaze to look for an increase in ptosis. The palpebral apertures can also be measured before and after a 30-minute nap, a 2-minute application of cool compresses to the lids, or an intravenous injection of edrophonium chloride (Tensilon). In MG, all of these procedures tend to cause a temporary reduction in the amount of ptosis. An acetylcholine-receptor antibody titer is a highly specific test for MG. Electromyography can be used in cases in which the diagnosis is in doubt.

Plan

The patient with suspected MG should be referred to a neurologist for further evaluation and treatment. Cholinesterase inhibitors used to treat the systemic manifestations often help reduce ptosis and extraocular muscle motility problems. The primary eye care provider can prescribe prisms, patches, and ocular lubricants for symp-

tomatic relief, as well as monitor the patient for ocular complications of systemic medications.

CEREBRAL PALSY

Subjective

Cerebral palsy (CP) is a term used to describe a broad range of motor disorders caused by prenatal, perinatal, or postnatal abnormalities or events. It is usually diagnosed before the age of 5. The primary symptoms are associated with impaired voluntary movement. Deafness and mental retardation occur in some cases.

Objective

The systemic signs include hypertonicity, weakness, and spasticity of the muscles. A scissorslike gait and toe walking are common. The degree of motor impairment ranges from mild impairment to quadriplegia. Seizures occur in approximately 25% of patients with CP. Ocular signs include strabismus, paralysis of upgaze, accommodative infacility, refractive errors, and occasional ptosis.

Plan

The primary eye care provider should prescribe lenses, prisms, and other types of therapy to CP patients when appropriate. In addition, patients with suspected CP should be referred to a pediatrician or neurologist for confirmation of the diagnosis. Anticonvulsant medications and physical therapy are commonly prescribed as supportive treatments.

MULTIPLE SCLEROSIS

Subjective

Multiple sclerosis (MS) is a demyelinating disease that primarily affects young adults. It is more prevalent in areas with cooler climates than in tropical zones. Systemic symptoms include paresthesia or weakness in the limbs, gait difficulties, and Lhermitte's sign (a tingling sensation in the back of the neck as the chin is bent toward the chest). Ocular symptoms include acute monocular vision loss, Uhthoff symptom (a worsening of vision associated with elevations in body temperature), and diplopia.

Objective

The acute vision loss in MS is associated with optic neuritis. The presence of an afferent pupillary defect, red desaturation, increased visual evoked potential latency, and central scotoma are confirmatory findings. Ophthalmoscopy may reveal papillitis; however, it is important to remember that in MS the optic neuritis is often retrobulbar. Other ocular signs of MS include extraocular motility disorders, ptosis, and uveitis.

MRI and cerebrospinal fluid analysis are used to diagnose MS.

Plan

Patients with suspected MS should be referred to a neurologist for further evaluation.

MUSCULAR DYSTROPHY

Subjective

Muscular dystrophy is a genetically determined disorder with an autosomal dominant mode of inheritance. It is characterized by muscle weakness, myotonia, and wasting. In addition to muscular involvement, it can affect the endocrine, cardiovascular, respiratory, gastrointestinal, genitourinary, and skeletal systems. The systemic symptoms vary with the organ systems involved. Ocular symptoms include blurred vision and irritation secondary to exposure keratopathy.

Objective

The astute clinician may observe the characteristic expressionless facial appearance of the patient with myotonic dystrophy. Ocular signs include ptosis, lagophthalmos, extraocular motility dysfunctions, convergence insufficiency, cataracts, hypotony, and pigmentary retinopathy.

Plan

Lid taping and lubricant therapy can be helpful in alleviating exposure keratopathy. Patients with suspected myotonic dystrophy should be referred to a neurologist for further evaluation. Genetic counseling is also in order.

TRAUMATIC PTOSIS

Subjective

Traumatic ptosis can be caused by damage to the eyelid muscles or lids or can be induced by toxins affecting the neuromuscular junction. It can also be a result of scarring. Patients with acquired ptosis should be questioned carefully about previous eye trauma, surgery, or botulinum toxin injection. Patients may be asymptomatic or may complain of the cosmetic appearance of the ptosis. Significant ptosis that blocks the visual axis can cause vision loss.

Objective

In addition to the ptosis, the clinician should look for scarring and other signs of trauma. Perimetry can be used to determine whether the ptosis is causing a significant visual field defect.

Plan

Ptosis induced by botulinum toxin usually resolves over several months. Other forms of traumatic ptosis may require surgical repair if they affect vision or are cosmetically unacceptable to the patient.

TUMOR

Subjective

A number of different types of tumor of the lids and orbit can cause the lids to have a deformed appearance. These include lymphoma, hemangioma, dermoid, leukemia, neurofibroma, rhabdomyosarcoma, and orbital pseudotumor. The lid lesions are usually asymptomatic; however, a lesion causing significant ptosis in a young child can lead to amblyopia.

Objective

These lesions vary in their shape and appearance. Most are flesh colored; hemangiomas tend to be red or purple. Associated proptosis or globe displacement suggests an orbital lesion. CT or MRI is helpful in the differential diagnosis of these lesions.

Plan

Most benign tumors can be monitored routinely; however, any tumor that has the potential to cause amblyopia in a young child requires removal. Patients with suspected malignancies should be referred to an oncologist for further evaluation and management.

BLEPHAROCHALASIS

Subjective

Blepharochalasis is a rare condition with an onset typically between the ages of 7 and 20. Patients with this condition are usually asymptomatic but may complain of the cosmetic appearance of the lids.

Objective

Blepharochalasis is characterized by recurrent episodes of bilateral lid and periorbital edema. The condition results in progressive damage to the lid tissues, which causes fat prolapse and ptosis. In some cases, exacerbations are triggered by fever or sun exposure. The episodes tend to diminish with age.

Plan

Surgical repair of the damaged lids may be attempted after the attacks diminish in frequency.

REACTIONS TO DRUGS AND OTHER ALLERGENS

Allergic reactions (type I, type IV, or mixed) can cause the lid to have a thickened, droopy appearance.

Type I hypersensitivity reactions (anaphylactic, immediate, IgE-mediated reactions) of the lid include hay fever blepharitis and angioneurotic edema. Pollens, molds, and animal dander are common causes of hay fever blepharoconjunctivitis, whereas reactions to foods, ingested medications, or insect stings can cause angioneurotic edema.

Type IV hypersensitivity reactions (delayed, cell-mediated reactions) require a previous sensitizing exposure to the offending agent. Common allergens that cause contact blepharitis include poison ivy, nail polish, dyes, nickel, preservatives, and topical medications.

Mixed reactions have some characteristics of both type I and type IV reactions. Vernal and atopic conditions are examples of this type of reaction.

Subjective

Itching is the classic symptom of allergic blepharitis.

Objective

Type I hypersensitivity blepharitis is characterized by significant lid edema. The lid is more erythemic in hay fever blepharitis than in angioneurotic edema. In type IV reactions, the lid is mildly edematous and often develops scaly eruptions. In mixed reactions, the lid often has a corrugated appearance. All of these conditions are usually found in association with conjunctivitis, and the eyes often have a serous or mucoid discharge.

Plan

Type I lid reactions are initially managed with the use of cool compresses and oral antihistamines. Type IV and mixed reactions are managed with the use of cool compresses and topical corticosteroid ointments for symptomatic relief. Mast cell stabilizers are useful in preventing subsequent histamine release in type I and mixed reactions. Avoidance of the offending allergen whenever possible is the best therapy to prevent recurrence of any type of allergic reaction.

INVOLUTIONAL PTOSIS

Subjective

Involutional ptosis is a type of acquired lid droop found in the elderly population. It is believed to be caused by stretching, thinning, or traumatic damage to the levator aponeurosis. It may be induced by cataract surgery. Patients with this condition often complain about the cosmetic appearance. If the lid impinges on the visual axis, it can cause vision loss.

Objective

The signs of this condition include unilateral or bilateral ptosis with a high or absent crease in the eyelid. There may be a visible thinning of the superior lid above the tarsal plate or a defect in the aponeurosis that can be detected with palpation. The levator function is usually normal.

Plan

Patients who complain of vision loss or the cosmetic appearance of involutional ptosis should be referred to an ophthalmic surgeon for further evaluation and management.

CICATRICIAL LID RETRACTION

Subjective

Scarring secondary to trauma, surgery, or other forms of severe inflammation can cause cicatricial lid retraction. Patients with this condition usually complain of irritation, pain, or blurred vision associated with exposure keratopathy.

Objective

The signs of cicatricial lid retraction include scarring of the anterior or posterior lid, lagophthalmos, and exposure keratoconjunctivitis.

Plan

Ocular lubricant drops and ointments can be prescribed for symptomatic relief. The patient should be referred for surgical repair when appropriate.

COMPENSATORY RETRACTION

Subjective

Compensatory retraction may occur in an eye when there is a ptosis in the other eye. The patient is usually asymptomatic.

Objective

The presence of ptosis in the contralateral eye and an elevated brow position in the affected eye are helpful clues in diagnosing compensatory retraction.

Plan

No specific treatment is indicated for this condition; however, it may be alleviated if the ptosis in the fellow eye can be resolved.

GRAVES' DISEASE (HYPERTHYROIDISM)

Subjective

Graves' disease is defined as hyperthyroidism plus proptosis, goiter, or pretibial myxedema. It is more common in females than in males and usually manifests between the ages of 30 and 50. The systemic symptoms include nervousness, heat intolerance, sweating, palpitations and tachycardia, increased appetite, increased gastrointestinal motility, weight loss, insomnia, and fatigue.

Ocular symptoms include lid retraction ("Graves' stare"), ocular irritation, photophobia, and diplopia. Reduced central or peripheral vision and changes in color perception can occur if the optic nerve is involved.

Objective

Systemic signs of Graves' disease include goiter, hypertension, tachycardia, tremor, sweating, and pretibial myxedema.

The most common ocular sign is proptosis (unilateral or bilateral). The proptosis can be quantified with an exophthalmometer. Lid retraction on downgaze is another frequent finding. This finding is in contrast to the lid retraction noted in primary gaze but absent in downgaze found in association with encephalitis, meningitis, syphilis, and certain midbrain tumors. The patient with Graves' disease may also exhibit lagophthalmos, exposure keratopathy, conjunctival injection, and periorbital edema. Diplopia is secondary to restrictions in extraocular muscle motility. The inferior rectus muscle is the most frequently involved. Occasionally, patients with Graves' disease develop a compressive optic neuropathy that causes an afferent pupillary defect, color desaturation, and central or peripheral visual field defects.

A number of laboratory tests are used in the diagnosis of hyperthyroidism. Tests commonly used in thyroid profiles include measurement of total serum thyroxine, thyroid-hormone-binding ratio (triiodothyronine resin uptake), and serum thyrotropin. It is important to remember that some patients with signs and symptoms of Graves' disease show normal test results on a thyroid profile. Orbital ultrasonography or CT can be used to demonstrate the orbitopathy and rule out orbital tumors.

Plan

The primary eye care provider can help the patient obtain symptomatic relief from exposure keratopathy by prescribing lubricant drops and ointments. Patients with Graves' ophthalmopathy should also be referred for medical or surgical management of the underlying systemic disease. Orbital decompression surgery may be indicated in cases with compression optic neuropathy to preserve vision.

BROWN'S SYNDROME

Subjective

Brown's syndrome is a condition characterized by a tight superior oblique tendon. It may be congenital or acquired. The patient should be questioned about previous ocular trauma, surgery, or inflammation. Patients with this condition may be asymptomatic or may complain of diplopia or blurred vision.

Objective

Signs of Brown's syndrome include decreased ability to elevate the eye during adduction. The affected eye may even turn downward slightly during adduction, and the lids may retract, widening the palpebral fissure. Some patients exhibit a compensatory chin-up, head-tilted posture.

Plan

If the patient is able to fuse well in primary gaze and does not have a compensatory anomalous head posture, routine monitoring is indicated. Otherwise, the patient should be referred for surgical management.

ABERRANT REGENERATION (MISDIRECTION) OF THE THIRD NERVE

Subjective

After the third nerve has been disrupted, it may sprout axons that have anomalous terminations. Aberrant regeneration may be primary (i.e., not associated with a preceding acute third nerve palsy) or secondary (i.e., associated with a previous traumatic or compressive acute third nerve palsy). It is important to note that aberrant regeneration does not occur secondary to an ischemic third nerve palsy.

Objective

Aberrant regenerations can be further classified as lid-gaze dyskinesis or pupil-gaze dyskinesis. In lid-gaze dyskinesis, the lid may retract on downgaze or adduction. In pupil-gaze dyskinesis, there may be an unusually large pupil constriction during convergence or the pupil may constrict on downgaze. See the earlier section on third nerve palsy for more information.

Plan

Patients with confirmed ischemic third nerve palsy can be monitored carefully. Most show recovery within 3 months. All other patients should be referred for further neurologic assessment and treatment.

DUANE'S SYNDROME

Subjective

Duane's syndrome (retraction syndrome) is a congenital condition in which abnormal innervation causes extra-ocular motility anomalies. The condition is unilateral in approximately 80% of cases, and it is more common in females than in males. Most patients with this condition are asymptomatic; however, a few may complain of diplopia or blurred vision.

Objective

Three subtypes of Duane's syndrome exist. In type 1, the patient has little or no ability to abduct and some reduction in the ability to adduct. During adduction, the globe retracts and the palpebral aperture narrows. Conversely, when abduction is attempted, the palpebral aperture widens. Esotropia in primary gaze is common with this type. In type 2, there is significant restriction of gaze and retraction when adduction is attempted, while abduction is affected to a lesser degree. Exotropia in primary gaze is associated with type 2. Both adduction and abduction are significantly restricted in type 3.

Plan

Patients who do not have strabismus in primary gaze and do not demonstrate a compensatory head turn can be monitored routinely. Other patients with Duane's syndrome should be referred for surgical management.

ENTROPION

Subjective

Entropion is an inward turning of the lower or upper lids. It can be unilateral or bilateral and can be further classified as congenital, cicatricial, involutional, or spastic. The latter two types are more common in the elderly population. If entropion is associated with trichiasis, a condition in which the cilia contact the globe, the patient usually complains of irritation.

Objective

Entropion is usually visible with gross observation. It may be exacerbated with forced lid closure. Sodium fluorescein staining can be used to identify areas of corneal or conjunctival disruption associated with trichiasis.

Plan

Lash epilation or eversion of the lid margin with tape may be used to provide temporary relief from the irritation caused by trichiasis. Electrolysis, cryotherapy, or laser ablation of the cilia follicle provides longer term relief. Various surgical procedures can be used to repair entropion.

ECTROPION

Subjective

Ectropion is characterized by an outward turning of the lower lid margin. It can be further classified as congenital, atonic (age-related or paralytic), cicatricial, or inflammatory (allergic). It is occasionally associated with seventh nerve palsy. Patients with this condition may complain of ocular irritation and photophobia secondary to exposure keratopathy.

Objective

Ectropion is usually evident with gross observation. Associated findings are injection of the inferior conjunctiva and punctate keratopathy of the inferior cornea.

Plan

Topical lubricating drops and ointments can be prescribed to temporarily alleviate the symptoms of exposure ker-

atopathy. Antihistamines may be helpful in managing inflammatory ectropion associated with allergy. Ectropion secondary to Bell's palsy usually improves spontaneously with resolution of the palsy. Patients with nonresolving ectropion should be referred for surgical repair when indicated.

SUGGESTED READING

Bajandas FJ, Kline LB. Neuro-ophthalmology Review Manual (3rd ed). Thorofare, NJ: Slack, 1988.

Bartlett JD, Jaanus SD. Clinical Ocular Pharmacology (3rd ed). Boston: Butterworth–Heinemann, 1995.

Berkow R, Fletcher AJ. The Merck Manual of Diagnosis and Therapy. Rahway, NJ: Merck, 1992.

Fraunfelder FT, Roy FH. Current Ocular Therapy 4. Philadelphia: Saunders, 1995.

Margo CE, Hamed LM, Mames RN. Diagnostic Problems in Clinical Ophthalmology. Philadelphia: Saunders, 1994.

Marks ES, Adamczyk DT, Thomann KH. Primary Eyecare in Systemic Disease. Norwalk, CT: Appleton & Lange, 1995.

Roberts DK, Terry JE. Ocular Disease: Diagnosis and Treatment (2nd ed). Boston: Butterworth–Heinemann, 1996.

Roy FH. Ocular Differential Diagnosis (5th ed). Philadelphia: Lea & Febiger, 1993.

van Heuven WAJ, Zwaan JT. Decision Making in Ophthalmology. St. Louis: Mosby–Year Book, 1992.

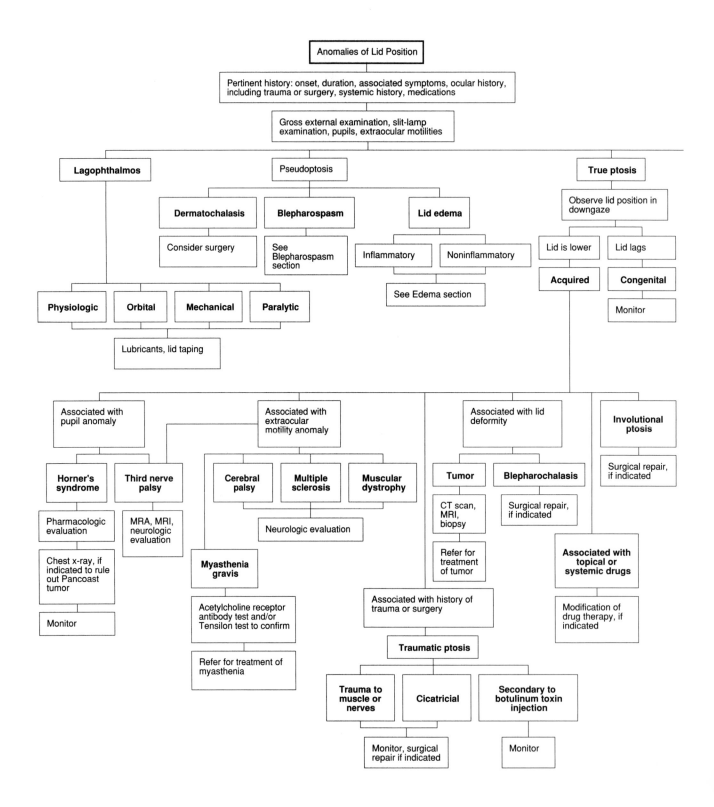

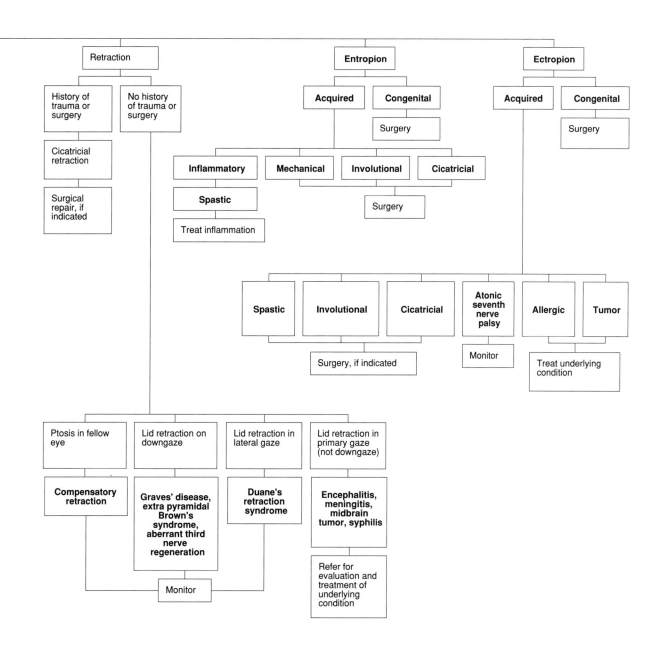

33

Injection of the Sclera or Episclera

FRANK P. LARUSSA

INJECTION OF THE SCLERA OR EPISCLERA AT A GLANCE

Scleritis
Episcleritis
Thyroid eye disease
Arteriovenous fistula (carotid cavernous or dural cavernous)
Cavernous sinus thrombosis
Polycythemia
Leukemia
Neoplasm (underlying uveal melanoma)
Right-sided heart failure

A patient with injection beneath the conjunctiva often is a clinically challenging case to diagnose. Scleritis and episcleritis are the most probable diagnoses, but distinguishing between these two can be difficult at times. When a patient is noted to have deep injection, the first step is to take a careful case history. The patient's symptoms often help the clinician make the diagnosis. A helpful test is to instill 2.5% epinephrine in the affected eye and observe whether it causes the affected vessels to blanch.

SCLERITIS

Subjective

Scleritis is a relatively rare inflammatory condition that can affect both the anterior and posterior sclera. Patients with anterior scleritis often complain of eye pain and redness. The pain is far more intense than that typically experienced by patients with episcleritis. Tearing, photophobia, and decreased vision may also be present. Patients with scleritis often have an associated connective tissue disease such as rheumatoid arthritis, systemic vasculitis, ankylosing spondylitis, or systemic lupus erythematosus.

Objective

Anterior scleritis can be classified as diffuse, nodular, or necrotizing. The necrotizing form may be further divided into inflammatory and noninflammatory (scleromalacia perforans). Biomicroscopy reveals purple or deep bluish red injection. Topical phenylephrine does not blanch the injection. There may be associated scleral thinning, particularly with necrotizing anterior scleritis. B-scan ultrasonography is useful in ruling out associated posterior scleritis.

Plan

Patients with scleritis may be treated with topical and oral nonsteroidal anti-inflammatory agents or topical and oral steroids. Immunosuppressive therapy may also be instituted in cases that do not respond well to other therapies. Scleral grafts may be used if perforation is impending. Patients with scleritis should also be referred to their internists or family practitioners for a systemic workup if the underlying cause is unknown.

EPISCLERITIS

Subjective

Episcleritis is a common condition with a sudden onset. Patients with episcleritis often complain of eye redness and mild discomfort. The eye is often described as feeling warm. Other symptoms include tearing and photophobia. A history of recurrence is common. Simple episcleritis is much less frequently associated with systemic disease than is scleritis. Nodular episcleritis, however, is often associated with an underlying systemic disorder such as Crohn's disease.

Objective

Episcleritis is typically unilateral. Biomicroscopy usually reveals a sectoral or diffuse area of vessel injection. Episcleritis occasionally can be nodular. The more superficial episcleral vessels blanch with 2.5% phenylephrine.

Plan

The patient with episcleritis can be treated with artificial tears or topical decongestants. If the patient is particularly symptomatic, topical steroids or oral nonsteroidal anti-inflammatory agents can be prescribed. The patient generally does not need a systemic workup unless the episcleritis is nodular or there are other significant systemic symptoms.

SUGGESTED READING

Bartlett JD, Jaanus SD. Clinical Ocular Pharmacology (3rd ed). Boston: Butterworth–Heinemann, 1995.
Roy FH. Ocular Differential Diagnosis (5th ed). Philadelphia: Lea & Febiger, 1993.

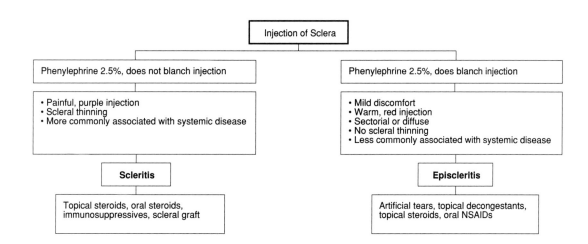

34

Lesions of the Iris

David P. Sendrowski

LESIONS OF THE IRIS AT A GLANCE

Pigmented lesions
  Adenoma
  Anterior staphyloma
  Congenital cyst
  Traumatic cyst
  Malignant melanoma
  Metastatic carcinoma
  Neurofibromatosis (Lisch nodules)
  Nevus
  Pigment epithelial tumor
  Ectropion uveae
  Foreign body
Nonpigmented lesions
  Amelanotic melanoma
  Fibrosarcoma
  Foreign body
  Hemangioma
  Iris cyst
  Iris nodules (Koeppe, Busacca)
  Metastatic carcinoma
  Sarcoid nodule
  Neuroglioma
  Tuberculosis (miliary, granulomatous)
  Fibrotic scar
  Brushfield's spots

Many lesions of the iris are asymptomatic. The diagnosis is often made on the basis of clinical examination and ancillary diagnostic procedures. The clinician should therefore be familiar with the clinical features and variations of iris lesions. This knowledge allows a more accurate referral to an ophthalmologist or ophthalmic oncologist, who may elect to obtain a biopsy of the lesion to gain additional information.

IRIS COLOBOMA

Subjective

A number of congenital anomalies arise from the localized failure of the fetal optic tissue to close. One of these anomalies is iris coloboma (coloboma iridis). The patient history should include questions regarding birth weight, term of pregnancy of the mother, and the presence of other congenital defects. Patients with isolated iris coloboma present with few complaints other than concern about the cosmetic appearance of the misshapen pupils. Patients who have a posterior segment coloboma in addition to an iris coloboma often have significant vision loss.

Objective

Visual acuity is unaffected by an iris coloboma. Pupils react normally in the region outside the coloboma. Transillumination through the coloboma can be noted during pupil examination. Dilation should be performed because iris colobomas may be associated with more extensive colobomas in the posterior segment of the eye. These associated colobomas may be visually significant and may be associated with other systemic anomalies. If there is an associated coloboma of the nerve head, threshold visual field testing should be carried out to evaluate the extent of the visual field defect.

Plan

Patients who are asymptomatic need only reassurance that the condition will not progress. If the cosmetic aspect is of concern, an opaque-iris contact lens may be used to improve the overall appearance. Routine follow-up for these patients should occur on a regular basis.

SIMPLE CONGENITAL HETEROCHROMIA

Subjective

Iris heterochromia (differently colored irides) can be congenital or acquired. It can be associated with conditions such as Horner's syndrome, iridocorneal epithelial syndrome, Fuchs' heterochromic iridocyclitis, and chronic uveitis. It can also be caused by intraocular foreign bodies and the monocular use of certain medications such as latanoprost. With congenital heterochromia, there are no subjective complaints other than the cosmetic appearance. Congenital heterochromia is not associated with glaucoma; however, in acquired cases of heterochromia, the patient may develop glaucoma.

Objective

The condition manifests as a lack of pigmentation in the affected eye. The condition may affect the entire iris of one eye or may be sectoral. The pupillary reactions, anterior chamber, and intraocular pressure should be carefully assessed to rule out heterochromia associated with other ocular conditions.

Plan

No treatment other than patient reassurance is indicated. If the patient is concerned about cosmetic appearance, the use of tinted contact lenses may be desirable.

HETEROCHROMIA FROM CONGENITAL HORNER'S SYNDROME

Subjective

Most cases of congenital Horner's syndrome are secondary to trauma. In rare instances, this condition may be caused by neuroblastoma, lymphoma, or metastasis. Patients with heterochromia due to congenital Horner's syndrome are typically asymptomatic but may be concerned about the cosmetic appearance of the heterochromia.

Objective

The clinician should pay close attention to the pupils and the lids. In Horner's syndrome, the pupil in the lighter iris may be smaller due to little or no sympathetic tone. Therefore, when the iris is stressed in dark and light environments, the asymmetry should increase in the dark. The lid on the affected eye may also show a slight ptosis. The amount of ptosis is usually 1–2 mm. The lid fold is usually lost, and this absence can be a confirmatory sign. The lower lid may be somewhat elevated as a result of the paresis of the smooth muscle. The side of the face with the lighter iris may also show anhydrosis. The practitioner can test for this sign by having the patient perform some physically exerting task for a short time and then looking for lack of perspiration on the affected side. After this exertion, talcum powder blown gently on each side of the face may fail to adhere to the affected side.

Testing with 10% topical cocaine and 1% hydroxy-amphetamine can be used to confirm the diagnosis of Horner's syndrome and to help localize the lesion.

Plan

Because the cause of heterochromia in children is usually disruption of sympathetic tone by trauma, no treatment is necessary. The parents and patient should be reassured of the benign nature of the heterochromia. A referral to a pediatrician or pediatric oncologist is not indicated.

ALBINISM

Subjective

In albinism, there is typically no subjective complaint about the iris itself. The iris condition is usually just one of the findings noted as the clinician is examining a patient with albinism. Patients with oculocutaneous albinism show macular hypoplasia and very poor vision with secondary nystagmus. They have a tendency toward high refractive errors, usually myopia. They are very photophobic due to the lack of pigmentation. Three common types of albinism exist: tyrosinase, or negative oculocutaneous albinism; positive oculocutaneous albinism; and ocular albinism.

Objective

In albinism, the eyebrows and eyelashes may be white. The irides appear light blue or red, and the pupils may appear to be red. The use of retroillumination from the retina almost always shows iris transillumination.

The fundus examination reveals a very visible choroidal vasculature, and hypoplasia of the macula is always present. The poorly developed macula is often associated with a searching nystagmus.

The visual acuity is usually poor if a nystagmus is present. The patient is usually photophobic as well.

Plan

The patient with poor visual acuity and a searching nystagmus should be referred to a low vision consultant, and should be prescribed UV-radiation protection for the eyes. Consultation with a dermatologist should also be recommended if the patient has not already been evaluated by such a specialist.

IRIS NEVUS

Subjective

An iris nevus is a pigmented lesion of the iris stroma. It may become more apparent during puberty and is more visible on lightly colored irides. Most commonly a patient with an iris nevus complains of the cosmetic appearance of a dark bump or spot on the iris.

Objective

The clinician should evaluate the lesion for elevation. Most nevi are flat and do not exceed 3 mm in diameter. The lesion should also be evaluated for vascularization. Most nevi are not vascularized.

Nevi are more common in the inferior half of the iris. If they are located close to the pupillary margin, they may cause ectropion uveae. Nevi may also be associated with a sectorial cataract or secondary glaucoma, but these occurrences are rare.

A dilated fundus examination should be performed to rule out additional nevi of the uveal tract and to evaluate changes in the lens. A visual field and optic nerve head evaluation should be performed to rule out secondary glaucoma. Gonioscopy should be considered to rule out any lesions in the ciliary body. Most nevi do not grow over time, and malignant transformation is very rare.

Plan

Photodocumentation is important to aid in noting any change over time. The patient can be monitored on a yearly basis if there has been no evidence of change after the initial finding. If there is change over time, the patient should be referred for a biopsy.

The patient should be educated about the importance of monitoring the lesion. Some practitioners advocate prescribing UV-radiation protection in an attempt to reduce potential abnormalities in the uveal tract.

LISCH NODULE

Subjective

Lisch nodules are usually found during examination of the iris of a patient with neurofibromatosis.

The nodules alone are not diagnostic of this disorder, and additional physical findings should be sought to confirm the diagnosis of neurofibromatosis. Although the Lisch nodules are congenital, they usually do not become clinically apparent until the individual has reached the second or third decade of life. Lisch nodules typically cause no symptoms.

Objective

Lisch nodules manifest as one or more discrete, pigmented stromal masses on the iris. They are often found bilaterally. There may be associated tumors on the lids or elsewhere on the skin that can be isolated cutaneous neurofibromas or plexiform ("bag of worms") neurofibromas. The patient may also have café-au-lait spots (small pigmented areas) on the skin, usually six or more. They are very significant when they occur on the axillary region of the body. In addition, the optic nerves may have a glioma, which is very suggestive of neurofibromatosis.

Plan

The patient should be referred to an internist for a systemic workup for neurofibromatosis if this has not already occurred. The patient needs to be followed closely for development of lesions in the optic nerve heads and visual pathways. A threshold visual field test should be performed to obtain baseline data and should be repeated periodically to look for changes. Dilated fundus examination should also be performed. When neurofibromas are confined to the skin, the prognosis is fairly good. When there are intracranial and intraspinal lesions, the prognosis is more guarded.

POSTINFLAMMATORY IRIS ATROPHY

Subjective

Herpes zoster is one of the primary causes of postinflammatory iris atrophy. Anterior segment surgery is another common cause. Patients who have herpes zoster uveitis are generally over age 50 or have a compromised immune system. They have a history of having a painful, red eye with the vesicular dermal changes that accompany herpes zoster. There may or may not be evidence of the dermal lesions of herpes zoster. The patient's history should include previous infection with chickenpox, usually as a child.

Objective

The iris shows an area of sectorial or diffuse atrophy. There may be ectropion uveae along with the atrophy.

Pigment is often scattered throughout tissues in the anterior segment, and the iris vessels are replaced with sclerosed white lines.

The finding that best distinguishes postinflammatory atrophies from normal senile atrophy is the presence of synechiae. They may be either posterior or peripheral anterior synechiae. Gonioscopy is a superb technique for locating peripheral anterior synechiae.

The intraocular pressure may be elevated, especially if the filtration angle was damaged during the inflammatory process. Neovascularization of the iris is uncommon because of the abrupt ischemic nature of the event.

Plan

The patient should be evaluated for changes in intraocular pressure, corneal infection, and retinal involvement. The patient should be instructed to return immediately for evaluation and treatment if the involved eye becomes red or painful.

IRIS METASTASIS

Subjective

The patient with iris metastasis has a primary cancer elsewhere in the body that may or may not have been previously diagnosed. The patient may observe bumps on the iris that the patient reports are new. This finding in association with a history of cancer should alert the clinician to the potential of iris metastasis.

Objective

The iris may show multiple metastatic tumors, in contrast to iris melanoma, in which there is typically a single lesion. The metastatic lesions may appear as irregular, vascularized, gray-white tumors and may also be bilateral. The superior and inferior portions of the iris may be affected equally. It is not uncommon for the metastasis to liberate cells and create a pseudohypopyon in the anterior chamber. Other features can include an irregular pupil, iridocyclitis, rubeosis iridis, secondary glaucoma, and hyphema.

A dilated fundus examination should be performed to rule out metastatic lesions in other areas of the uveal tract.

Plan

The patient should be referred to an oncologist or internist immediately, and the findings reported. If the patient is already undergoing treatment for the primary cancer, external beam irradiation may be used as a local measure for the iris metastasis. The patient should be followed

very closely for development of any new iris tumors and dilated for evaluation of the posterior uveal tract.

IRIS CYST

Subjective

An iris cyst is found most often during a routine eye examination. The patient usually is unaware of its presence and has no ocular complaints related to the cyst.

Objective

Biomicroscopic examination reveals that part or all of the middle to peripheral portion of the iris bulges forward. There is no pigment change over the bulge. The clinician should suspect iris cysts if there is an abrupt, localized area of bulging in one or more locations. If the pupil can be widely dilated, use of a gonioscopy lens may help in visualizing the iris cyst.

The cyst is usually clear or very slightly pigmented. It may wobble with eye movement. In contrast, ciliary body melanomas are heavily pigmented and do not wobble with eye movement. The gonioscopy lens should also be used to visualize the filtration angle. The iris cyst may narrow the iris/angle approach and predispose the patient to an angle-closure attack. Such an occurrence is more common if the cyst is present circumferentially around the angle. B-scan ultrasonography or ultrasonic biomicroscopy should show the cyst to be fluid filled. Transillumination of the cyst should demonstrate that it transmits light, unlike solid pigmented tumors.

Plan

If the cyst puts the patient at risk for angle closure or obscures part or all of the visual axis, the patient should be referred for disruption of the cyst. This treatment is accomplished using an argon laser.

If the cyst is localized, the clinician should photodocument it and monitor for changes such as glaucoma and cataract formation.

The patient should be reassured as to the benign nature of the lesion and educated about the need to watch for changes over time.

IRIS MELANOMA

Subjective

In iris melanoma, the patient may suddenly become aware of a pigmented spot on the iris, or it may be found as part of a routine eye examination. The clinician's suspicion should be raised if the patient has a light complexion, because iris melanomas are most common among whites and are rare in blacks.

Included in the patient history should be questions concerning previously diagnosed cancer, ocular surgery, trauma, weight loss, and anorexia.

Objective

An iris melanoma is a slow-growing lesion. It is dark brown or amelanotic. It is usually raised and greater than 3 mm in diameter at the base, and a prominent feeder vessel may course throughout the lesion. The melanoma can produce ectropion uveae and extend into the chamber angle, possibly producing secondary glaucoma. It may produce a pseudohypopyon by seeding tumor cells into the anterior chamber. Clinicians should use high magnification in the slit lamp to evaluate the characteristics of the cells. A dilated fundus examination, gonioscopy, ultrasonography, and transillumination of the lesion should all be performed.

Plan

Photodocumentation is an excellent way to monitor changes in a lesion. The patient with a suspicious lesion should be referred to an ophthalmologist or ophthalmic oncologist for biopsy and evaluation of the lesion.

SUGGESTED READING

Bartlett JD, Jaanus SD. Clinical Ocular Pharmacology (3rd ed). Boston: Butterworth–Heinemann, 1995.

Char CH. Intraocular Masquerade Syndromes. In TD Duane (ed), Clinical Ophthalmology. Vol 4. Philadelphia: Lippincott, 1993;1–12.

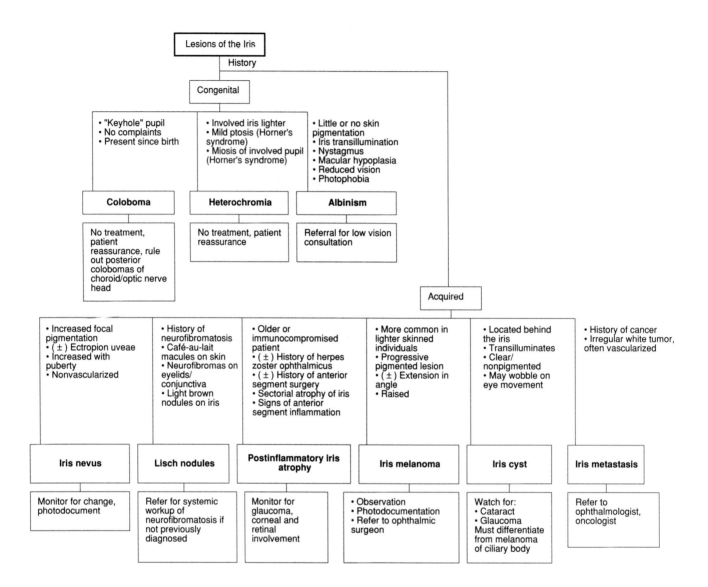

35

Acute Iritis and Iridocyclitis

DAVID P. SENDROWSKI

ACUTE IRITIS AND IRIDOCYCLITIS AT A GLANCE

Iritis and iridocyclitis
  Idiopathic anterior uveitis
  Ankylosing spondylitis
  Inflammatory bowel disease
  Behçet's syndrome
  Sarcoidosis
  Candidiasis
  Coccidioidomycosis
  Cysticercosis
  Cytomegalovirus
  Post–laser surgery
  Fuchs' heterochromic iridocyclitis
  Herpes simplex
  Herpes zoster
  Reiter's disease
  Rubella syndrome
  Juvenile rheumatoid arthritis
  Syphilis
  Tuberculosis
  Vogt-Koyanagi-Harada syndrome
  Sympathetic ophthalmia
  Posner-Schlossman syndrome
  Trauma
  Lens induced
  Lyme disease
Masquerade syndromes
  Adenocarcinoma
  Adenoma
  Glioneuroma
  Medulloepithelioma
  Ciliary body cyst
  Malignant melanoma
  Melanocytoma
  Post-traumatic pigmentary migration

Acute anterior segment inflammation is characterized by a rapid onset of symptoms of pain, redness, photophobia, and blurring of vision, although these symptoms can exist to varying degrees. Acute iridocyclitis is an anatomic diagnosis with inflammatory activity that primarily involves the anterior uvea. Some systemic disorders affect both the anterior and posterior uveal tissues. There are also some noninflammatory conditions that mimic uveitis; these are termed *masquerade syndromes.*

Anterior uveitis is most commonly of unknown origin; however, some types of anterior uveitis are associated with systemic disease. Certain laboratory and radiologic tests can be valuable aids to the clinician in searching for the cause of uveitis.

IDIOPATHIC ANTERIOR UVEITIS

Subjective

The patient with acute idiopathic anterior uveitis is commonly between the ages of 18 and 50. The patient typically complains of a sudden onset of eye pain, redness, and photophobia. There is no history of trauma or previous similar episodes. Acute idiopathic iritis is almost always unilateral. Other associated symptoms that the patient may have are decreased vision and tearing.

If the uveitis is recurrent, thorough medical and ocular histories should be obtained to rule out underlying systemic disease.

Objective

The first goal of the examination is to rule out other causes of red eye such as an infectious or inflammatory conjunctivitis and acute glaucoma. The entrance testing should include a pupillary examination. In iritis, the pupil in the affected eye is miotic, whereas in acute glaucoma it is fixed and dilated. Conjunctivitis does not affect pupillary response. Externally, the vasculature in the limbal area is engorged so that there is circumlimbal flush. The patient may also show ptosis or blepharospasm in the affected eye as a result of photophobia. Confrontation field testing usually suffices for screening the visual field and should reveal no defects.

The biomicroscope should be used with conical beam illumination to evaluate the inflammatory reaction in the anterior chamber. In idiopathic iritis, the clinician may note cells and flare. Cells are usually the more prominent feature in the early stages of the inflammation. The intraocular pressure is often lowered secondary to ciliary body inflammation, but may rise as time passes.

The patient should have a binocular indirect ophthalmoscopic examination of the fundus to rule out a posterior inflammatory cause for the anterior chamber reaction.

Plan

The patient should be given a long-acting cycloplegic agent (e.g., homatropine) to reduce synechia formation. The inflammation should be treated with topical steroids (e.g., prednisolone acetate) every 1–4 hours depending on the severity of the reaction. A topical beta blocker (e.g., timolol) can be used to reduce the intraocular pressure if it is elevated.

A follow-up visit should occur between 24 and 48 hours after the initial examination so the clinician can evaluate the effect of the topical steroid and make sure the patient is complying well with the treatment regimen. The intraocular pressure and cornea should be checked at each follow-up visit. Administration of the topical steroids should be based on the anterior chamber reaction. If the anterior chamber reaction shows improvement, the steroid can be tapered. The patient should be seen several months after the inflammation has resolved to determine whether there are residual ocular effects.

ANKYLOSING SPONDYLITIS

Subjective

The patient with ankylosing spondylitis is typically a young man between the ages of 20 and 40. Whites are more commonly affected than any other race. Patients with this condition usually present with complaints of ocular pain, photophobia, tearing, and a mild decrease in visual acuity.

The history should include questions about lower back pain, particularly pain that occurs in the morning and goes away with time. The lower back pain is usually present for more than 3 months. Chest pain on full chest expansion may also be a complaint. Information regarding any family history of arthritis, rheumatoid disease, or ankylosing spondylitis should be obtained as well.

Objective

Entrance testing should reveal a miotic and less reactive pupil in the involved eye. There may be a circumlimbal flush around the corneal limbal area. A mild to severe blepharospasm may also be present as a result of the pain and light sensitivity of the eye.

The diagnosis of anterior uveitis is based on the presence of cells and flare in the anterior chamber. The quantity of cells defines the severity of the inflammation. The intraocular pressure may be decreased initially from ciliary body inflammation. A dilated examination should reveal no or few cells in the posterior segment. A predominance of white cells in the vitreous suggests a posterior uveitis. The ophthalmoscopic appearance of the retina is usually normal.

The anterior lens should also be examined for the presence of synechiae, which form fairly quickly in this disorder. Gonioscopy is usually reserved until the patient is in less pain and the inflammation has resolved.

Additional tests that can be helpful in confirming the diagnosis of ankylosing spondylitis are radiographs of the sacroiliac region of the back, complete blood count (CBC), erythrocyte sedimentation rate (ESR), and an HLA-B27 antigen test.

Plan

The ocular treatment typically consists of a strong cycloplegic agent (e.g., homatropine) instilled two times a day and a topical steroid (e.g., prednisolone acetate) instilled every 1–4 hours initially to reduce the inflammation. In some cases, the steroid may need to be continued for up to 4–5 weeks. The steroid should be tapered according to the cellular response in the anterior chamber. Oral anti-inflammatory agents (e.g., indomethacin) may also be helpful in reducing ocular and systemic inflammation. Oral analgesics (e.g., codeine) may be used on a short-term basis to reduce ocular pain, if the patient is in extreme discomfort.

The patient should be referred to a rheumatologist or internist for evaluation and potential treatment of the underlying systemic disorder. In addition, the patient should be educated regarding the seriousness of a sudden onset of pain and redness in the eye and the need to seek immediate care if such symptoms occur.

INFLAMMATORY BOWEL DISEASE

Subjective

Patients with acute or chronic bowel disease have a slight risk of developing a secondary iritis. The clinician should question the patient about an onset of diarrhea or constipation concurrent with the iritis. Abdominal pain, weight loss, vomiting, dehydration, and low-grade fever signal the onset of a flare up. The patient should specifically be asked about Crohn's disease, Whipple's disease, and colitis.

The ocular complaints are very similar to those of idiopathic iritis: There is a sudden onset of pain, photophobia, and redness with secondary tearing and mild visual acuity loss. If these symptoms are coupled with the recent diagnosis of bowel disease or exacerbation of a previously diagnosed bowel disease, the clinician should be highly suspicious of a secondary iritis.

Objective

Entrance testing should reveal a miotic and less reactive pupil in the affected eye. There may be some blepharospasm of the eye from ocular pain. A circumlimbal flush around the corneal limbal area may also be noted.

The clinician should look for cells and moderate flare in the anterior chamber. Early formation of posterior synechiae are not uncommon and they are easily broken. Intraocular pressure readings may be lower in the affected eye.

After dilation, a binocular indirect ophthalmoscopic examination should be performed to rule out posterior segment inflammation. Gonioscopy is usually performed after symptoms have subsided to rule out peripheral anterior synechiae. Additional testing may include a CBC, ESR, radiographs of the hands, and an HLA-B27 antigen test.

Plan

The ocular treatment is similar to that described for ankylosing spondylitis. The patient should be referred to a gas-

trointestinal specialist or internist for evaluation and treatment of the underlying systemic condition. The patient should be educated regarding the association between the ocular inflammation and exacerbation of the inflammatory bowel disease. Patients should also be warned about developing hypovitaminosis A. Supplemental vitamin A may be recommended as adjunct therapy.

TUBERCULOSIS

Subjective

The individuals at greatest risk of developing tuberculosis are African-Americans, Hispanic Americans, Native Americans, the elderly, and persons who have resided in areas where the disease is prevalent, such as Asia, Africa, and Mexico. Alcoholics, prison inmates, intravenous drug users, and acquired immunodeficiency syndrome patients are also at high risk.

The patient should be asked about productive cough, hemoptysis, night sweats, weight loss, chest pain, and anorexia. The history should include questions regarding recent travel, intravenous drug use, indwelling catheters, skin lesions or rashes, systemic diseases, and blood-borne diseases. The ocular symptoms more commonly encountered are blurred vision, floaters, pain, and photophobia.

Objective

The anterior segment may show phlyctenules, conjunctival nodules, episcleritis, and scleritis. Iritis can appear as a granulomatous or nongranulomatous smoldering low-grade inflammation. The clinician should look for the presence of synechiae, cataracts, glaucoma, and iris nodules.

The dilated fundus examination may occasionally reveal choroidal granulomas. In miliary tuberculosis, choroidal tubercles may be present. These are small, white lesions with blurred borders that have an appearance similar to that of histoplasmotic spots. Additionally, optic neuritis may be present and associated with the chronic inflammation.

Additional testing includes a purified protein derivative (PPD) skin test. A skin reaction suggests that the uveitis may be a result of tuberculosis. It should be noted that the PPD test can elicit either a false-negative or false-positive result. Results of an anergy panel can help in the interpretation of a false-negative result. If the skin test is positive, chest radiography and sputum culture can help confirm the diagnosis.

Isoniazid may also be used diagnostically as well as therapeutically. If the ocular inflammation responds to a 2- to 3-week trial of the drug, it is strongly suggested that tuberculosis is the underlying cause.

Plan

The patient should be referred to an internist for treatment of the systemic disease. Therapy may include isoniazid, rifampin, ethambutol, and pyrazinamide for the resistant strains.

The uveitis usually responds to topical cycloplegics (e.g., homatropine) used two to three times a day and topical steroids (e.g., prednisolone acetate) used every hour to four times a day, depending on the severity of the inflammation. Concurrent systemic therapy helps resolve the anterior and posterior segment inflammation.

BEHÇET'S DISEASE

Subjective

Behçet's disease is a multisystem disease that most commonly affects young males of Japanese or Mediterranean origin. The patient with anterior uveitis due to Behçet's disease typically complains of a very rapid onset of bilateral eye pain and photophobia. Unlike the other iridocyclitic syndromes, bilateral onset is more commonly seen in this disease. Ocular symptoms also include redness, tearing, and vision loss if there is posterior segment involvement.

Patients may also complain of (or should be asked about) oral aphthous ulcers, a very common finding in Behçet's disease. Genital ulcerations, erythema nodosum–like lesions on the anterior aspect of the legs, and arthritis of the weight-bearing joints are other systemic signs. Patients may also complain of cough, chest pain, dyspnea, and hemoptysis. Occasionally, associated central nervous system involvement may manifest as confusion, meningomyelitis, and local ischemic effects.

Objective

Entrance testing may reveal good to poor visual acuity depending on the involvement of the posterior pole. Amsler grid testing should be performed to help rule out macular involvement. Pupillary testing reveals bilateral miotic pupils. Biomicroscopic examination shows a severe anterior chamber reaction, often with a hypopyon. The hypopyon has been shown to be transient and is usually formed because of the explosive onset of the inflammation.

Dilated fundus examination may show the posterior pole and retina to be normal, or it may reveal a retinal vasculitis. Posterior segment involvement usually presents with vitreous inflammatory cells from an underlying retinal or choroidal vasculitis. The vasculitis may lead to retinal edema and/or retinal hypoxia, which in turn could result in neovascularization of the retina. Additionally, testing might include a CBC, ESR, and an HLA-B27 or HLA-B5 antigen test. A Behçet's skin puncture test might be considered if the active systemic disease is present.

Plan

Topical steroids (e.g., prednisolone acetate) and oral steroids (e.g., prednisone) are the mainstays of the initial treatment. The topical steroids should be prescribed every 1–4 hours in accordance with the severity of the anterior chamber reaction. Oral steroids are given at a dosage of 60–80 mg per day depending on the degree of the inflammation. A long-acting cycloplegic agent (e.g., homatropine) should be used to reduce the chance of posterior synechia formation.

The patient should be comanaged with a rheumatologist or internist. Treatment may include the use of immunosuppressive agents if the patient does not respond well to corticosteroid therapy. The long-term prognosis varies depending on the severity of the inflammatory process and secondary complications. The ocular inflammation becomes harder to control with each subsequent attack.

HERPES SIMPLEX

Subjective

Herpes simplex anterior uveitis is the result of corneal irritation from a herpes simplex ulcerative keratitis. It can also be caused by active virus inside the anterior chamber. The ulcerative keratitis is present concurrently with the iritis. The patient may complain of foreign body sensation, photophobia, tearing, and decreased vision. It is sometimes possible to uncover a history of previous episodes of herpes simplex keratitis. Approximately 500,000 cases of ocular herpes simplex are reported in the United States each year.

Objective

The eye may show a miotic pupil if the anterior chamber reaction is present. Biomicroscopic examination should reveal an epithelial lesion with a dendritic or geographic pattern that stains centrally with sodium fluorescein and stains peripherally with rose bengal. Drawing a cotton wisp over the involved area may reveal corneal hypoesthesia. Use of conical beam illumination to investigate the anterior chamber reveals a mild cellular response with little or no flare. The iris should be checked for posterior synechiae formation. A dilated fundus examination should also be performed to rule out any posterior segment inflammation, which, if present, requires immediate treatment.

Corneal scrapings may be collected for Giemsa staining and viral culture if there is doubt as to the type of keratitis present.

Plan

The keratitis should be treated with a topical antiviral agent (e.g., trifluridine), which is usually administered nine times a day. The iritis is best treated with a topical cycloplegic agent (e.g., homatropine) administered two or three times a day. There is usually no need for a topical steroid. Steroid therapy should be considered if the uveitis is still present after 1 week. The patient should be re-evaluated 24–48 hours after initiation of topical therapy. The course of the keratitis and uveitis is variable, but most cases resolve in 10–14 days.

The use of an oral antiviral (e.g., acyclovir) should be considered if the uveitis fails to respond to the topical therapy.

FUCHS' HETEROCHROMIC IRIDOCYCLITIS

Subjective

Fuchs' heterochromic iridocyclitis occurs in both males and females, usually in the third or fourth decade of life. There are few symptoms with this type of uveitis, and it is sometimes detected during a routine eye examination. The patient may notice a decrease in visual acuity from secondary cataract formation. Additional complaints include floaters, fluctuating vision, and metamorphopsia.

Objective

The hallmark of this disease is the heterochromia, with a lighter colored iris in the affected eye. Pupillary abnormalities may exist if posterior synechiae are present.

Biomicroscopic examination should reveal a diffuse endothelial distribution of fine keratitic precipitates. There is no spindle formation on the inferior corneal endothelium as is found in other types of uveitis. A mild anterior chamber reaction and a few, if any, posterior synechiae are present. The astute clinician may notice a blunting of

the iris architecture. Iris transillumination is present and is best seen as the pupil reaches a mid-dilated state. The intraocular pressure may be elevated from a neovascular glaucoma, which is common in this disorder. Gonioscopy should be performed to confirm the presence of neovascular involvement of the chamber angle.

The dilated fundus examination may reveal cataract formation and glaucoma, which are the result of a chronic inflammatory reaction in the eye. Vitreous cells and other vitreal opacities may be found in these patients as well.

Plan

Because uveitis is often chronic in Fuchs' heterochromic iridocyclitis, a topical steroid (e.g., prednisolone acetate) is indicated only for exacerbations of the inflammatory state. Topical cycloplegics (e.g., homatropine) can also be prescribed to reduce the chance of posterior synechia formation. The clinician should be very careful not to overtreat the uveitis. The clinician may have to accept the presence of a few cells in the anterior chamber, because it may be impossible to eradicate all the cells. Long-term use of topical steroids (e.g., prednisone acetate) may hasten cataract and glaucoma development. Topical beta blockers and topical or oral carbonic anhydrase inhibitors may be indicated if the intraocular pressure is elevated secondary to neovascular glaucoma.

In more severe cases, the patient should be comanaged with a rheumatologist. Cataract extraction may be indicated if the visual acuity is reduced to a level that impedes the performance of normal or required visual tasks.

SARCOIDOSIS

Subjective

In the United States, sarcoidosis is a disease that is more prevalent among African-Americans. The condition presents bilaterally and occurs more frequently in females. Therefore, an African-American woman in the third or fourth decade of life with a complaint of mild to moderate photophobia, pain, and redness should be suspected of having sarcoidosis. Other ocular symptoms may include watery eyes, irritation, and decrease in visual acuity.

The pulmonary system is frequently affected by sarcoidosis; therefore, the patient should be asked about difficulty in breathing, hemoptysis, wheezing, and coughing spells. Other systemic symptoms include weight loss, anorexia, and fever. The liver and central nervous system may also be involved.

Objective

Entrance testing should include a thorough examination of the periocular and facial skin to evaluate the areas for sarcoid nodules. Pupillary testing may or may not be normal depending on the length and severity of the ocular inflammation. If possible, Amsler grid testing should be done to rule out macular involvement.

A biomicroscopic examination should begin with evaluation of the palpebral and bulbar conjunctiva for evidence of sarcoid granulomas. The lacrimal gland, if involved, may be enlarged. Lacrimal gland enlargement or dacryoadenitis may be an early finding in sarcoidosis. The corneal endothelium should be evaluated for large, greasy keratitic precipitates usually referred to as *mutton fat*. The anterior chamber should be evaluated for cells and flare. The anterior surface of the lens may reveal evidence of previous or present posterior synechiae formation. The iris should be evaluated near the pupillary frill for Koeppe nodules and in the midperiphery for larger Busacca nodules. The intraocular pressure may be elevated from glaucoma, which sometimes occurs with sarcoidosis.

A dilated fundus examination should be performed, and the lens, vitreous, and retina should be thoroughly evaluated. The lens may show evidence of cataract formation from chronic inflammatory insult. The vitreous may show evidence of inflammation in the form of vitreous "snowballs," or large accumulations of inflammatory cells. The optic nerve head should be evaluated to rule out optic disc edema and neovascularization. The retinal vasculature should be evaluated for retinal periphlebitis in the midperiphery. Other entities that should be ruled out are nodules at the level of the choroid (Dalen-Fuchs nodules) and macular edema. Yellow-white, waxy retinal exudates (termed *candle-wax drippings*) may appear adjacent to retinal veins and are very diagnostic of the disease.

A test used to confirm the diagnosis of sarcoidosis is chest radiography, which demonstrates hilar adenopathy of the lungs. A biopsy of conjunctival granulomas may also be helpful in confirming the diagnosis. Blood testing may show elevations of angiotensin-converting enzyme (ACE), serum lysozyme, and serum calcium. A PPD test should be performed to rule out tuberculosis, and antinuclear antibody (ANA) testing can be also be used to rule out an autoimmune etiology.

Plan

The uveitis is treated with a topical cycloplegic agent (e.g., homatropine) and a topical steroid (e.g., prednisolone acetate). The use of periocular steroid injections may be required in those cases in which the uveitis does not respond to the topical therapy.

If there is concurrent posterior segment involvement, the use of oral steroids (e.g., prednisone) at 60–100 mg per day is indicated as the initial treatment to reduce the inflammatory reaction. If there is any evidence of neovascularization of the retina or optic nerve head, the patient should be referred to a retinologist. If there is associated glaucoma, a topical antiglaucoma medication (e.g., timolol) should be prescribed.

The patient should be followed every 3–5 days to evaluate the therapeutic response, and the steroid therapy should be adjusted accordingly. After the inflammation has subsided, the patient should be evaluated every 4–6 months. The time between office visits should be reduced for children with sarcoidosis. Comanagement with an internist or pediatrician is strongly recommended.

PARS PLANITIS

Subjective

The patient with pars planitis does not usually complain of redness or pain. The patient usually complains of floaters or a decrease in visual acuity. The complaints are almost always bilateral. The patients are young and usually present between the ages of 14 and 30. Visual acuity may be affected by ciliary body involvement, lens opacification, vitreous floaters, or macular edema. The patient should be questioned very specifically about loss of visual acuity and the onset of the floaters. To rule out other etiologies of the ocular inflammation, the clinician should ask the patient about residence in the Ohio/Missouri/Mississippi River valley areas as well as about a history of tick bites, recent ocular trauma, ocular surgery, blood-borne diseases, systemic diseases, and intravenous drug use.

Objective

Entrance testing usually reveals normal findings for confrontation fields and motility tests. Acuity loss from suspected macular involvement should be investigated with an Amsler grid test, followed by a photostress test.

Biomicroscopic examination may reveal a mild cellular response in the anterior chamber, with a greater response in the anterior vitreous or retrolental space. Pupil dilation and examination using a three-mirror gonioscopy lens may reveal a buildup of white cells at the inferior ora serrata, called *snowbanking*. This finding is very suggestive of pars planitis. If the three-mirror lens fails to provide an adequate view of the inferior ora, scleral indentation with binocular indirect ophthalmoscopy may be helpful.

A dilated fundus examination may also reveal posterior subcapsular cataracts, clumps of white blood cells or snowballs in the vitreous, posterior vitreous detachment, vitreous hemorrhage, cystoid macular edema (CME), sheathing of the retinal vessels, and retinal tears. Extended ophthalmoscopy and fluorescein angiography may be used to confirm the presence of macular edema.

The diagnosis of pars planitis is based primarily on the clinical appearance. If the diagnosis is in question, laboratory testing may include blood tests to rule out other forms of uveitis (i.e., fluorescent treponemal antibody absorption test [FTA-ABS], ESR, ANA test, *Toxoplasma* titer, and ACE levels). Additionally, chest radiography and diagnostic vitrectomy should be considered.

Plan

If the patient is experiencing discomfort, a topical steroid (e.g., prednisolone acetate) may be used to reduce the anterior chamber reaction. If CME is causing reduced acuity (>20/40), periocular repository steroid injections may be needed to reduce the edema. Alternatively, topical nonsteroidal anti-inflammatory agents (e.g., ketorolac tromethamine) may be used to reduce the CME. If local therapy is ineffective, oral steroids (e.g., prednisone) may be used over several weeks to reduce the CME. If steroid therapy is ineffective, cryotherapy, pars plana vitrectomy, or use of immunosuppressive agents may be necessary.

The patient should be followed every 5–7 days while under local or systemic treatment. The clinician should watch for secondary complications from long-term steroid use. The patient should be comanaged with a retinologist when there is CME or retinal vascular involvement. The patient can be followed every 4–6 months after the inflammation has subsided.

GLAUCOMATOCYCLITIC CRISIS (POSNER-SCHLOSSMAN SYNDROME)

Subjective

Patients with glaucomatocyclitic crisis are usually between 20 and 50 years of age. These patients typically present complaining of unilateral, mild to moderate ocular pain. They may also complain of colored haloes around lights if corneal edema is present. Unless this is the very first event, the patient may remember similar episodes in the past.

Objective

Entrance testing may show a mild decrease in visual acuity. Pupillary testing may reveal a larger or mid-dilated pupil with diminished light response.

Slit-lamp evaluation may show a few keratic precipitates on the endothelium and trace to 1+ cells in the anterior chamber. The intraocular pressure is a very useful diagnostic finding. It is markedly elevated, usually in the range of 35–60 mm Hg. Gonioscopy shows a wide-open angle without evidence of peripheral anterior synechiae and perhaps some mild debris in the trabecular meshwork. The presence of a wide-open angle rules out an angle-closure type of glaucoma. In contrast to patients with glaucomatocyclitic crisis, patients with pigmentary glaucoma usually manifest a Krukenberg spindle on the corneal epithelium and transillumination defects in the iris. Patients with Fuchs' heterochromic iridocyclitis do not show the marked elevation in intraocular pressure that is seen in glaucomatocyclitic crisis. The optic nerve head and visual fields should be evaluated for signs of glaucomatous damage, but normal findings are not uncommon.

Plan

The patient should be started on a topical antiglaucoma medication (e.g., timolol) administered twice a day, along with a topical steroid (e.g., prednisolone acetate) administered approximately four times a day. The steroid helps to reduce the inflammation of the trabecular meshwork, which in turn helps to reduce the pressure. Oral or topical carbonic anhydrase inhibitors (e.g., acetazolamide or dorzolamide hydrochloride) during the active episode are also beneficial in reducing the intraocular pressure.

Patients should be followed every 3–5 days initially to make sure the pressure is responding to therapy and the symptoms are diminishing. After resolution, the patient should be followed every 6 months. Patients may be given topical and oral medications to have on hand to counter future attacks.

JUVENILE RHEUMATOID ARTHRITIS

Subjective

The typical patient profile for this disease is that of a young girl with the diagnosis of pauciarticular-type juvenile rheumatoid arthritis. The anterior uveitis associated with this disease is frequently bilateral and causes very little pain, photophobia, or redness. It is possible for the ocular disease to precede, coincide with, or follow the onset of the arthritis. Pauciarticular arthritis (fewer than five joints involved) more frequently shows associated ocular involvement than do the other forms of juvenile rheumatoid arthritis. Children may be more sedentary because of joint inflammation. Occasionally, the parent may bring in the child with the complaint of leukocoria, which is secondary to a cataract formation in the lens.

Objective

Pupillary testing may show less reactive pupils secondary to chronic inflammation or posterior synechiae. An Amsler grid test may help to rule out macular edema. The conjunctiva is white or mildly injected. This finding is in contrast with the typical presentation of anterior uveitis in which circumlimbal injection is a prominent sign. Biomicroscopy may reveal band keratopathy and cataracts that result in leukocoria in more advanced cases. Biomicroscopy of the anterior chamber reveals few cells and mild flare.

Gonioscopy should be attempted to rule out peripheral anterior synechiae. Tonometry should be performed to monitor intraocular pressure, as glaucoma is common in these patients. A dilated fundus examination helps to evaluate the vitreous for the presence of white blood cells and to inspect the fundus for macular edema.

Laboratory and radiologic testing should include CBC, ESR, ANA tests, and radiography of joints with suspected arthritis, such as the knees. Additional tests to rule out other systemic etiologies might include rapid plasma reagin (RPR), microhemagglutination assay–*Treponema pallidum* (MHA-TP), PPD with anergy panel, Lyme titer (in areas where Lyme disease is more endemic), HLA-B27 antigen, and chest radiography.

Plan

If an anterior chamber angle reaction is present, a topical cycloplegic agent (e.g., homatropine) should be administered two to three times a day and a topical steroid (e.g., loteprednol etabonate) should be administered every 1–6 hours, depending on the severity of the inflammation. If topical steroids are ineffective, periocular repository steroids (e.g., methylprednisolone) may be effective. If periocular injections are ineffective, administration of oral steroids (e.g., prednisone) should be initiated. The clinician should be very conservative in the use of steroids in the pediatric population, and comanagement with a rheumatologist and a pediatrician is highly recommended. A major pitfall in the management of the juvenile rheumatoid arthritis patient is the desire to rid the anterior chamber of all cells and flare when that may not be possible. Long-term cycloplegic therapy may be the best treatment for the patient. The clinician may have to accept treating the inflammatory exacerbations of the disease.

If secondary glaucoma is present in association with the anterior chamber reaction, a topical nonselective beta blocker (e.g., timolol) usually brings the pressure under control. Additional topical glaucoma medications may occasionally be necessary.

If a cataract is present, the clinician should keep in mind that there is a moderate complication rate with cataract surgery in these patients. The benefits of visual rehabilitation must be weighed carefully against the possible deleterious effects of surgical complications.

TRAUMATIC IRITIS

Subjective

Trauma to the eye can result in abrasion or laceration of the external ocular structures, perforation of the globe, cataract, and damage to the chamber angle, retina, and choroid. Iritis can result from either sharp or blunt trauma to the anterior segment of the eye.

Objective

External examination may show evidence of the trauma, such as ecchymosis, subconjunctival hemorrhage, or abrasions or lacerations of the ocular and periocular tissues. The pupil is usually miotic as a result of inflammation or trauma to the sphincter muscle of the iris. The intraocular pressure may initially be low because of traumatic compression of aqueous fluid out of the eye. After several days, the intraocular pressure may be elevated as a result of inflammation or the presence of debris in the trabecular meshwork.

Biomicroscopic examination of the anterior chamber may show cells and possibly flare. The anterior chamber should also be evaluated for hyphema. A dilated fundus examination should be performed to rule out traumatic retinal detachment, commotio retinae, choroidal rupture, and other forms of posterior segment involvement.

Plan

The initial treatment of traumatic iritis consists of administering a long-acting cycloplegic agent (e.g., homatropine) two to three times a day. If the anterior chamber reaction is severe or if cellular activity does not diminish within a few days of initiating cycloplegic therapy, a topical steroid (e.g., 1% prednisolone acetate) should be added. The frequency of administration of steroid therapy is every 1–4 hours depending on the severity of the reaction. The patient may also benefit from the use of an oral non-steroidal anti-inflammatory medication (e.g., ibuprofen) to relieve the ocular pain and inflammation.

The patient should be followed every 2–3 days to evaluate resolution of the anterior chamber reaction. Referral to a retinal surgeon is indicated if there is any evidence of retinal detachment.

SUGGESTED READING

Kanski JJ. Uveitis: A Colour Manual of Diagnosis and Treatment. Oxford: Butterworth–Heinemann, 1996.

Rothova A. Uveitis and systemic disease. Br J Ophthalmol 1992;76:137.

Sheppard JD, Nozik RA. Practical Diagnostic Approach to Uveitis. In W Tasman, EA Jaeger (eds), Duane's Clinical Ophthalmology. Philadelphia: Lippincott, 1997.

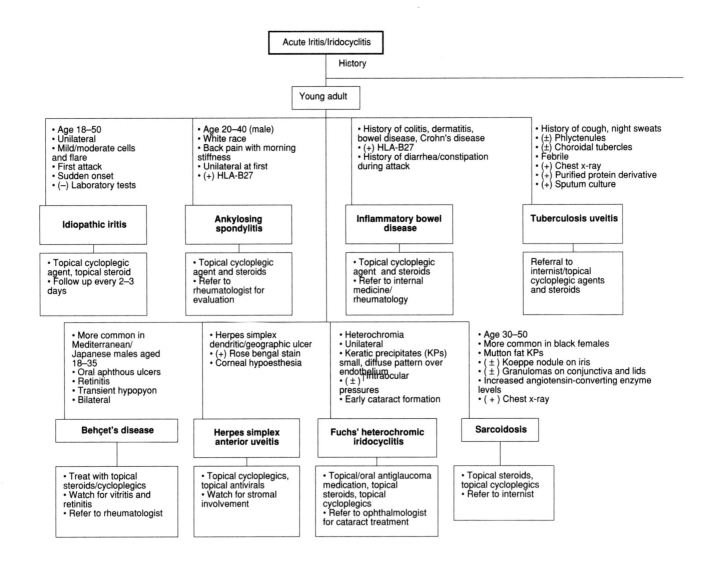

Young adult/child

- Age 18–30
- Bilateral
- Snowbanking at inferior ora serrata
- Floaters↓visual acuity
- Cystoid macular edema, cataract formation
- Vitreous cells (snowballs)

- High intraocular pressure
- Trace cells
- Open chamber angles
- Unilateral
- History of similar episodes

- Young child
- Female > male
- Band keratopathy
- Cataract formation
- "Quiet" uveitis
- Trace cells

- Trauma
- Ecchymosis
- Subconjunctival hemorrhage
- (±) Corneal abrasion

Pars planitis

Glaucomato-cyclitic crisis (Posner-Schlossman syndrome)

Juvenile rheumatoid arthritis

Traumatic iritis

- 1/3 No treatment
- 1/3 Periocular steroids
- 1/3 Oral steroids, immunosuppressive medications

Topical steroids, oral antiglaucoma, topical antiglaucoma agents

Refer to rheumatologist, treat with topical steroids, should treat only the exacerbations of the inflammation

Topical cycloplegic agent, topical antibiotic if epithelial damage, steroids if needed after 7 days

Refer to immunologist, retinologist

36

Debris in the Anterior Chamber

FRANK P. LARUSSA

DEBRIS IN THE ANTERIOR CHAMBER AT A GLANCE

Postsurgical debris in the anterior chamber
  Post–laser procedures
    White inflammatory cells
    Flare
    Pigment cells
    Red blood cells
  Post–cataract extraction, post–penetrating keratoplasty, post–radial keratotomy
    Debris from crystalline lens (cataract extraction)
    White inflammatory cells, hypopyon
    Flare
    Red blood cells, hyphema
    Vitreous
Debris in the anterior chamber not related to surgery
  Post-trauma
    Small white cells
    Flare
    Red blood cells, hyphema
    Pigment cells
    Metallic foreign body
  Nontraumatic
    White cells
    Flare
    Pigmented cells

Debris in the anterior chamber is always of clinical significance. However, a certain degree of debris in the anterior chamber is considered normal after intraocular surgery. When viewing debris in the anterior chamber with the slit-lamp biomicroscope, the clinician should use a conical beam or a 1 mm ↔ 3 mm parallelepiped with high magnification to note the size, color, and amount of debris.

POSTSURGICAL DEBRIS IN THE ANTERIOR CHAMBER

Post–Laser Procedure (Peripheral Iridotomy, Argon Laser Trabeculoplasty, Nd:YAG Capsulotomy)

Subjective
Patients who develop inflammation after laser procedures may complain of dull eye pain. They may describe their eye as sore.

Objective
Biomicroscopy reveals small white cells that indicate an iritis secondary to the laser procedure. The clinician may also note small pigment cells that are dispersed into the chamber secondary to the laser trauma. Occasionally, the clinician may note small red blood cells, which indicate that there was a small amount of bleeding secondary to the laser procedure.

Plan
In most cases, the condition of debris secondary to laser procedures resolves without treatment. Use of topical steroids such as prednisolone acetate can be beneficial to reduce inflammation and reduce anterior cellular debris. Whenever there is debris in the chamber, the clinician should monitor frequently for elevation of the patient's intraocular pressure.

Post–Cataract Extraction, Post–Penetrating Keratoplasty, Post–Radial Keratotomy

Subjective

The patient may have no complaints or may complain of soreness of the operated eye.

Objective

Small white cells (1–2 +) are more common during the first few days after surgery and represent a mild iritis in response to the surgical procedure. In the vast majority of cases the condition resolves without treatment.

The practitioner may occasionally see red cells floating in the anterior chamber. The presence of such cells represents a microhyphema. When red cells are present, the practitioner should have the patient gaze downward and carefully perform biomicroscopy to rule out a larger hyphema.

During the first couple of days after cataract extraction, the clinician may see small clumps of floating white debris that represent cortical matter from the cataractous lens. Occasionally after cataract extraction a clear jelly-like material may be seen in the anterior chamber. This material may be retained viscoelastic agent or prolapsed vitreous secondary to posterior capsule rupture. Prolapsed vitreous can cause endothelial damage if it touches the cornea. It also can cause increased intraocular pressure if the vitreous gets into the angle.

On very rare occasions, a patient may have a hypopyon in the inferior part of the chamber. This condition is usually associated with the presence of a tremendous number of white cells in the anterior chamber. The patient usually has reduced vision and pain in the eye that was operated on. When a hypopyon is present, the clinician should assume that the patient has an endophthalmitis until proved otherwise.

Plan

Patients with cortical debris, small white cells, or pigment cells in the anterior chamber during the first few days after surgery need no specific treatment other than the typical postsurgical protocol, including monitoring IOP.

Patients with red cells in the anterior chamber should be carefully examined to rule out a hyphema. The patient's intraocular pressure should be checked regularly until the condition has resolved. If a hyphema is present, the patient should be referred back to the surgeon. The surgeon may consider an anterior chamber wash if the intraocular pressure becomes elevated.

Patients with vitreous in the anterior chamber should have intraocular pressure monitored closely. If there are signs of increased intraocular pressure or vitreal touch to the cornea, the patient should be referred back to the surgeon. The surgeon may consider an anterior vitrectomy.

If significant numbers of white cells or a hypopyon is present, the patient should be referred back to the surgeon, because this condition is suggestive of endophthalmitis. The patient with endophthalmitis should be hospitalized and treated with oral, subconjunctival, or intravitreal antibiotics. Vitrectomy also may be used as a treatment option.

POST-TRAUMA, NONSURGICAL

Subjective

Patients with a recent history of ocular trauma may complain of dull pain in the eye. This pain is often associated with an anterior chamber reaction.

Objective

Small white cells and flare in the anterior chamber after trauma are manifestations of iritis or iridocyclitis. Small red cells indicate a microhyphema. A large red globular mass in the anterior chamber represents a hyphema. A patient with a recent history of metal grinding or other metal work involving small high-velocity particles may have a foreign body that has perforated the globe.

Plan

Post-traumatic iritis may be treated initially with a cycloplegic agent such as homatropine. If further control of inflammation is needed, a steroid such as prednisolone acetate may be added.

If red blood cells are present in the anterior chamber, the practitioner should look carefully for a hyphema. In general, gonioscopy should not be performed during the acute stages. If the hyphema is a microhyphema, the patient should be advised not to be active and not to use aspirin or similar products. The patient should be monitored daily until resolution is complete. If a larger hyphema is present, intraocular pressure should be monitored closely and the patient may require hospitalization. The patient may be confined to bed rest and should lie with the head elevated at a 30-degree angle. Aminocaproic acid or oral corticosteroids may be prescribed to prevent rebleeding. If the pressure rises and cannot be controlled medically, an anterior chamber wash procedure is advised. Black patients with hyphema should be screened for sickle-cell disease. Those with sickle-cell disease or sickle cell trait should be treated more aggressively because they are at risk for developing complications.

If a foreign body is noted in the anterior chamber or elsewhere within the globe, the patient should be referred to an ophthalmic surgeon for its removal.

NONSURGICAL, NONTRAUMATIC

Subjective

Nontraumatic iritis may be idiopathic or may be caused by one of a large number of underlying systemic diseases, including ankylosing spondylitis, sarcoidosis, or Behçet's disease. Patients with nontraumatic iritis often complain of dull pain in the eye and photophobia.

Objective

The patient has white cells and flare in the anterior chamber. The patient may have circumlimbal flush and a miotic pupil in the involved eye. These signs represent an iritis. The clinician should note whether the iritis is granulomatous or nongranulomatous, unilateral or bilateral, isolated or recurrent, and whether it is associated with significant systemic signs and symptoms.

Plan

The patient with iritis should be treated with a topical steroid such as prednisolone acetate and a cycloplegic such as 5% homatropine. If the patient has bilateral, recurrent, chronic, or granulomatous iritis, or if the iritis is associated with suggestive systemic symptoms, the clinician should order pertinent laboratory tests and consider having the patient evaluated by an internist or family practitioner to rule out systemic disease. Iritis in a pediatric patient that is not secondary to trauma also warrants an evaluation for systemic disease.

PIGMENT DISPERSION SYNDROME

Subjective

Patients with pigment dispersion syndrome usually have no symptoms, although they may occasionally complain of blurred vision and eye pain after exercise. Those patients who develop pigmentary glaucoma note glaucomatous field losses in the advanced stages of the disease.

Objective

In this condition, pigmented cells may be seen in the anterior chamber. The iris may show spoked transillumination. The posterior corneal surface often has heavy pigmentation (Krukenberg's spindle), and gonioscopy reveals heavy pigmentation of the angle. Intraocular pressure is often normal but may be elevated. Elevated pressure suggests pigmentary glaucoma. The pressure in this condition often spikes from normal to abnormally high.

Plan

The patient with pigment dispersion syndrome should be monitored closely for pigmentary glaucoma. Intraocular pressure should be checked every 3 months, and visual fields should be monitored annually. Patients with pigment dispersion syndrome associated with reverse pupillary block often respond well to laser peripheral iridotomy.

PIGMENT RELEASED AFTER DILATION

Subjective

The use of adrenergic mydriatics such as phenylephrine hydrochloride to dilate the eyes can cause a small amount of pigment release in some patients. This release may be significant in patients with pigment dispersion syndrome. Patients usually have no symptoms related to the pigment release but experience the symptoms of photophobia, glare, and blurred near vision in association with the pharmacologic dilation.

Objective

A few pigmented cells may be visible in the anterior chamber within approximately 30 minutes of dilation. The intraocular pressure may become elevated in patients with pigmentary glaucoma.

Plan

This effect is transient and no treatment is indicated.

SUGGESTED READING

Bartlett JD, Jaanus SD. Clinical Ocular Pharmacology (3rd ed). Boston: Butterworth–Heinemann, 1995.

Catania LJ. Primary Care of the Anterior Segment. Norwalk, CT: Appleton & Lange, 1995.

Murrill CA, Stanfield DL, VanBrocklin MD. Primary Care for the Cataract Patient. Norwalk, CT: Appleton & Lange, 1994.

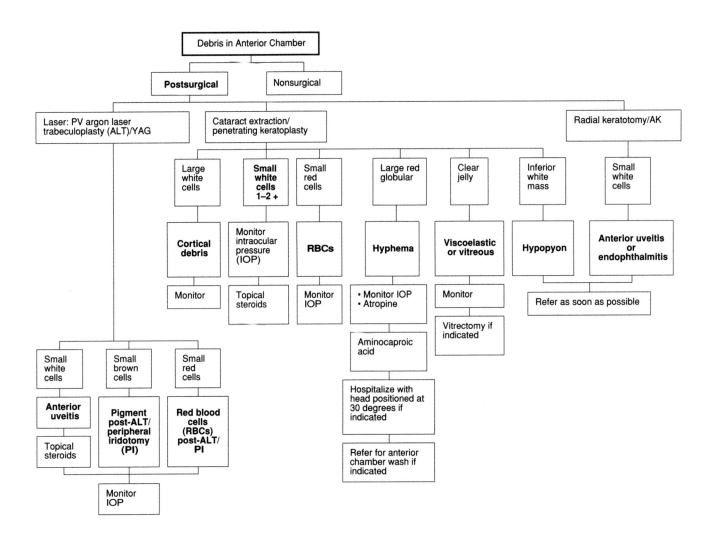

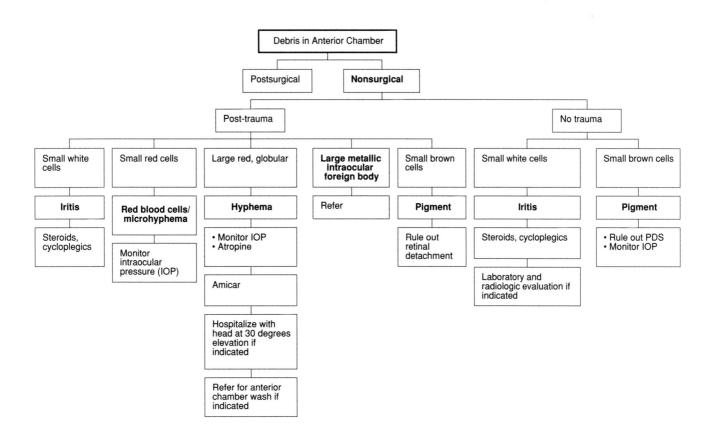

37

Increased Intraocular Pressure

Frank P. LaRussa

INCREASED INTRAOCULAR PRESSURE AT A GLANCE

Usually monocular
  Acute angle-closure glaucoma, pupillary block
  Uveitic glaucoma
  Angle-recession glaucoma
  Glaucoma secondary to hyphema
  Neovascular glaucoma
  Plateau iris syndrome
  Malignant glaucoma
  Phakolytic glaucoma
  Posner-Schlossman syndrome
  Steroid response glaucoma
Usually binocular
  Chronic open-angle glaucoma
  Pigment dispersion glaucoma
  Pseudoexfoliation glaucoma
  Primary congenital glaucoma
  Ocular hypertension

Increased intraocular pressure is always a significant finding during an eye examination. The practitioner must always investigate the cause of the rise in intraocular pressure to determine the exact diagnosis and the proper treatment. The first step is to determine whether the elevated intraocular pressure is monocular or binocular. After this initial determination, the practitioner must perform a comprehensive glaucoma evaluation.

INCREASED INTRAOCULAR PRESSURE, USUALLY MONOCULAR

Acute Angle-Closure Glaucoma

Subjective
Patients with acute angle-closure glaucoma usually complain of eye pain or brow pain on the affected side. They also often complain of blurred vision and haloes around lights; they are also frequently nauseated.

Objective
Biomicroscopy reveals a steamy, edematous cornea. The conjunctiva is often mildly injected, and the pupil is fixed in a mid-dilated position. The intraocular pressure is significantly elevated, usually above 40 mm Hg. Gonioscopy reveals a closed angle.

Plan
The initial management of acute pupillary-block angle-closure glaucoma involves reducing the intraocular pressure through medical means. If the intraocular pressure is above 50 mm Hg, a topical beta blocker and/or alpha-agonist should be tried initially. Concurrent therapy with oral acetazolamide or isosorbide is often needed to reduce the pressure. An antiemetic may be needed before initiating oral therapy if the patient is nauseated. Once the intraocular pressure is below 50 mm Hg, topical 2% pilocarpine is effective in lowering intraocular pressure. The use of pilocarpine should be avoided in aphakic, pseudophakic, secondary mechanical, neovascular, or uveitic (synechia) angle closure. In some cases, corneal indentation can be effective in breaking an angle-closure attack. Once the intraocular pressure is brought under reasonable control, a peripheral iridotomy is indicated for long-term management of acute angle closure that is a result of a papillary block.

Uveitic Glaucoma

Subjective
Patients with uveitic glaucoma usually complain of pain in the affected eye. They are also usually very light sensitive and may have decreased or foggy vision.

Objective
Biomicroscopy reveals the typical signs of anterior uveitis (cells and flare in the anterior chamber, and circumlim-

bal injection). A posterior uveitis may also be present. The pupil on the affected side is usually miotic. There may be keratic precipitates or posterior synechiae. The intraocular pressure is elevated in the affected eye. Gonioscopy reveals an open angle.

Plan
Topical steroids such as 1% prednisolone acetate or rimexolone are the best initial treatment option. If synechiae are present, mydriatics should be used to try to break the adhesion. Mydriatics may also be used to prevent synechia formation. Topical beta blockers, brimonidine tartrate, or dorzolamide hydrochloride may be used to lower the pressure. Miotics such as pilocarpine should not be used because their cholinergic activity tends to increase the uveitic response. Latanoprost should also be avoided because it may exacerbate the inflammation.

Angle-Recession Glaucoma

Subjective
Patients with angle-recession glaucoma usually have no complaints unless the trauma that caused the recession is recent.

Objective
Intraocular pressure is elevated in the affected eye. Gonioscopy reveals a recessed angle in at least one quadrant. There may be visual field loss or a larger cup-to-disc ratio in the affected eye.

Plan
Treatment is similar to that for open-angle glaucoma. Topical antiglaucoma drops such as timolol (Betimol) are generally used initially. Topical carbonic anhydrase inhibitors, prostaglandins, and alpha-agonists may also be considered. Miotics may not be as effective as in primary open-angle cases. Oral antiglaucoma carbonic anhydrase inhibitors or surgical trabeculectomy may be used in nonresponsive cases.

Glaucoma Secondary to Hyphema

Subjective
Patients with a hyphema usually have a recent history of trauma.

Objective
Biomicroscopy reveals blood in the anterior chamber. Intraocular pressure is elevated in the affected eye.

Plan
Many patients with hyphema are confined to bed rest with their heads elevated at a 30- to 45-degree angle. Hospitalization may be necessary to insure compliance. A Fox eye shield is recommended to protect the eye, and topical atropine is recommended to immobilize the pupil. Oral aminocaproic acid may be used to reduce the risk of rebleeds. The patient should avoid aspirin products. If the intraocular pressure is elevated, topical beta blockers or carbonic anhydrase inhibitors are recommended. If intraocular pressure cannot be reduced or endothelial stain is forming on the visual axis, an anterior chamber wash is recommended. Surgical intervention should be avoided or delayed if possible because of the increased risk of causing a rebleed. Black patients with hyphema should be screened for sickle-cell disease, because patients with this disease are more susceptible to complications.

Neovascular Glaucoma

Subjective
The patient with neovascular glaucoma usually has a history of diabetes, central or branch retinal vein occlusion, or ocular ischemic syndrome.

Objective
Biomicroscopy or gonioscopy reveals rubeosis iridis and neovascularization of the chamber angle. Intraocular pressure is elevated in the affected eye.

Plan
The intraocular pressure may be lowered with a beta blocker, dorzolamide hydrochloride, dipivefrin hydrochloride, or a carbonic anhydrase inhibitor. Miotics should not be used. The patient should be referred to a retinologist for panretinal photocoagulation as soon as possible if retinal ischemia is thought to be the underlying cause. Other therapies include goniophotocoagulation and trabeculectomy. In addition, steroids and cycloplegic agents may be used to help decrease pain.

INCREASED INTRAOCULAR PRESSURE, USUALLY BINOCULAR

Chronic Open-Angle Glaucoma (May Be Monocular in Early Stage)

Subjective
Patients with open-angle glaucoma usually have no symptoms until the condition is in the advanced stages.

Later in the disease, loss of visual field is noticeable to the patient.

Objective

In most cases of chronic open-angle glaucoma, the intraocular pressure is elevated. There is often asymmetry between the two eyes in intraocular pressure, and there may be a large diurnal variation in the intraocular pressures. There is usually a visual field loss. The most common field defects are paracentral scotomas, enlarged blind spots, arcuate scotomas, and nasal steps. The optic nerve may show an enlarged cup-to-disc ratio or neuroretinal rim notches. Corresponding nerve fiber defects may also be visible on retinal examination. Gonioscopy reveals an open angle.

Plan

The first line of treatment typically is the use of one or more topical antiglaucoma medications, including beta blockers, prostaglandins, alpha-agonists, dipivefrin hydrochloride, topical carbonic anhydrase inhibitors, and miotics. Oral carbonic anhydrase inhibitors, argon laser trabeculoplasty, and surgical trabeculectomy are used in nonresponsive cases.

Pigment Dispersion Glaucoma

Subjective

Patients with pigment dispersion glaucoma usually are asymptomatic. However, occasionally a patient may experience eye pain or blurred vision after exercise. The condition is most common in young males.

Objective

Biomicroscopy usually reveals pigment on the posterior surface of the cornea (Krukenberg's spindle). There is spoked iris transillumination. Gonioscopy reveals an open angle with excessive pigment in the angle. The intraocular pressure has a tendency to spike during dispersion episodes. On rare occasions, the clinician may see pigment floating in the anterior chamber. There are often visual field defects and optic nerve damage as are typical of open-angle glaucoma.

Plan

Pigmentary glaucoma is best treated with miotics. If the miotic alone does not reduce pressure adequately or if the patient is intolerant of miotics, other medications typically used in open-angle glaucoma, such as beta blockers or carbonic anhydrase inhibitors, are recommended. These patients also tend to respond well to argon laser trabeculoplasty. In cases of pigmentary dispersion associated with reverse pupillary block, laser peripheral iridotomy may be the initial treatment of choice.

Pseudoexfoliation Glaucoma

Subjective

Patients with pseudoexfoliation glaucoma usually have no complaints.

Objective

Postdilation biomicroscopy reveals white flakes on the anterior surface of the lens. Intraocular pressure is elevated. Gonioscopy reveals an open angle with white flakes or excessive pigment on the angle structures. There are usually visual field defects and optic nerve damage similar to those seen in open-angle glaucoma.

Plan

The therapeutic regimen is similar to that for open-angle glaucoma.

Steroid Response Glaucoma

Subjective

Patients with this condition typically have a history of topical steroid use; however, the condition may also occur secondary to the use of systemic steroids. There may be a personal or family history of chronic open-angle glaucoma.

Objective

The clinical findings are very similar to those for chronic open-angle glaucoma.

Plan

The steroids should be tapered initially and discontinued as soon as possible, or the patient should be switched to a steroid that is less likely to elevate intraocular pressure or to a nonsteroidal anti-inflammatory agent. Antiglaucoma medications may be needed if the intraocular pressure remains elevated. If steroids cannot be discontinued because of a medical condition, the clinician should consider adding a topical beta blocker to the therapy.

SUGGESTED READING

Alexander LA. Primary Care of the Posterior Segment (2nd ed). Norwalk, CT: Appleton & Lange, 1994.

Bartlett JD, Jaanus SD. Clinical Ocular Pharmacology (3rd ed). Boston: Butterworth–Heinemann, 1995.

Cullom RD, Chang B. The Wills Eye Manual: Office and Emergency Room Diagnosis and Treatment of Eye Disease (2nd ed). Philadelphia: Lippincott, 1994.

Eskridge JB, Amos J, Bartlett JD. Clinical Procedures in Optometry. Philadelphia: Lippincott, 1995.

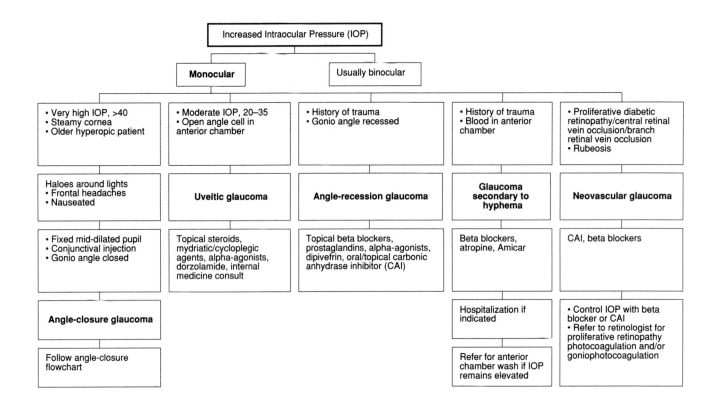

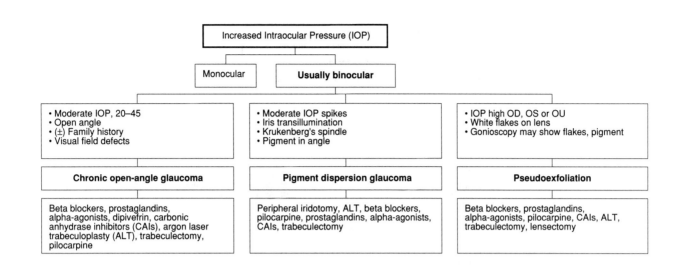

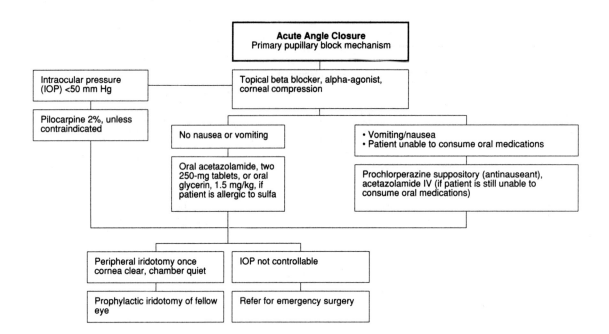

38

Decreased Intraocular Pressure (Hypotony)

CARL H. SPEAR

DECREASED INTRAOCULAR PRESSURE (HYPOTONY) AT A GLANCE

Postsurgical or post-traumatic
  Wound leak
  Retinal detachment
  Choroidal detachment
  Global perforation
  Iridocyclitis
  Cyclodialytic cleft
Other
  Unilateral
    Central retinal vein occlusion
    Temporal arteritis
    Ocular ischemic syndrome
    Central retinal artery occlusion
  Bilateral
    Pharmacologic agents
    Systemic disease
    Uremia
    Myotonic dystrophy
    Dehydration
    Diabetes

A patient with ocular hypotony may be asymptomatic or may present with mild to severe pain and reduced vision. Objective findings include an intraocular pressure of less than 6 mm Hg and a shallow anterior chamber. Taking a comprehensive patient history can help to identify the cause of the hypotony. Ocular history should include detailed questioning about recent surgeries or incidents of trauma. A thorough evaluation of both the anterior and posterior segments is essential to determine the appropriate treatment, because surgical repair is indicated in many instances.

WOUND LEAK

Subjective

Patients with hypotony due to a wound leak present with a history of recent trauma or surgery. They are typically symptomatic and report ocular pain and decreased vision.

Objective

Intraocular pressure is lower than normal and usually measures less than 6 mm Hg. The presence of a wound leak can be confirmed by a positive Seidel's sign. The anterior chamber is shallow, and the pupil may be irregularly shaped, either from trauma or after intraocular surgery. If a penetrating injury is the cause of the hypotony, signs of global rupture should be apparent.

Plan

If the globe is ruptured or a penetrating injury is known to have occurred, pressure to the eye should be avoided. The eye should be patched with a protective shield, and intravenous antibiotic therapy should be initiated. Diagnostic imaging may be indicated to localize the rupture site and to rule out an intraocular or intraorbital foreign body. Surgical repair as soon as possible is indicated for wound leaks due to a penetrating injury.

RETINAL DETACHMENT

Subjective

Patients with retinal detachments present reporting flashes of light, a large number of floaters, and the appearance of a shadow or curtain in either the peripheral or central field of view. History includes recent ocular trauma, a prior retinal detachment, or a previous diagnosis of a peripheral retinal degeneration.

Objective

Visual acuity is variable depending on the location of the retinal detachment. Likewise, a relative afferent pupillary defect may be present depending on the extent of the detachment. Slit-lamp examination reveals pigmented cells in the anterior chamber or in the vitreous. Intraocular pressure is lower than normal and measures less than 6 mm Hg. Elevated retina with or without the presence of a flap tear or break is observed during a dilated fundus evaluation. A vitreous hemorrhage may also be present.

Plan

A patient with a retinal detachment should be referred immediately to a retinal specialist for surgical repair.

CHOROIDAL DETACHMENT

Subjective

Patients with choroidal detachments may be asymptomatic, or they may present reporting a decrease in vision. History typically includes recent ocular surgery.

Objective

An anterior chamber reaction is present, and intraocular pressure is less than 6 mm Hg. If the choroidal detachment is associated with a wound leak or a leaking filtering bleb, a positive Seidel's sign is present. There is an orange-brown elevation of the retina and choroid. The choroidal detachment may or may not be associated with a retinal detachment.

Plan

If the wound or bleb leak is minimal, the eye should be patched for 24 hours to allow the leak to seal spontaneously. If the leak is larger and more advanced, it should be sutured or sealed with cyanoacrylate glue. The anterior uveitis should be treated appropriately.

GLOBE PERFORATION

Subjective

A patient that has experienced a globe perforation presents reporting pain and a decrease in vision. Ocular history includes recent trauma.

Objective

The degree of vision loss varies. During slit-lamp examination, an obvious scleral or corneal laceration may be present with or without intraocular contents visible. An extensive subconjunctival hemorrhage and a hyphema typically are also apparent, as are other signs of blunt trauma.

Plan

Diagnostic imaging (B-scan ultrasonography, computed tomography, radiography, or magnetic resonance imaging) should be considered to rule out the presence of an intraorbital or intraocular foreign body. The patient should be informed not to eat, and, if the patient is nauseated, an antiemetic such as promethazine hydrochloride (Phenergan) or prochlorperazine maleate (Compazine) should be administered, either in the form of a suppository or as an intramuscular injection. A Fox shield should be used to protect the eye from further trauma. Patients diagnosed with globe perforation should be referred for surgical repair as soon as possible.

TRAUMATIC UVEITIS

Subjective

Patients with traumatic uveitis present with ocular redness and pain and complain of photophobia and blurred vision. History includes recent blunt ocular trauma or corneal trauma.

Objective

Visual acuity varies in patients experiencing traumatic uveitis. An anterior chamber reaction is noted; however, it may be mild in comparison to the patient's symptoms. The pupil may be miotic. The intraocular pressure may be lower than normal but not as reduced as in the other conditions covered in this chapter.

Plan

The uveitis should be treated with a cycloplegic agent. A steroid may also be included if the corneal epithelium is intact. The associated ocular conditions resulting from the trauma should also be managed appropriately.

CYCLODIALYTIC CLEFT

Subjective

Patients with cyclodialytic clefts present with a recent history of ocular surgery or trauma.

Objective

The intraocular pressure is lower than normal and typically is less than 6 mm Hg. A visible detachment of the ciliary body from the scleral spur can be seen during gonioscopy. However, in the presence of hypotony, gonioscopy should be performed carefully, and a good view may not be possible due to corneal deformation.

Plan

A patient diagnosed with a cyclodialytic cleft should be referred for surgical intervention to reattach the ciliary body to the sclera. Surgical repair may be accomplished with sutures, laser photocoagulation, diathermy, or endocyclophotocoagulation.

PHARMACOLOGICALLY INDUCED HYPOTONY

Subjective

Patients presenting with pharmacologically induced hypotony are asymptomatic. History is essential in making this diagnosis. The patient's recent or current medications include an agent known to reduce intraocular pressure, such as a beta blocker or a carbonic anhydrase inhibitor.

Objective

Objective findings are unremarkable except for the presence of bilateral shallow anterior chambers and bilateral reduced intraocular pressures.

Plan

The medication causing the hypotony should be discontinued or the dosage reduced after careful evaluation of the risks versus benefits of medical therapy. Comanagement of the case may be required if the medication was prescribed for a nonocular condition, such as prescription of an oral beta blocker for the treatment of hypertension.

VASO-OCCLUSIVE DISEASE

Subjective

Patients with vaso-occlusive disease present with a unilateral decrease in vision of either an acute or insidious onset. Symptoms may or may not include ocular pain. No history of recent ocular surgery or trauma is reported.

Objective

Objective findings include a decrease in vision. An afferent pupillary defect may or may not be noted. A shallow anterior chamber angle is present, and there is a mild decrease in intraocular pressure. The fundus shows the characteristic appearance of a central retinal vein occlusion, a central retinal artery occlusion, or ocular ischemic syndrome. Associated vasoproliferation may also be noted, and iris neovascularization may be present. Another cause for this type of hypotony is temporal arteritis.

Plan

The underlying retinal and systemic vaso-occlusive disorders should be managed appropriately.

OTHER SYSTEMIC DISEASE

Subjective

Taking a thorough history is essential in diagnosing hypotony due to a systemic disease other than a vaso-occlusive disorder. The patient's history includes uremia, myotonic dystrophy, severe dehydration, or diabetes. Absent from the history is recent ocular trauma, recent ocular surgery, or vaso-occlusive disease. Medical therapy does not include agents known to lower intraocular pressure.

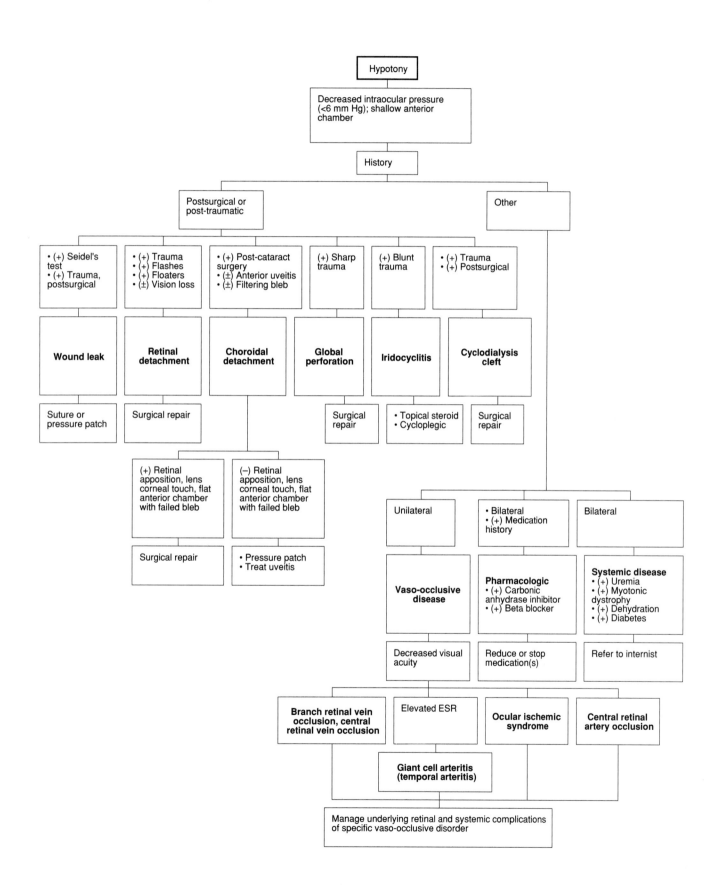

39

Opacities of the Lens

DAVID P. SENDROWSKI

OPACITIES OF THE LENS AT A GLANCE

Cataracts
  Epicapsular
  Anterior subcapsular
  Polar
  Lamellar
  Stellate
  Zonular
  Cortical
  Nuclear
  Sutural
  Coronary
  Punctate
  Posterior subcapsular
  Iridescent crystalline deposits

Careful evaluation of the lens is an essential part of a complete eye examination. Cataracts are among the most common ocular findings in older patients. With the prolongation of human life, increasing numbers of patients with age-related disorders, especially cataracts, are to be expected.

The cataract evaluation should include a careful inquiry into the patient's occupational, leisure, and social activities, and any related visual impairment that the patient perceives in the pursuit of these activities. A thorough history allows the practitioner to recommend an appropriate course of action.

PSEUDOEXFOLIATION

Subjective

Patients with pseudoexfoliation are asymptomatic. Pseudoexfoliation is usually discovered during the routine dilated biomicroscopic examination or when the patient presents with unilateral elevated intraocular pressure. True exfoliation of the lens capsule secondary to infrared light exposure may present as a sharp pain in the affected eye, but it is rarely seen in practice today.

Patients with pseudoexfoliation tend to be white or of Scandinavian descent; however, not all patients fit this profile. Pseudoexfoliation should be ruled out as a possible cause of secondary glaucoma in older patients.

Objective

Visual acuity, ocular motility, and pupillary responses are usually normal. The pseudoexfoliative material may be seen in an undilated eye on the pupillary frill under high magnification with the biomicroscope. It appears as a whitish, pale material and can be easily missed without close scrutiny. Gonioscopy is very helpful in establishing the presence of material or pigment in the anterior chamber angle. It is often necessary to dilate the eye to see the full clinical spectrum of the pseudoexfoliation syndrome. Tonometry, threshold visual field testing, and stereoscopic photographs of the optic nerve heads are helpful in detecting early or progressive glaucomatous changes.

Plan

If there is no evidence of glaucoma, the patient can be followed on a regular basis for an increase in intraocular pressure and nerve head cupping.

If there is evidence of glaucomatous changes, the patient should be started on beta blockers (e.g., timolol maleate) twice a day. The intraocular pressure should be evaluated 2–4 weeks after initiation of therapy.

Consideration should be given to argon laser trabeculoplasty for patients who have compliance problems with topical therapy. Trabeculectomy should be considered when both medical and laser therapies fail.

GLAUKOMFLECKEN

Subjective

Glaukomflecken are produced during the intraocular pressure spikes of transient acute angle-closure attacks. Patients with *Glaukomflecken* are not symptomatic from the lens changes but may be symptomatic from the intraocular pressure spikes. The patient should be questioned about previous ocular pain, blurred vision, appearance of colored haloes around lights, frontal headaches, nausea, and vomiting.

The patient should also be questioned about a family history of glaucoma, a personal history of glaucoma, the use of topical or oral antiglaucoma medications, and recent laser or surgical treatments.

Objective

Visual acuity, ocular motility, and pupillary responses are normal. Biomicroscopy reveals a shallow anterior chamber and narrow chamber angles. The anterior chamber should be inspected for posterior synechiae and peripheral anterior synechiae. The *Glaukomflecken* appear as focal lens opacities under the anterior capsule of the lens. They appear whitish and separate from one another. The intraocular pressure is usually within normal limits, unless the patient is having an attack at the time of presentation.

The definitive diagnosis is made with gonioscopy. Both eyes should exhibit very few visible angle structures, and peripheral anterior synechiae may be present.

Dilation should be deferred until the patient has had a peripheral iridotomy or a provocative pressure test is attempted. The dilation can be considered a provocative pressure test.

Plan

Because the angle closure in these patients is subacute, they should be treated as nonemergent cases and referred for laser peripheral iridotomy (argon or Nd:YAG). Surgical iridectomy should be performed if special circumstances make laser peripheral iridotomy impossible.

After the procedure, the patient should be followed with gonioscopy to make sure that the angles are open and angle structures are visible.

PIGMENT ON THE LENS SURFACE

Subjective

Patients rarely, if ever, have complaints arising from pigment on the lens. The finding is one that suggests old inflammatory disease, a congenital condition (epicapsular stars), trauma, pigment dispersion syndrome, use of oral psychoactive drugs (e.g., chlorpromazine hydrochloride [Thorazine]), or ocular surgery.

Objective

Pigment on the lens surface does not affect the entrance testing except for visual acuity. The acuity may be diminished slightly if the pigment is located centrally and is fairly dense. Otherwise, pupils, motility, confrontation field findings, and intraocular pressures are usually normal.

If the pigment is the result of posterior synechiae, the pupil may be misshapen. Synechiae adhere the iris to the anterior surface of the lens and allow no movement in that section of the iris. If synechiae are present 360 degrees around the pupillary frill, the intraocular pressure is extremely high secondary to pupil block. Pigment remaining on the lens after synechiae have been broken appear as a pseudo–Vossius' ring or crescent.

A circular distribution of pigment (Vossius' ring) may indicate old or recent blunt trauma to the eye. If the trauma is recent, the retina should be evaluated for breaks or tears, and the chamber angle should be evaluated for angle recession. A change in astigmatic correction could indicate damage to the zonule fibers.

Pigment located centrally in a stellate pattern indicates the use of an oral psychotropic agent such as chlorpromazine hydrochloride. In such cases, the pigment is bilateral and is located on the front surface of the lens. Systemic medications that can cause pigment deposition on the lens include chloroquine, chlorpromazine, diethylcarbamazine citrate, fluphenazine, mesoridazine, methotrimeprazine, penicillamine, prochlorperazine, promethazine hydrochloride, thioridazine hydrochloride, and trimeprazine tartrate. The posterior pole should be thoroughly evaluated for pigment changes as well.

Pigmentary dispersion syndrome is a form of secondary glaucoma in which there is bilateral elevation of intraocular pressure, open chamber angles, accumulation of pigment within the trabecular meshwork, Krukenberg's spindle on the corneal endothelium, and occasionally pigment on the lens. The disease characteristically occurs in young myopic males.

Plan

If the pigment deposition is secondary to a recurrent inflammatory disease, an underlying systemic disorder should be suspected.

Pigment deposition caused by oral medication is usually not a concern unless visual acuity is affected. If so, the patient's physician should be contacted and made aware of the medication's side effect. In certain cases, alternative medications may be prescribed.

If trauma is the cause of the pigment deposition, the patient should be evaluated for anterior and posterior damage from the trauma. If, for example, the patient has sustained an angle recession, yearly follow-up is advisable to monitor for secondary glaucoma.

ANTERIOR AND POSTERIOR CORTICAL CATARACTS

Subjective

Patients with cataracts complain of a gradual decrease in visual acuity. Cortical cataracts are usually found in older people; however, they can occur at a younger age in persons with diabetes. The history should help determine whether the patient is a good candidate for surgery. The patient should be questioned regarding eye injuries, amblyopia or strabismus, past and present eye diseases, eye surgeries, and the use of topical medications. The practitioner should inquire about specific visual tasks that are performed by the patient and should elicit a thorough history of any medical problems such as diabetes, elevated blood pressure, heart disease, respiratory problems, and allergies.

Objective

Distance and near acuities should be tested with the patient's habitual spectacle prescription. Ocular motility and pupillary responses are usually normal. Cataracts, even dense ones, do not typically affect pupillary reactions. Refraction is very important, because changes in sphere and cylinder power may result in better visual acuity. Intraocular pressure is unaffected by cataracts unless, as the lens diameter increases with age, it begins to narrow the anterior chamber angle. Contrast sensitivity testing (i.e., Vistech) and glare testing (i.e., Mentor BAT) may provide additional information for those patients who have significant glare complaints.

Dilated biomicroscopy is extremely helpful in confirming the diagnosis of anterior or posterior cortical cataracts. The use of an optic section allows a quick assessment of the level of lens opacity. The integrity of the corneal endothelium should also be assessed before surgery. A fundus examination can help to rule out peripheral retinal degenerations that may result in postoperative retinal detachment. During the dilation, a macular evaluation should be performed to assess potential postoperative acuity. This assessment can be done with a potential acuity meter or an interferometer. These tests also help to differentiate visual acuity loss from the cataract and loss caused by macular disease.

Additional testing might include A-scan ultrasonography and keratometry to determine the required intraocular lens power for the ophthalmic surgeon. B-scan ultrasonography is useful when the cataract is too dense to allow visualization of posterior structures. No laboratory tests are required for this ocular diagnosis.

Plan

If a change in spectacle correction does not satisfy the patient's visual requirements, surgery should be considered as an option. The optometrist should review various options with the patient and allow the patient time to consider them.

If surgery is agreed on, an ophthalmic surgeon should be given the preoperative data. A postoperative follow-up schedule should be worked out with the surgeon.

Any chronic ocular or systemic health problems should be treated and stable before surgical referral.

NUCLEAR SCLEROTIC CATARACTS

Subjective

Patients with nuclear sclerotic cataracts complain of a gradual loss of visual acuity, generally over months to years. Patients are usually older. Glare, particularly from oncoming headlights while driving at night, is a common complaint. These patients may also observe a reduction of color perception along with the loss in their acuity. Patients may report that their distance vision is reduced to a greater degree than their near vision. Patients report that they have better near vision without their reading glasses. This effect is due to the myopic shift caused by the increase in the index of refraction of the lens nucleus.

During the history taking, the patient should be questioned concerning visual tasks that may be more difficult to perform with loss of acuity. The ocular history should elicit information regarding any ocular surgeries, injuries, infections, or use of topical medications. The medical history should make note of any ongoing health problems such as diabetes, hypertension, pulmonary problems, and cardiovascular disease. The past ocular and medical histories help in assessing the patient's preoperative status if surgery is indicated.

Objective

Results of ocular motility and pupil testing are normal. Acuities and color vision are reduced in proportion to the density of the nuclear sclerotic cataract. Refraction shows a myopic shift from the patient's present spectacle correction.

Dilation allows a thorough biomicroscopic examination of the lens. Using an optic section, the lens nucleus is delineated or separated away from the lens cortex. The cortex and nucleus may have a yellow or brown discoloration.

Nuclear sclerotic cataracts can be graded objectively with modified slit-lamp photography or imaging. There are various systems for grading the lens changes. The lens opacities classification system II is as follows:

The lenses are graded for opalescence from 0 to 4. Opalescence is graded by comparing the opalescence of the nuclear region itself with that in standard photographs. If the average opalescence of the patient's nucleus is less than or equal to the nuclear opalescence standard for a given grade, it is assigned that opalescence grade. Average opalescence across the entire nuclear region is used in comparing the patient's lens to the photographs.

Nuclear color is determined by assessing the degree of yellowing of the posterior cortex and posterior subcapsular reflex. Dilated fundus examination of the posterior pole is normal. Visual field screening commonly shows a generalized depression, but cataracts can manifest many types of field defects.

Additional testing might include a glare test (i.e., Mentor BAT) if the patient complains of glare. Presurgical testing might also include A-scan ultrasonography and keratometry for intraocular lens calculations. B-scan ultrasonography is reserved for those rare cases in which the nuclear sclerotic cataract is too dense to allow visualization of the posterior pole.

Laboratory testing is not indicated for the ocular diagnosis of nuclear sclerotic cataracts.

Plan

Cataract surgery is an option for those patients in whom visual function does not improve with refraction. It should also be considered for patients with a disease such as diabetes or glaucoma, in which a cloudy media no longer allows adequate monitoring of the retina or optic nerve head.

If the patient does not want or require surgery, follow-up visits are usually scheduled every 6 months to re-evaluate vision changes.

POSTERIOR SUBCAPSULAR CATARACTS

Subjective

Unlike the other types of cataracts discussed in this chapter, posterior subcapsular cataracts cause a rapid loss of visual acuity. In addition, patients with these cataracts may be younger, usually younger than 50. Such an early onset is not found with the other types of cataracts. The rapid loss of acuity is attributable to the location of the cataract, which is near the visual axis and nodal point. Therefore, patients may complain of a loss of acuity at both distance and near over several weeks to months. Patients may also complain of glare and difficulty with reading. These symptoms are worse in bright, sunny conditions due to the pinhole effect of the pupil and the position of the cataract.

The patient should be questioned about a history of chronic ocular inflammation, prolonged use of topical and oral steroids, diabetes, ocular trauma, or exposure to radiation. Information should be obtained regarding cardiovascular disease, pulmonary disorders, recent surgeries, allergies, and hypertension. In addition, patients should be questioned about specific visual tasks and their ability to perform these tasks with their present spectacle correction.

Objective

Visual acuity is diminished at both distance and near. The acuity may deteriorate further when a pinhole is introduced in front of the eye with the cataract. Entrance testing is usually normal, because posterior subcapsular cataracts do not affect confrontation field findings, pupillary response, color vision, or motility testing. Retinoscopy and distance ophthalmoscopy may reveal a black opacity in the lens seen in the retroillumination of the retina. Dilation and a biomicroscopic examination should be performed. The posterior subcapsular cataract appears as a centrally or peripherally located, red or black ground-glass opacity in retroillumination. An optic section helps to localize the opacity in the posterior subcapsular portion of the lens. A posterior subcapsular cataract appears yellow or white in direct illumination. The fundus should be evaluated with the binocular indirect ophthalmoscope for evidence of any peripheral retinal degenerations or macular disease before referral for surgical removal. The posterior segment is usually normal.

Additional testing might include contrast sensitivity testing, glare testing (i.e., Mentor BAT), potential acuity meter, interferometry, and A-scan ultrasonography.

Plan

If the patient's spectacle correction is not effective, the option of cataract surgery should be considered.

Alternatively, if the cataract is small, a trial of mydriasis (e.g., 0.25% scopolamine two times a day) may be successful in some patients if they choose not to have the surgery performed. The cycloplegic effect and spectacle correction should be taken into consideration if this alternative therapy is used.

Patients who do not initially select surgery as an option should be examined every 6 months.

CONGENITAL CATARACTS

Subjective

A wide variety of congenital lens opacities exist. These opacities may be genetic, traumatic, or metabolic in origin.

Maternal infection (with rubella, herpes zoster, syphilis, etc.) or maternal exposure to certain drugs or radiation can cause congenital cataracts. Fetal trauma is another source of lens opacification. A good history of the prenatal health care of the patient is an important part of the workup for a suspected congenital cataract.

Congenital cataracts can be caused by a number of enzymatic disorders (e.g., galactosemia, homocystinuria) and can be associated with other ocular or systemic anomalies.

Congenital cataracts can cause significant vision loss and, if not treated at an early age, can lead to amblyopia ex anopsia. Additionally, many congenital cataracts do not cause a decrease in vision and need only to be followed over time.

Objective

Visual acuity loss from congenital cataracts ranges from none to severe. Congenital opacities may appear black when seen with a direct ophthalmoscope or retinoscope in retroillumination. They usually appear white or yellow in the direct illumination of the biomicroscope and are more easily seen when the pupil is dilated. The types of congenital cataract most commonly encountered are polar, cortical, subcapsular, zonular, sutural, and membranous, or total. A dilated fundus examination should be performed to rule out any posterior segment anomalies. Additional laboratory testing is based on the etiology of the congenital cataract.

Plan

Patients with a suspected metabolic disorder should be referred to a pediatrician for further evaluation. Patients with significant vision loss due to a congenital cataract should be referred to a pediatric ophthalmologist for a surgical consultation.

Proper postsurgical vision correction to prevent amblyopia is an important component of the management of congenital cataracts.

SUGGESTED READING

Brown N, Bron A, Sparrow J. Methods of evaluation of lens changes. Int Ophthalmol 1988;12:229.

Chylack LT, Leske MC, McCarthy D, et al. Lens opacities classification system II (LOCS II). Arch Ophthalmol 1989;107: 991.

Young R. Age-Related Cataract. New York: Oxford, 1991.

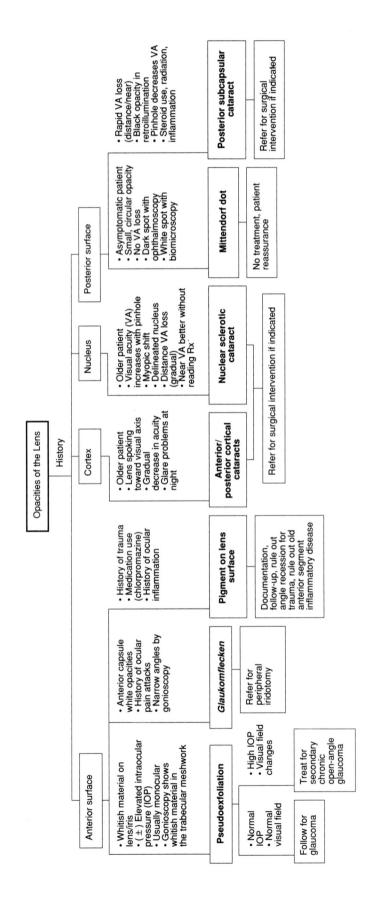

40

Anomalies of Lens Position

DAVID P. SENDROWSKI

ANOMALIES OF LENS POSITION AT A GLANCE

Dislocated lens
   Marfan syndrome
   Apert's syndrome
   Ehlers-Danlos syndrome
   Pseudoxanthoma elasticum
   Homocystinuria
   Weill-Marchesani syndrome
   Rieger's syndrome
   Spontaneous dislocation
   Syphilis
   Trauma
Microspherophakia
   Alport's syndrome
   Marfan syndrome
   Homocystinuria
   Weill-Marchesani syndrome
   Rubella syndrome

Ectopia lentis is a dislocation, malposition, or subluxation of the crystalline lens. It may occur as an isolated disorder; accompany other ocular abnormalities; be associated with systemic syndromes, many of which involve skeletal dysplasia; or be caused by trauma. Heritable abnormalities or acquired disruption of zonular support may allow the lens to decenter within the normal plane of its equator or to migrate anteriorly or posteriorly.

Several signs may be helpful in identifying subtle lens subluxation. Progressive myopia or noncorneal astigmatism can be clues to anterior displacement or tilting of the lens. Phacodonesis, a tremulous movement, is appreciated by observing the lens while delivering a firm downward rap to the slit-lamp table or having the patient change position of gaze.

SIMPLE ECTOPIA LENTIS

Subjective

Patients with simple ectopia lentis present without a history of trauma, ocular surgery, or systemic disorders that predispose the lens to dislocation. Patients with the condition may complain of monocular diplopia. The degree of diplopia varies with the severity of the dislocation. The patient may also complain of decreased central acuity if there is a sudden increase in astigmatism from lenticular tilt.

Patients are generally middle-aged to older adults. The disorder is passed on as an autosomal dominant trait, and family ocular history should be investigated. The patient should be asked about cardiovascular disease, skeletal abnormalities, visual disturbances, mental retardation, and early family deaths to help rule out systemic causes of ectopia lentis, such as Marfan syndrome, homocystinuria, or Weill-Marchesani syndrome.

Objective

Visual acuity may be decreased from acquired astigmatism. Retinoscopy may reveal abnormal reflexes.

The anterior segment should be examined for corneal diameter, anterior chamber depth, iridocorneal angle anomalies, lens position, and iris configuration. The practitioner should specifically look for iridodonesis and transillumination defects in evaluating the iris.

A dilated fundus examination should be performed to rule out retinal detachment. A-scan ultrasonography may help in evaluation of the axial length of the globe.

Additional testing to rule out associated systemic diseases might include cardiac ultrasonography, urinalysis for amino acids, and radiography of the hands to look for skeletal changes or abnormalities.

Plan

When the lens dislocates into the vitreous cavity, it can attach to the retina or float freely in the vitreous body. The other ocular tissues tolerate the intact lens very well, and surgery may not be indicated. The patient should still be evaluated for systemic conditions that may cause lens dislocation.

A free-floating lens in the vitreous, particularly if it leaks proteins, may also produce lens-induced uveitis and glaucoma. If the patient shows ocular signs of an inflammatory disease, surgical referral is indicated.

MARFAN SYNDROME

Subjective

Marfan syndrome is a disorder that affects both sexes equally and shows no difference in incidence among different racial or ethnic groups. The major organ systems affected by this disorder are cardiovascular, skeletal, and ocular. The disorder is inherited as an autosomal dominant trait.

Patients with Marfan syndrome often present with a bilateral loss of vision or onset of diplopia. It usually occurs in late adolescence or early adulthood. Axial myopia is often cited as a common cause of decreased vision in these patients as well. Mental retardation is rare in individuals with Marfan syndrome.

Objective

The corneal curvature is often flattened, and the corneal diameter decreased. The pupils are usually small and difficult to dilate in these patients.

The refractive error commonly shows a high degree of myopia, and the lens is subluxated in approximately 80% of cases. The lens commonly displaces upward and outward. The lens zonules usually remain intact so that accommodation is normal.

Arachnodactyly (long fingers) is a common feature of Marfan syndrome. Patients are tall, and the upper body is usually shorter than the lower body. Scoliosis may also be present. The wrist sign test can be performed on these patients. If the patient is asked to wrap the distal phalanges of the first and fifth digits around the opposite wrist and the two fingers overlap, the wrist sign is positive.

Laboratory testing may include a urinalysis for cyanide-nitroprusside reaction, which helps to rule out homocystinuria.

Dilated fundus examination should be performed to rule out a retinal detachment. The risk of retinal detachment increases with longer axial lengths.

Plan

The patient should be referred for a cardiovascular evaluation if one has not been performed. Cardiovascular complications account for a high percentage of the early deaths associated with Marfan syndrome.

If lens dislocation is present, surgical referral is indicated, especially if the lens dislocates into the anterior chamber or there is evidence of lens-induced glaucoma or uveitis. Follow-up is warranted every year to evaluate the retina for peripheral degeneration and possible detachment.

HOMOCYSTINURIA

Subjective

The profile of a patient with homocystinuria resembles that of a Marfan syndrome patient. Homocystinuria is an inborn error of metabolism of the sulfur-containing amino acids. Mental retardation is more common in this disorder than in Marfan syndrome. The physical findings are usually present by age 10, but it is possible for the signs to be delayed until the third decade.

The patient or parent should be asked about malar rash, mental retardation, osteoporosis, decreased joint mobility, and eczema.

Objective

Patients with homocystinuria may have a tall, thin stature, but arachnodactyly is present to a much lesser degree in homocystinuria than in Marfan syndrome. Skeletal deformities are also common in homocystinuria.

The ocular signs are similar to those in Marfan syndrome. The lens dislocation is more commonly downward and nasal rather than upward and temporal as in Marfan syndrome. The lens zonules are usually abnormal, and the lens cannot accommodate. The lens more commonly dislocates into the anterior chamber or vitreous in homocystinuria cases. A dilated fundus examination should be performed to evaluate for peripheral retinal abnormalities as well as retinal detachment.

Plan

Ocular management of patients with a subluxated lens is similar to management of Marfan syndrome patients. Patients with homocystinuria are at increased risk of thromboembolic events, especially during anesthesia; therefore, a more conservative approach to any surgery is warranted for these patients.

Patients should be referred to an internist for treatment with pyridoxine and dietary therapy involving reduced intake of methionine.

WEILL-MARCHESANI SYNDROME

Subjective

Weill-Marchesani syndrome is a rare disease with unclear inheritance patterns. Both sexes are affected equally. Patients with this disorder have ocular complaints similar to those of patients with Marfan syndrome and homocystinuria because of the associated ectopia lentis. Decreased vision and double vision are the more common complaints. These patients are also at risk for pupillary-block glaucoma and may also present with a complaint of ocular pain.

Objective

The lens is usually very small (microspherophakia) in these patients. Because the lens is small and steep, a lenticular myopia results. Dislocation of the lens occurs in almost all cases. If the lens dislocates anteriorly, it may result in a pupillary-block glaucoma, and the intraocular pressure will be markedly elevated.

The patient is short with broad hands and fingers (brachydactyly). There may be joint stiffness, joint prominence, and decreased joint mobility. The hypoextendible joints are in direct contrast to those of the Marfan syndrome patient.

Plan

The most important concern is to prevent pupillary-block glaucoma, which can result in angle obstruction and lead to a chronic glaucoma that is very difficult to treat.

Many patients have a prophylactic laser peripheral iridotomy and are then managed on topical miotics. Without a peripheral iridotomy, the risk of developing angle-closure glaucoma is high for these patients.

There is no specific systemic therapy indicated at this time for Weill-Marchesani syndrome.

TRAUMA OR CHILD ABUSE

Subjective

Trauma is a major cause of lens displacement. The history is usually positive for some forceful trauma to the ocular region. Thus, there are usually other signs of trauma

as well. These may include ecchymosis; lacerations of the lids, conjunctiva, or cornea; abrasions of the dermal or corneal areas; and subconjunctival or anterior chamber hemorrhages.

Physical abuse can occur at any age, but many cases are seen in children under the age of 4. Warning signs of child abuse include an injury that is not compatible with the alleged accidental trauma, delay in presentation of the child, multiple visits to the physician's office or hospital for various traumatic events, soft-tissue injuries at different stages of healing, tears to the floor of the mouth that may indicate forced feedings, and skin burns. An unexplained or poorly explained traumatic history should prompt further investigation.

Objective

Examination should be focused on the globe to rule out perforation from trauma. Visual acuity assessment, Seidel's test, and biomicroscopic evaluation of the anterior chamber angle structure should all be performed.

The lids, periorbital tissues, and ocular tissues should be evaluated for abrasions, lacerations, evulsions, and contusions. The fracture of the lamina papyracea may result in orbital emphysema and crepitus. A soft, crackling sound may be heard, and there may be a popping sensation under the fingertips when the lids are palpated.

In children, a dilation should be performed, and lens position and zonular integrity should be evaluated. The anterior chamber and retina should be thoroughly examined as well. As with adults, computed tomographic (CT) scans or orbital radiographs should be ordered if the presence or degree of damage is uncertain.

In adults, dilation should be performed, and lens position evaluated. Gonioscopy may be helpful in assessing zonular damage. The retina should be thoroughly examined to rule out retinal detachment. Forced duction tests should be attempted if there are signs of muscle entrapment or complaints of diplopia. A CT scan or orbital radiograph should be obtained if the diagnosis is uncertain.

Plan

Patients should be seen every 1–2 weeks post-trauma and evaluated for monocular diplopia or persistent enophthalmos. The presence of these findings may indicate a persistent entrapment of the extraocular muscles or orbital contents, and surgical repair may be required.

Patients should also be monitored for secondary complications, including cataract, choroidal rupture, retinal detachment, and angle-recession glaucoma. Gonioscopy and scleral depression can usually be performed 3–4 weeks post-trauma. If the patient has a traumatic lens dislocation or cataract formation, surgery may be indicated.

If child abuse is suspected, the eye care practitioner should immediately report the case to the authorities. Failure of the practitioner to report a suspected nonaccidental injury could result in misdemeanor charges as well as a civil lawsuit.

HYPERMATURE CATARACT

Subjective

When a cataract reaches a hypermature state, the patient is more commonly older, usually over the age of 70. The patient typically complains of decreased visual acuity at all distances because of the uniformity of the lens involvement. Other complaints may include glare, reduced color perception, and visual field loss.

The history should include questions regarding medication use, systemic diseases, trauma, and ocular diseases.

A morgagnian cataract is a mature cataract in which the lens cortex becomes liquefied to the extent that the dark brown nucleus sinks to the bottom of the capsule, creating an internal subluxated lens. In extreme cases, the cortex may become so liquefied that it becomes clear, and vision is relatively good through the pupil superior to the sunken lens. These patients are at high risk for phacoanaphylactic anterior uveitis and secondary glaucoma.

Objective

A complete ocular examination should be attempted, including visual acuity testing, pupil examination, and refraction. Dilation should be attempted in these patients, but the lenticular changes may be sufficiently dense to totally obscure the view of the posterior part of the lens as well as the posterior segment of the eye. If the posterior segment can be viewed, the macular area should be assessed for its integrity to rule out other causes of visual acuity loss. Interferometry or a potential acuity meter should be used to evaluate postoperative visual potential.

B-scan ultrasonography is very useful in assessing retinal integrity in those cases in which the posterior segment is obscured because of the cataract.

Plan

The patient should be referred for surgical intervention. If liquefied cortex is present, extracapsular cataract surgery is very difficult to perform. The zonules are usually weak in these eyes. An intracapsular cataract extraction is usually more successful.

DISLOCATED INTRAOCULAR LENS

Subjective

The posterior intraocular lens may become malpositioned. Downward displacement is referred to as a *sunset sign*. Upward displacement is referred to as a *sunrise sign*. The intraocular lens may also be displaced horizontally; such displacement usually occurs when one haptic is in the capsular bag and the other is outside the bag.

Patients present postoperatively with the complaint of flare, glare, or diplopia. The patient may also report marked blur or distortion. Pain is an uncommon complaint in these patients unless the dislocation is associated with active inflammation.

Objective

The patient should first be examined with the biomicroscope. This examination allows the clinician to evaluate the appearance of the intraocular lens under normal conditions (i.e., no pharmacologic dilation). Dilation should then be performed to allow further observation of the lens location, haptic position, and integrity of the lens capsule.

Plan

The patient should be sent back to the ophthalmic surgeon for surgical repair of the dislocation. The surgeon usually repairs the lens by securing the superior haptic to the iris; or the haptics may be repositioned for better alignment.

The patient should be followed periodically to monitor for additional symptoms or complications after the repositioning procedure.

SUGGESTED READING

Cross HE. Ectopia lentis in systemic heritable disorders. Birth Defects 1974;10:113–119.

Jaffe NS, Jaffe MS, Jaffe GS. Cataract Surgery and Its Complications (6th ed). St. Louis: Mosby, 1998.

Maumenee IH. The eye in Marfan syndrome. Trans Am Ophthalmol Soc 1981;79:684–733.

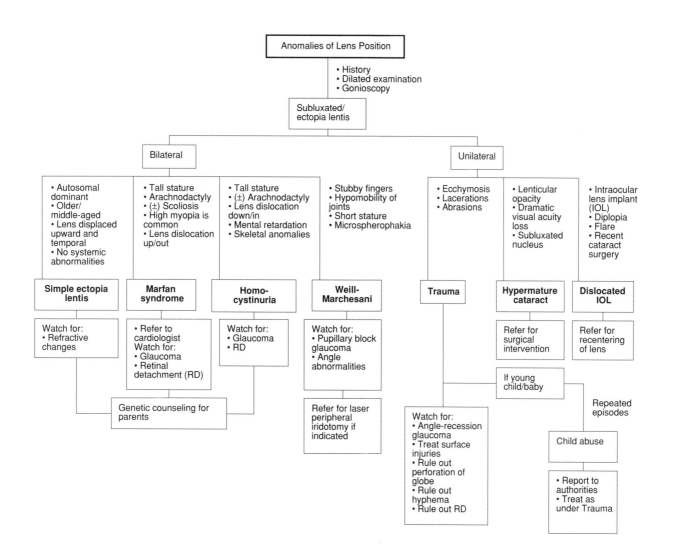

41

Leukocoria (White Pupil)

DEBRA J. BEZAN

LEUKOCORIA (WHITE PUPIL) AT A GLANCE

Cataract
Persistent hyperplastic primary vitreous
Organized vitreous hemorrhage
Falciform fold
Retinal detachment
Retinoschisis
Retinopathy of prematurity
High myopia
Coloboma
Medullated nerve fibers
Chorioretinitis
Coats' disease
Familial exudative vitreoretinopathy
Retinoblastoma
Reticulum cell sarcoma
Astrocytoma
Glioma
Hemangioma
Norrie's disease
Retinal dysplasia
Incontinentia pigmenti
Trisomy 13–15 (trisomy D)

Leukocoria, or white pupil, is usually associated with decreased vision. Pertinent information to elicit from the patient who presents with leukocoria includes age of onset of the condition, history of ocular trauma or infection, and history of systemic disease. The initial evaluation of leukocoria should include measurement of best-corrected visual acuity, pupil assessment, and dilated examination of the lens, vitreous, and retina.

CATARACT

Subjective

Cataracts can be congenital or acquired. Acquired cataracts are most commonly age related; however, they may be associated with infection, inflammation, or trauma. Cataracts usually cause blurred vision and increased sensitivity to glare.

Objective

Cataracts have different appearances depending on the layers of the lens that are affected. Congenital cataracts and acquired cortical cataracts tend to be white, and nuclear cataracts tend to be yellow or brown.

Plan

Cataracts are managed by lens extraction, usually accompanied by implantation of an intraocular lens. Congenital cataracts should be extracted and postsurgical vision corrected at as early an age as possible to prevent the development of amblyopia.

DICTYOMA (MEDULLOEPITHELIOMA)

Subjective

A dictyoma is a neuroectodermal tumor of the ciliary body. It may cause vision loss depending on its location and size.

Objective

A dictyoma is a unilateral tumor of the ciliary body that, if it extends posteriorly, can cause leukocoria. Evaluation with a three-mirror contact lens can be helpful in localizing this type of lesion.

Plan

Management involves local resection or enucleation, because the tumor can extend into the orbit.

PERSISTENT HYPERPLASTIC PRIMARY VITREOUS

Subjective

Persistent hyperplastic primary vitreous (PHPV) is a congenital condition caused by failure in the normal regression of the primary vitreous. Both the anterior and the posterior forms cause unilateral vision loss.

Objective

In addition to leukocoria, anterior PHPV is associated with microcornea, cataract, vitreous membrane, congenital glaucoma, and a normal-appearing retina. The posterior form is associated with microcornea, leukocoria, vitreoretinal membranes, retinal folds, retinal pigmentary changes, and optic nerve hypoplasia. Norrie's disease, an inherited X-linked condition, has a similar ocular appearance to PHPV, but it also has symptoms of deafness and mental retardation.

Plan

Surgical treatment of anterior PHPV, if performed early enough, can improve vision in some cases. Patients with posterior PHPV should be monitored for development of retinal detachment; however, little can be done to improve the visual prognosis.

ENDOPHTHALMITIS

Subjective

Endophthalmitis can be either sterile or infectious. Infectious endophthalmitis is most commonly associated with ocular trauma, including intraocular surgery. Symptoms include mild to severe eye pain and blurred vision.

Objective

The leukocoria caused by endophthalmitis is due to the presence of inflammatory debris in the vitreous. It is usually found in association with corneal edema and conjunctival chemosis. The presence of lid edema is one of the signs used to help differentiate infectious endophthalmitis from other forms of postoperative uveitis. Culture of vitreous aspirate can be used to confirm the diagnosis of infectious endophthalmitis.

Plan

Aggressive therapy with antibiotics administered topically, subconjunctivally, orally, intravenously, or intravitreously is used to treat the underlying infection in infectious endophthalmitis. Agents used include gentamicin, tobramycin, clindamycin, vancomycin, cefazolin sodium, and ceftriaxone sodium. In addition, cycloplegic agents and corticosteroids are used to manage the inflammatory component of either sterile or infectious endophthalmitis.

POSTERIOR UVEITIS

Subjective

Significant spillover of inflammatory debris into the vitreous from a posterior uveitis can cause leukocoria. Organisms that most commonly cause a pronounced vitritis include *Toxoplasma*, *Toxocara*, and *Candida*. Vitritis is also a sign of acute retinal necrosis secondary to a herpes simplex or herpes zoster infection. All of the above organisms can cause opportunistic infections in patients with acquired immunodeficiency syndrome. In these infections, if the visual axis is involved, the patient typically complains of blurred or reduced vision.

Objective

The vitreous response may range from mild to severe ("headlight-in-a-fog" appearance). It is associated with retinal vasculitis, macular edema, and chorioretinitis, which may be focal or diffuse. Culture of vitreous aspirate and other laboratory studies may be helpful in the differential diagnosis of vitritis associated with posterior uveitis. These tests include anti-*Toxoplasma* antibody titer, enzyme-linked immunosorbent assay (ELISA) for *Toxocara*, complement fixation titer for *Candida*, and Western blot test for human immunodeficiency virus (HIV).

Plan

Appropriate antimicrobial therapy combined with oral or injected corticosteroids is used to treat the underlying infection causing the vitritis. (See specific disease entities listed under Chorioretinitis, later.)

ORGANIZED VITREOUS HEMORRHAGE

Subjective

Hemorrhage into the vitreous is usually caused by a ruptured neovascular vessel or a retinal tear. Initially, patients may complain of a red haze, blurred vision, or floaters.

Objective

As a vitreous hemorrhage begins to resolve, it changes in color from red to yellow to white. It may eventually clear, or whitish fibrous sheets may remain. Vitreous hemorrhage is often seen in association with proliferative retinopathies, retinal tears, or retinal or vitreous detachment. B-scan ultrasonography may be helpful in identifying a vitreous hemorrhage when a direct view is obscured.

Plan

Vitrectomy is the primary treatment for a long-standing vitreous hemorrhage that interferes with vision.

MASQUERADE SYNDROME (TUMORS)

Subjective

Certain tumors can seed into the vitreous and mimic inflammatory debris; thus, they may be classified as masquerade syndromes. These malignancies include reticular cell sarcoma, retinoblastoma, lymphoma, melanoma, metastatic carcinoma, and leukemia. The primary symptoms are floaters or vision loss reflecting the degree of vitreous opacification.

Objective

Vitreous opacities associated with tumors are often linearly or radially oriented, unlike opacities associated with inflammation, which tend to form clusters or clumps. There is also less vitreous syneresis associated with tumor than with inflammation. Evidence of a tumor in the retina or choroid helps to support the diagnosis of vitreous seeding. A diagnostic vitrectomy provides confirmatory information.

Plan

Radiation and enucleation are the most common therapies used to treat intraocular tumors. Patients with suspected tumors should also be referred for an oncologic evaluation and management of systemic malignancies.

CONGENITAL FALCIFORM FOLD

Subjective

Congenital falciform fold is a condition that occasionally has an autosomal recessive pattern of inheritance. It may cause reduced vision depending on the area of the retina involved.

Objective

Falciform fold appears as a whitened fold in the retina that extends from the peripheral retina to the optic disk. It may be associated with other ocular conditions such as PHPV or retinopathy of prematurity.

Plan

Routine monitoring is sufficient to manage falciform folds.

RETINAL DETACHMENT

Subjective

Risk factors for the development of retinal detachment include ocular trauma and intraocular surgery, vitreous degeneration or detachment, high myopia, retinal breaks or degenerations, retinal vascular disease, and a positive history of detachment in the opposite eye. Symptoms of retinal detachment include flashes of light, floaters, or decreased vision in the field corresponding to the detached area. It is important to note, however, that some retinal detachments are asymptomatic.

Objective

Detachments can be rhegmatogenous (associated with retinal tear), tractional (associated with traction bands between the retina and vitreous), or exudative (associated with subretinal fluid exudation). They appear as a translucent area of elevated retina that undulates slightly with movement. Long-standing detachments become more opaque. Large, centrally located detachments can cause leukocoria.

Plan

Retinal reattachment surgery is indicated for most cases of retinal detachment.

RETINOPATHY OF PREMATURITY

Subjective

Retinopathy of prematurity (ROP) occurs in premature, low-birth-weight infants. Oxygen therapy given to these infants is thought to cause vaso-obliteration of the peripheral retina. When the infant is removed from oxygen supplementation, the relative hypoxia of the retina stimulates the development of peripheral neovascularization. Advanced ROP can cause significant vision loss.

Objective

ROP begins as a whitish demarcation zone followed by proliferative retinopathy in the peripheral retina. Other signs include fibrous band formation, dragged disc, vitreous hemorrhage, retinal detachment, and white retrolental mass. Advanced cases can cause leukocoria.

Plan

Management of ROP includes cryotherapy or photocoagulation of the peripheral retina and reattachment surgery in the event of a detachment.

COATS' DISEASE (RETINAL TELANGIECTASIA)

Subjective

Coats' disease is typically a unilateral condition found in young boys. It is usually diagnosed between the ages of 2 and 10. It can cause vision loss, particularly if the macula is affected.

Objective

Massive exudation from retinal telangiectasias and aneurysms is the hallmark of Coats' disease. Either the exudate alone or an exudative retinal detachment can cause leukocoria. Fluorescein angiography is helpful in highlighting the vascular abnormalities characteristic of this disease.

Plan

The treatment of Coats' disease consists of photocoagulation or cryotherapy to seal leaking vessels. In some cases, retinal reattachment surgery may be indicated.

DEGENERATIVE MYOPIA

Subjective

Degenerative myopia begins in childhood and is a progressive bilateral disease. Vision loss can result, particularly if macular hemorrhaging or retinal detachment occurs.

Objective

High refractive error is one of the signs of degenerative myopia. Lacquer cracks and Fuchs' spots indicate breaks in Bruch's membrane. Myopic conus, staphyloma, and generalized retinal pigment degeneration associated with degenerative myopia can cause leukocoria.

Plan

Correction of refractive error and frequent monitoring for the development of retinal breaks, detachments, and subretinal neovascularization are indicated in the management of patients with degenerative myopia. Neovascular nets can sometimes be treated successfully with photocoagulation.

COLOBOMA

Subjective

Coloboma is a congenital condition caused by incomplete closure of the fetal fissure. Vision loss can range from mild to severe depending on the extent of the coloboma.

Objective

Colobomas can be unilateral or bilateral, and can involve the iris, retina, choroid, or optic nerve head. They appear as well-demarcated, rounded areas of bare sclera in the inferior fundus. Morning-glory syndrome, a condition characterized by an enlarged optic nerve head covered with whitish glial tissue, is considered by some to be a variation of optic nerve coloboma. B-scan ultrasonography can be helpful in the diagnosis of these conditions.

Plan

Patients with coloboma should be informed of the symptoms of retinal detachment and should be monitored annually.

MEDULLATED (MYELINATED) NERVE FIBERS

Subjective

This condition is a congenital anomaly caused by myelination of the retinal nerve fibers extending beyond the lamina cribrosa sclerae. It is usually asymptomatic but occasionally can cause a relative scotoma.

Objective

The condition manifests as a feathery white patch that follows the pattern of the nerve fiber layer. Unusually large areas of medullation can cause leukocoria.

Plan

Medullated nerve fibers require no treatment other than routine observation.

CHORIORETINITIS

Subjective

Trauma, infection, or other sources of inflammation can cause chorioretinitis. Chorioretinitis or posterior uveitis, unlike anterior uveitis, is rarely painful. It can be associated with blurred vision or scotoma depending on the location and extent of inflammation.

Objective

The pronounced accumulation of inflammatory debris in the vitreous associated with some types of active chorioretinitis can cause leukocoria. An example is the headlight-in-a-fog appearance associated with active toxoplasmosis. Inactive chorioretinitis typically presents as one or more focal white chorioretinal scars surrounded by a rim of retinal pigment epithelium hyperplasia. Large chorioretinal scars can also cause leukocoria.

A number of laboratory and radiologic tests are available to aid in the differential diagnosis of posterior uveitis. These include the herpes simplex virus serum antibody test for herpes simplex, fluorescent treponemal antibody absorption test for syphilis, anti-*Toxoplasma* antigen titer for toxoplasmosis, ELISA for toxocariasis, cytomegalovirus serum antibody test for cytomegalovirus, angiotensin-converting enzyme test and chest radiography for sarcoidosis, and HLA-B5 for Behçet's disease.

Plan

Management of posterior uveitis involves treating the underlying cause whenever possible and controlling inflammation. The first line of therapy for syphilis is penicillin. Sulfonamides, pyrimethamine, and clindamycin are used for toxoplasmosis. Foscarnet sodium, ganciclovir, fomi-versen, and cidofovir, along with systemic HIV therapy, are used to treat cytomegalovirus chorioretinitis. For conditions with an unknown mechanism, such as sarcoidosis or Behçet's disease, the primary goal is control of inflammation. Agents used to control inflammation in posterior uveitis include corticosteroids, nonsteroidal anti-inflammatories, cytotoxic immunosuppressives, and antimetabolites.

TUMORS

Subjective

A number of different tumors, including retinoblastoma, astrocytoma, glioma, and hemangioma, can cause leukocoria. Vision loss and strabismus can result depending on the location and extent of the tumor.

Objective

As mentioned previously, tumor cells seeding into the vitreous can mimic uveitis (masquerade syndrome) and cause leukocoria. The primary retinal tumor can cause leukocoria as well. Ultrasonography, computed tomography (CT) and fluorescein angiography are useful procedures in the differential diagnosis of retinal tumors. For example, the calcific nature of a retinoblastoma is highlighted with ultrasonography or CT, whereas the highly vascular nature of a hemangioma is quite evident with fluorescein angiography.

Plan

Retinoblastoma can be life-threatening. In unilateral cases, the treatment of choice is enucleation; in bilateral cases, the worst eye is usually enucleated and the better eye irradiated. All other retinal tumors should be carefully monitored and referred for surgical excision or other treatment if indicated.

SUGGESTED READING

Alexander LA. Primary Care of the Posterior Segment (2nd ed). Norwalk, CT: Appleton & Lange, 1994.

Margo CE, Hamed LM, Mames RN. Diagnostic Problems in Clinical Ophthalmology. Philadelphia: Saunders, 1994.

Roy FH. Ocular Differential Diagnosis (5th ed). Philadelphia: Lea & Febiger, 1993.

Tabbara KF. Posterior uveitis—part I. Int Ophthalmol Clin 1995;35:1–29.

van Heuven WAJ, Zwaan JT. Decision Making in Ophthalmology. St. Louis: Mosby–Year Book, 1992.

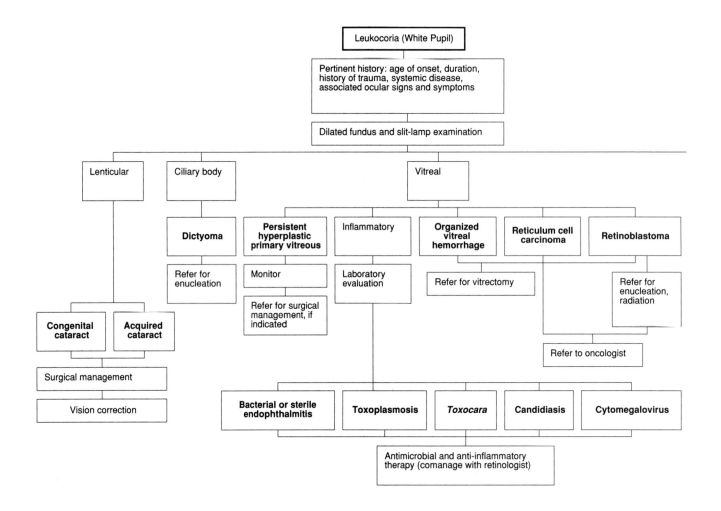

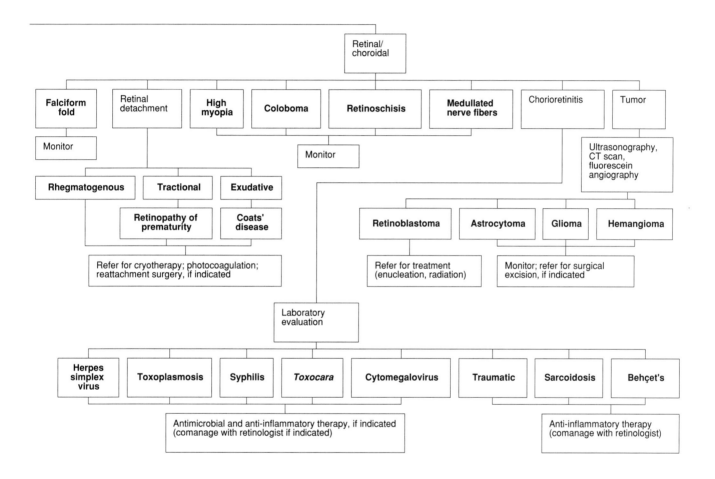

42

Vitreous Opacities

Debra J. Bezan

VITREOUS OPACITIES AT A GLANCE

Vitreous strands or condensation
Vitreous detachment
Retinal detachment
  Rhegmatogenous detachment
  Trauma
  Diabetic retinopathy
  Sickle cell retinopathy
  Retinopathy of prematurity
  Eales' disease
  Coats' disease
  Tumor
Vitreous hemorrhage
Fibrovascular proliferation
Asteroid hyalosis
Synchesis scintillans
Persistent hyperplastic primary vitreous
Amyloidosis
Tumor
  Retinoblastoma
  Reticular cell sarcoma
  Melanoma
  Lymphoma
  Metastases
Intermediate or posterior uveitis
  Pars planitis
  Toxoplasmosis
  Toxocariasis
  Cytomegalovirus infection
  Syphilis
  Candidiasis
  Sarcoidosis
  Behçet's disease
  Vogt-Koyanagi-Harada syndrome
  Traumatic inflammation

Endophthalmitis
Acute retinal necrosis

Vitreous opacities are associated with a number of conditions ranging from benign degenerative changes to severe sight-threatening pathologies. Vitreous opacities may be asymptomatic or may cause the patient to perceive floaters or experience blurred vision.

The evaluation of the vitreous typically consists of a slit-lamp examination with and without the aid of a fundus lens, direct ophthalmoscopy, and binocular indirect ophthalmoscopy. A three-mirror lens or scleral indentation may be needed to adequately view the peripheral vitreous near the ora serrata. Occasionally, culturing or histologic evaluation of an aspirate of vitreous material is required for definitive diagnosis. In addition, laboratory and radiologic tests can provide useful information in the differential diagnosis of vitreous opacities associated with posterior uveitis.

VITREOUS STRANDS OR CONDENSATIONS

Subjective

Focal condensations of vitreous protein and collagen are the most common type of benign degenerative vitreous opacity. Remnants of the fetal vascular system suspended in the vitreous can also cause the patient to experience floaters. Floaters of both these types are chronic, relatively stable in size, and tend to shift with changes in fixation.

Objective

Focal vitreous condensations sometimes can be visualized with the slit-lamp biomicroscope as wispy strands that drift and then settle back to their original position with eye movements.

Plan

No treatment beyond reassurance and routine monitoring is indicated for these vitreous floaters.

POSTERIOR VITREOUS DETACHMENT

Subjective

Posterior vitreous detachment (PVD) is one of the most common types of vitreous opacity. It is associated with degenerative changes in the aging vitreous and thus is found primarily in patients over the age of 45. However, certain conditions—including trauma, inflammation, diabetic retinopathy, degenerative myopia, and other inherited vitreoretinal degenerations—can cause an earlier onset of PVD.

The floaters noted by patients with PVD typically have a sudden onset and appear as well-defined shapes that shift with fixation. The flashes occur as movements of the vitreous cause traction on the retina at areas of firm vitreoretinal attachment, such as the vitreous base. Cessation of the flashes usually indicates progression of the PVD and release of traction on the retina.

Objective

Centrally located PVDs can often be observed with a direct ophthalmoscope. Fundus biomicroscopy and binocular indirect ophthalmoscopy are two other techniques for viewing a PVD through a dilated pupil. The PVD often appears as a ring or crescent-shaped opacity just anterior to the optic nerve head (Weis' ring). Large PVDs may appear as a corrugated veil suspended in the vitreous cavity.

Plan

When a patient presents with a recent onset of PVD, the practitioner should carefully evaluate the peripheral retina for the presence of breaks using scleral indentation or a three-mirror lens. Such breaks occur in 15–30% of symptomatic PVD cases. Patients should be educated about the condition and the symptoms of retinal detachment. They should be monitored closely for the first 1–2 months after the onset of symptoms and then routinely thereafter.

RETINAL DETACHMENT

Subjective

Three basic types of retinal detachment exist: rhegmatogenous, tractional, and exudative. Rhegmatogenous detachments are caused by breaks in the retina and are often associated with trauma, degenerations, or high myopia. Tractional detachments are usually associated with proliferative vasculopathies or trauma. Exudative detachments are associated with conditions causing massive exudation (such as Coats' disease), inflammation (such as Vogt-Koyanagi-Harada syndrome), or tumors (such as choroidal melanoma). Each of these types of detachment has specific vitreous opacities associated with it.

Symptoms of retinal detachment include flashes, floaters, and vision loss. The lightning streak-like flashes caused by vitreoretinal traction are similar to those experienced in PVD. The floaters associated with a retinal break, however, are often multiple and resemble a swarm of gnats.

Objective

Peripheral breaks in the retina, either round holes or linear tears, and rhegmatogenous retinal detachments are often associated with small tobacco dust-like pigment particles in the anterior vitreous (Shaffer's sign). Retinal holes are round, whereas tears are linear or horseshoe shaped. There may be an adjacent vitreoretinal adhesion forming a flap tear. A white cuff surrounding a retinal break indicates the accumulation of fluid under the sensory retina, forming a retinal detachment. Larger retinal detachments have a milky appearance that obscures underlying details and often have an elevated, corrugated surface. They tend to undulate slightly with movements of the eye.

In proliferative retinopathies, exudation from neovascular vessels forms opaque fibrovascular adhesion strands that attach the vitreous to the retina. Tractional forces on these strands can cause a tractional detachment. Inflammatory cells, exudative debris, or tumor seeds can cause vitreous opacities associated with exudative detachments.

All proliferative retinopathies require a thorough evaluation for underlying systemic disease. A specific health history should be taken that includes questions about any history of premature birth, trauma, or systemic diseases in the patient or patient's family members. Laboratory tests can provide additional diagnostic information. Useful tests include fasting blood sugar for diabetes; Sickledex for sickle-cell disease; purified protein derivative (PPD) for Eales' disease; and complete blood count (CBC), lipid profile, and blood pressure assessment for occlusive vascular disease.

Plan

Retinal breaks should be monitored carefully or treated prophylactically with a laser procedure when appropriate. Surgical repair of detached retinas is performed using scleral buckling, pneumatic retinopexy and laser photocoagulation, or cryotherapy procedures.

Patients with retinal detachment secondary to systemic disease should be referred for management of the underlying systemic condition.

DIABETES MELLITUS

Subjective

Diabetes mellitus affects approximately 6% of the general population. Patients with diabetes may be asymptomatic or may complain of blurred or fluctuating vision. They may also report other symptoms associated with systemic diabetes, including polyuria, polydipsia, polyphagia, weight loss, fatigue, neuropathies, and frequent infections.

Objective

Diabetic retinopathy can be subdivided into nonproliferative diabetic retinopathy (NPDR) and proliferative diabetic retinopathy (PDR). The signs of NPDR include dot and blot hemorrhages, microaneurysms, exudates, intraretinal microvascular anomalies, cotton-wool spots, venous beading, and capillary nonperfusion. PDR has all of these signs plus neovascularization, which may lead to fibrovascular proliferation, vitreous hemorrhage, and retinal detachment. Macular edema may be associated with either NPDR or PDR and may or may not affect visual acuity.

The fasting blood sugar, 2-hour postprandial glucose, and oral glucose tolerance tests are helpful in the diagnosis of diabetes. Fluorescein angiography is useful in delineating microaneurysms, capillary nonperfusion, macular edema, and neovascularization.

Plan

Patients with NPDR should be examined at least yearly and more frequently if they show signs of increased retinal hypoxia. Patients with high-risk PDR usually benefit from panretinal photocoagulation, and those with clinically significant macular edema usually benefit from focal or grid photocoagulation. Vitrectomy can be used to prevent further neovascularization or to treat poorly resolving vitreous hemorrhages. Diabetic patients should also be referred for management of their systemic disease.

SICKLE CELL RETINOPATHY

Subjective

Sickle cell retinopathy is associated with sickling hemoglobinopathies, which are found in approximately 10% of blacks. The ocular lesions of sickle cell retinopathy are usually asymptomatic unless they are associated with retinal detachment. Nonocular signs and symptoms of sickle-cell disease include pain, fatigue, frequent infections, dehydration, hypoxia, congestive heart failure, organ infarction, gallstones, and skin ulcers.

Objective

Sickle cell retinopathy can be subdivided into nonproliferative and proliferative. Signs of nonproliferative retinopathy include salmon-patch intraretinal hemorrhages, refractile spots, black sunbursts, venous tortuosity, and angioid streaks. Signs of proliferative retinopathy include arteriovenous anastomoses, neovascular sea fans, fibrovascular bands, vitreous hemorrhage, and retinal detachment.

CBC, Sickledex, and hemoglobin electrophoresis are useful tests in the differential diagnosis of the sickle cell retinopathy.

Plan

Patients with signs of nonproliferative sickle cell retinopathy should be monitored for the development of proliferative retinopathy. If this should occur, photocoagulation or cryotherapy may be used to manage the proliferation. Vitrectomy may be indicated for poorly resolving vitreous hemorrhages. If retinal detachment occurs, scleral buckling procedures may be used for reattachment; however, patients with sickle-cell disease are at high risk for developing anterior segment necrosis secondary to buckling procedures. Patients with sickle cell retinopathy should also be referred for management of the systemic manifestations of sickle-cell disease.

OCCLUSIVE RETINAL VASCULAR DISEASE

Subjective

Occlusive retinal vascular disease is commonly associated with underlying systemic disease, including carotid artery disease, hypertension, diabetes, hyperlipidemia, chronic lung disease, and blood dyscrasias. The patient with a branch retinal vein occlusion (BRVO) often complains of vision loss corresponding to the area of hemorrhage or macular edema. The patient with a central retinal vein occlusion (CRVO) has a more generalized vision loss.

Objective

A BRVO presents as a wedge-shaped area of flame or dot-and-blot hemorrhages and exudates. The apex of the wedge points to the occlusion. Flame hemorrhages and cotton-wool spots are more commonly found in the ischemic form, as opposed to the nonischemic form, of BRVO. Retinal neovascularization is also more likely in ischemic than in nonischemic BRVO. If the occlusion involves the superior temporal retina, macular edema is likely to result.

The manifestation of a CRVO is similar to that of a BRVO except that the entire retina is involved. The development of retinal neovascularization is uncommon in CRVO, but neovascularization of the iris and angle are more common.

Patients who present with a BRVO or CRVO should be evaluated for underlying systemic disease. Useful tests in the initial evaluation include blood pressure assessment, carotid bruit auscultation, fasting blood sugar level, lipid profile, erythrocyte sedimentation rate, and CBC with differential and platelets. Fluorescein angiography is useful in differentiating nonischemic from ischemic occlusive disease and for pinpointing areas of leakage.

Plan

Patients with macular edema should be monitored monthly after the initial presentation. If the edema does not resolve within 4–6 months, grid photocoagulation may be indicated. This procedure is more effective in BRVO than in CRVO. Patients with ischemic venous occlusive disease should also be monitored closely for the development of neovascularization and, particularly in the case of ischemic CRVO, for neovascular glaucoma.

RETINOPATHY OF PREMATURITY

Subjective

Retinopathy of prematurity (ROP) is a condition found primarily in premature, low-birth-weight infants. It is thought to be caused by a failure in normal vascularization of the peripheral retina in a high-oxygen environment. When the infant is removed from oxygen supplementation, the retina becomes relatively hypoxic and forms peripheral neovascular vessels. Patients with this condition may experience vision loss as a result of tractional misalignment of the macular photoreceptors, vitreous hemorrhage, or retinal detachment.

Objective

The objective findings of ROP observable with a dilated fundus examination or fluorescein angiography vary with the severity of the disease. They include a peripheral demarcation line between vascularized and nonvascularized retina, neovascularization, vitreous hemorrhage, ridge of fibrovascular tissue, dragged disc, and partial or complete retinal detachment. The appearance of dilated, tortuous vessels in the posterior pole that is occasionally found in ROP is termed *plus disease*.

Plan

Infants at risk for ROP should be evaluated before leaving the hospital and should be examined frequently during the first 6 months. If ROP is detected, laser photocoagulation or cryotherapy can be used to stop its progression. Vitrectomy or detachment repair may be indicated in more advanced forms of the disease.

EALES' DISEASE (RETINAL PERIPHLEBITIS)

Subjective

Eales' disease is most commonly found in young adult males. In some cases it may be the result of a tubercular hypersensitivity reaction. Patients with Eales' disease may complain of floaters and blurred vision.

Objective

Eales' disease is characterized by inflammatory perivascular sheathing and vitritis. Peripheral neovascularization can develop in areas of nonperfusion and lead to vitreous hemorrhage. Edema from perimacular telangiectasia can also cause reduced vision.

The PPD test and chest radiography are useful adjunct tests in determining exposure to or active infection with tuberculosis. Fluorescein angiography is also helpful in determining areas of nonperfusion and leakage.

Plan

Patients with Eales' disease should be monitored carefully. Areas of nonperfusion or edema may be treated with laser photocoagulation. These patients should also be referred for management of tuberculosis if indicated.

TRAUMATIC HEMORRHAGE

Subjective

Intraocular foreign bodies and retinal breaks are the most common causes of vitreous hemorrhage secondary to trauma; however, blunt trauma to the eye or head can also cause this type of hemorrhage. Traumatic vitreous hemorrhaging has even been reported in association with subarachnoid hemorrhaging. The patient with vitreous hemorrhage may complain of floaters, blur, or a red haze over vision. The vision loss may be more profound depending on the location and extent of the injury.

Objective

Vitreous hemorrhage appears as a red patch or diffuse red cells within the vitreous body. It often obscures the underlying structures so that retinal evaluation is difficult. B-scan ultrasonography, orbital radiography, or computed tomography (CT) can assist in diagnosing a penetrating foreign body if the posterior segment cannot be adequately visualized.

Plan

It is important to determine the exact nature of the trauma to manage these cases appropriately. Metallic penetrating foreign bodies should be surgically removed. Vitreous hemorrhages typically resolve spontaneously over time; however, vitrectomy may be indicated for a poorly resolving hemorrhage that impairs visual function. Patients should also be monitored frequently for other sequelae of trauma, such as retinal detachment or angle-recession glaucoma.

ASTEROID HYALOSIS

Subjective

Asteroid hyalosis is a vitreous condition typically found in patients over the age of 60. It is usually unilateral and may be found in association with certain systemic diseases, particularly diabetes mellitus. Although most patients with asteroid hyalosis are asymptomatic, some report floaters or blurred vision.

Objective

Asteroid hyalosis appears as multiple small white spheres composed of calcium soaps suspended in the vitreous. They are visible with ophthalmoscopy or slit-lamp biomicroscopy and can be observed to shift slightly and then return to their original position after eye movements.

Plan

In most cases, asteroid bodies are benign and require only routine observation. Patients with this condition should be evaluated for diabetes mellitus and hypertension if these conditions have not already been diagnosed. If vision is significantly affected by asteroid bodies, or if they prevent adequate visualization of the retina needed to monitor diabetic retinopathy, vitrectomy may be indicated.

SYNCHESIS SCINTILLANS (CHOLESTEROLOSIS BULBI)

Subjective

Synchesis scintillans is a rare vitreous disorder associated with vitreous hemorrhage secondary to trauma or diabetes. It is usually found in blind or severely damaged eyes.

Objective

Synchesis scintillans is characterized by multiple refractile crystals of cholesterol found within liquefied vitreous. As the eye moves and then stabilizes, the particles swirl around and then sink down to the bottom of the liquefied vitreous. This finding is in contrast to that for asteroid hyalosis, in which the particles remain suspended.

Plan

Treatment is rarely indicated for synchesis scintillans alone, although vitrectomy may be performed to treat concurrent pathology.

PERSISTENT HYPERPLASTIC PRIMARY VITREOUS

Subjective

Persistent hyperplastic primary vitreous (PHPV) is a congenital condition caused by a failure in the normal regression of the primary vitreous during embryonic development. Acuity is often reduced in this condition due to traction on the macula, retinal detachment, or cataract.

Objective

PHPV has both anterior and posterior forms. A retrolental membrane can cause a vitreous opacity in the anterior form; remnants of the fetal vascular system and vitreoretinal adhesions can cause vitreous opacities in the posterior form. Other ocular findings in PHPV include leukocoria, congenital glaucoma, microcornea, strabismus, cataract, retinal pigmentary degeneration, and optic nerve pallor.

Plan

Patients with PHPV should be monitored carefully for retinal detachment. Vitrectomy is sometimes performed when the visual axis is occluded or when there is significant traction on the retina. A careful evaluation to rule out other serious causes of leukocoria, including retinoblastoma, should be performed on all children with suspected PHPV.

AMYLOIDOSIS

Subjective

Amyloidosis has a primary noninherited form that is limited to the eye and a secondary form with both ocular and systemic manifestations that is inherited as an autosomal dominant trait. Ocular symptoms include diplopia, photophobia, blepharospasm, and progressive loss of vision. Systemic symptoms of the secondary form include fatigue, weight loss, and symptoms caused by infiltration of the gastrointestinal, cardiac, renal, endocrine, and nervous systems.

Objective

Cotton candy–like vitreous opacities are found in both forms of amyloidosis. Other ocular findings include ophthalmoplegia, exophthalmos, and retinal hemorrhages and exudates. Vitreous biopsy and serum protein electrophoresis are useful tests to confirm a tentative diagnosis of amyloidosis.

Plan

Vitrectomy has a poor prognosis for providing long-term visual improvement in patients with amyloidosis due to the tendency of amyloid to re-form after this procedure. Patients with suspected secondary amyloidosis should be referred for further evaluation and supportive therapy.

TUMORS (MASQUERADE SYNDROME)

Subjective

Certain tumors can seed into the vitreous and mimic inflammatory debris; thus, they are sometimes classified as masquerade syndromes. These malignancies include retinoblastoma, lymphoma, melanoma, reticular cell sarcoma, metastatic carcinoma, and leukemia. The primary symptoms are floaters or vision loss reflecting the degree of vitreous opacification.

Objective

Vitreous opacities associated with tumors are often linearly or radially oriented, unlike opacities associated with inflammation, which tend to form clusters or clumps. There is also less vitreous syneresis associated with a tumor than with inflammation. Evidence of a tumor in the retina or choroid helps to support the diagnosis of vitreous seeding. A vitreous biopsy provides confirmatory information.

Plan

Radiation and enucleation are the most common therapies used to treat intraocular tumors. Patients with suspected tumors should also be referred for an oncologic evaluation and management of systemic malignancies.

TOXOPLASMOSIS

Subjective

Toxoplasmosis caused by the protozoan *Toxoplasma gondii* is the most common cause of posterior uveitis in the United States. The infection is acquired through contact with cat feces or ingestion of poorly cooked meat, and it can be transmitted transplacentally. The disease has both congenital and acquired forms. In the acute phase, the main ocular symptom is blurred vision due to vitreous debris. Subsequent permanent vision loss can occur due to chorioretinal scarring.

Objective

The congenital form classically affects the macula and results in large chorioretinal scars. The acquired form affects other areas of the retina as well. Reactivation due to immune suppression often causes secondary or satellite lesions to bud off adjacent to the primary lesion. During the acute phase, significant amounts of white blood cells and other inflammatory debris are released into the vitreous so that often there is only a hazy view of the retina. This condition is termed *headlight in a fog*. There may be a concurrent anterior uveitis.

Although the diagnosis is often made from the clinical appearance, a serum anti-*Toxoplasma* antibody titer is sometimes used for confirmation.

Plan

A common initial treatment of active toxoplasmosis is oral sulfadiazine combined with oral pyrimethamine. Folinic acid is added to reduce bone marrow toxicity. Oral prednisone may be added to antimicrobial therapy to control inflammation. Alternative therapies include oral clindamycin, tetracycline, or sulfamethoxazole-trimethoprim. Newer antimicrobial therapies include azithromycin and atovaquone. Laser photocoagulation and vitrectomy have also been used as supplemental therapy in some cases.

TOXOCARIASIS

Subjective

Toxocariasis is caused by the larvae of the dog roundworm (*Toxocara canis*). It has both an ocular and a visceral form. Toxocariasis is found most commonly in children who have a history of contact with dogs or who have eaten contaminated dirt. The primary symptom is vision loss. The loss is dependent on the area of the retina affected.

Objective

Ocular toxocariasis is generally a unilateral condition that classically presents as one or more focal retinal granulomas with white, fibrotic bands. These bands may extend from the optic nerve to the granuloma. Strabismus, cataract, and leukocoria are associated findings. A significant positive *Toxocara* enzyme-linked immunosorbent assay (ELISA) titer helps to confirm the diagnosis.

Plan

An oral antihelminthic, thiabendazole, combined with prednisone to control inflammation, is used to treat toxocariasis. Vitrectomy is occasionally used to release vitreous traction bands, and reattachment surgery is indicated in the case of retinal detachment.

CYTOMEGALOVIRUS RETINOPATHY

Subjective

Cytomegalovirus (CMV) is an opportunistic organism that typically infects an immunocompromised host, for example, one with acquired immunodeficiency syndrome (AIDS). The symptoms of CMV retinopathy vary according to the location and extent of the tissue damage. Some patients may be totally asymptomatic, whereas others may complain of floaters and central or peripheral vision loss.

Objective

CMV retinopathy begins as a focal area of necrosis, often at the site of a cotton-wool spot representing human immunodeficiency virus (HIV) retinopathy. The necrosis spreads over a period of weeks to months, usually in a "brush-fire" pattern. Other signs of ocular CMV infection include vitreous opacities, microaneurysms, hemorrhages, perivascular sheathing, and ischemic areas due to capillary nonperfusion. This condition has been called the "mustard and catsup fundus" or the "pizza fundus" because of the large yellow and red patches caused by hemorrhaging and necrosis. CMV retinopathy can lead to retinal detachment.

A laboratory evaluation for HIV infection (ELISA for HIV or Western blot test) should be performed on patients with suspected CMV retinopathy. A serum CMV antibody screen can be used to confirm the diagnosis of CMV. A CD4 lymphocyte count may also be useful in monitoring the progression of AIDS. CMV retinopathy is usually associated with a low CD4 count.

Plan

The primary drugs currently available to treat CMV retinopathy are ganciclovir, foscarnet sodium, cidofovir, and fomiversen. These drugs do not cure the condition but can cause it to stabilize or regress. Patients who develop retinal detachments may require reattachment surgery.

SYPHILIS

Subjective

Although syphilitic vitritis is uncommon, it is occasionally found in secondary acquired syphilis. Patients may be asymptomatic or may complain of floaters or vision loss.

Objective

Ocular signs of secondary syphilis include conjunctivitis, episcleritis, scleritis, dacryoadenitis, interstitial keratitis, anterior uveitis, vitritis, retinal vasculitis, chorioretinitis, and optic neuritis.

Tests commonly used to confirm the diagnosis of syphilis include VDRL test, rapid plasma reagin test, fluorescent treponemal antibody absorption test, and microhemagglutination assay-*Treponema pallidum*. Patients with syphilis should also be tested for HIV infection.

Plan

The management of syphilis consists of treating the patient with penicillin injections. Anterior segment inflammation is treated with topical corticosteroids and cycloplegic agents; however, these are relatively ineffective for posterior segment inflammation.

CANDIDIASIS

Subjective

Candidiasis is an infection by a yeast of the *Candida* genus. Posterior segment candidiasis is usually caused by spread of systemic infection; anterior segment infection can also occur from local inoculation. Systemic candidiasis is uncommon, and most often occurs in intravenous drug abusers or debilitated or immunocompromised patients. There may be no symptoms, or the patient may complain of floaters and vision loss, depending on the location and degree of inflammation.

Objective

Candidiasis occasionally presents as fluffy white abscesses and exudates in the vitreous. Other posterior segment manifestations include chorioretinitis, perivasculitis,

endophthalmitis, optic neuritis, and exudative detachment. Serum anti-*Candida* antibody testing and culture of vitreous aspirate are used to confirm the diagnosis of candidiasis.

Plan

Antifungal agents such as flucytosine and miconazole are used to treat intraocular candidiasis. Some also advocate the use of therapeutic vitrectomy, although this therapy is controversial.

BACTERIAL ENDOPHTHALMITIS

Subjective

Bacterial endophthalmitis can be caused by the endogenous spread of systemic infection, particularly in an intravenous drug abuser or an individual who is generally debilitated or immunocompromised. It can also come from an exogenous source through ocular trauma, including surgery. Symptoms include floaters and vision loss.

Objective

Signs of bacterial endophthalmitis revealed through biomicroscopic and ophthalmoscopic examination include lid and corneal edema, conjunctival injection, hypopyon, cells and inflammatory debris in the vitreous, and retinal hemorrhages and exudates. Cultures of blood, urine, or vitreous aspirate aid in identifying the causative organism.

Plan

Broad-spectrum antibiotics delivered systemically, periocularly, topically, or intravitreously are used initially, until the treatment can be modified based on the culture and sensitivity results. Topical corticosteroids and cycloplegic agents are used to manage anterior segment inflammation. Therapeutic vitrectomy has also been advocated for some cases.

PARS PLANITIS

Subjective

Pars planitis is an intermediate uveitis or retinal vasculitis that occurs most frequently in adolescents and young adults. The most common symptoms associated with this condition are floaters and blurred vision.

Objective

Cells and snowball-like opacities in the anterior inferior vitreous can be observed with biomicroscopy or ophthalmoscopy. Scleral depression or three-mirror evaluation is often needed to view the "snowbanks" of inflammatory debris in the far periphery. Other signs sometimes associated with pars planitis are anterior uveitis, posterior subcapsular cataract, glaucoma, cystoid macular edema, vitreous detachment, vitreous hemorrhage, retinal neovascularization, and retinal detachment. Fluorescein angiography is a useful adjunct test if cystoid macular edema is suspected.

Plan

Pars planitis typically has periods of exacerbation and remission, then ultimately subsides after many years. Patients with mild vision loss are simply monitored, but those with acuity of less than 20/40 may be treated with topical or injected corticosteroids. Oral acetazolamide has also been used in an attempt to improve vision in cases that do not respond to steroid therapy.

SARCOIDOSIS

Subjective

Sarcoidosis is a systemic inflammatory disease that affects primarily young adult blacks. It is also relatively common among certain Scandinavian populations. Females are affected more commonly than males. Ocular symptoms include photophobia, pain, and blurred vision. Systemic symptoms may include cough and pulmonary discomfort, as well as fever, fatigue, and malaise.

Objective

Sarcoidosis can affect both the anterior and posterior eye. Extraocular muscle palsies and proptosis may be noted during gross observation. Slit-lamp examination may reveal lacrimal gland enlargement, conjunctival granuloma, keratitis sicca, band keratopathy, granulomatous uveitis, cataract, and vitritis. The peripheral fluffy white clumps of inflammatory debris in the vitreous may take on a "string-of-pearls" appearance and can be better viewed with indirect ophthalmoscopy and scleral depression. Other posterior signs are perivascular sheathing, "candle-wax dripping" exudates, retinal neovascularization, cystoid macular edema, glaucoma, and optic neuritis.

Systemic signs include hilar adenopathy, skin nodules, salivary gland enlargement, hepatomegaly, splenomegaly, arthritis, lymphadenopathy, seventh nerve palsy, and other central nervous system changes.

The primary tests used to confirm the diagnosis of sarcoidosis are chest radiography and angiotensin-converting enzyme test. Supplemental testing includes gallium scan, PPD with anergy panel, tissue biopsy, serum lysozyme level, and Kveim skin test.

Plan

Patients with sarcoidosis should be comanaged with an internist. Oral corticosteroids are often given to manage systemic symptoms. Ocular manifestations such as anterior uveitis or glaucoma are treated accordingly.

BEHÇET'S DISEASE

Subjective

Behçet's disease is a vasculitis that most commonly affects young adult males of Japanese or Mediterranean descent. Ocular symptoms include pain, photophobia, and vision loss. Systemic symptoms are variable but may include cough, chest pain, tender oral or genital lesions, fever, malaise, joint pain, gastrointestinal disturbances, and deafness or other neurologic disorders.

Objective

The ocular signs of Behçet's disease are numerous. They include lid lesions, conjunctivitis, keratitis, episcleritis, scleritis, granulomatous anterior uveitis (often with hypopyon), iris neovascularization with secondary glaucoma, cataract, vitritis, vitreous hemorrhage, retinal vasculitis and sheathing, pigment epithelium hypertrophy, venous occlusion, macular edema, retinal detachment, papillitis, optic atrophy, and cranial nerve palsies.

Systemic manifestations include oral and genital aphthous ulcers, erythematous skin lesions, epididymitis, arthritis, colitis, thrombophlebitis, hemoptysis, fever, anemia, and central nervous system abnormalities.

Tests to aid in the diagnosis of Behçet's disease include HLA-B5, erythrocyte sedimentation rate, and behçentine skin test.

Plan

Behçet's disease runs a chronic course with exacerbations and remissions. Referral to a rheumatologist for management of the systemic disease is indicated. Care of the patient with Behçet's disease consists of attempting to control systemic and ocular inflammation through the use of corticosteroids and immunosuppressive agents. Anticoagulant therapy has also be used in cases in which anti-inflammatory agents are ineffective.

TRAUMATIC INFLAMMATION

Subjective

Ocular trauma, including surgical trauma, often causes inflammation. The presence of cells and other inflammatory debris in the vitreous is among the manifestations of intraocular inflammation. Patients with vitritis may complain of floaters or blurred vision.

Objective

The goal of the diagnostic evaluation is to determine the nature and location of the trauma. In addition to vitritis, other signs of ocular trauma include conjunctival injection, subconjunctival hemorrhage, perforation of the globe, hypotony, positive Seidel's sign, anterior chamber reaction, angle recession, cataract, vitreous hemorrhage, retinal pigment epithelium migration and hyperplasia, retinal hemorrhage, commotio retinae, retinal breaks, retinal detachment, choroidal rupture, choroidal detachment, and choroidal neovascularization. These signs vary with the type and extent of injury. If the posterior segment of the eye cannot be viewed adequately, B-scan ultrasonography, radiography, or CT scanning is indicated.

Plan

Management of ocular injuries consists of surgical repair of the damaged tissues when indicated and control of inflammation through the use of topical or systemic corticosteroids and nonsteroidal anti-inflammatory agents. In perforating injuries, antimicrobial agents are also used to treat or prevent infection.

SUGGESTED READING

Alexander LA. Primary Care of the Posterior Segment (2nd ed). Norwalk, CT: Appleton & Lange, 1994.

Cullom RD, Chang B. The Wills Eye Manual: Office and Emergency Room Diagnosis and Treatment of Eye Disease (2nd ed). Philadelphia: Lippincott, 1994.

Fraunfelder FT, Roy FH. Current Ocular Therapy 4. Philadelphia: Saunders, 1995.

Henahan JL. Treatment of cytomegalovirus retinitis in AIDS. Clin Eye Vis Care 1993;5:139–145.

Loeb S (ed). Clinical Laboratory Tests: Values and Interpretation. Springhouse, PA: Springhouse, 1991.

Marks ES, Adamczyk DT, Thomann KH. Primary Eyecare in Systemic Disease. Norwalk, CT: Appleton & Lange, 1995.

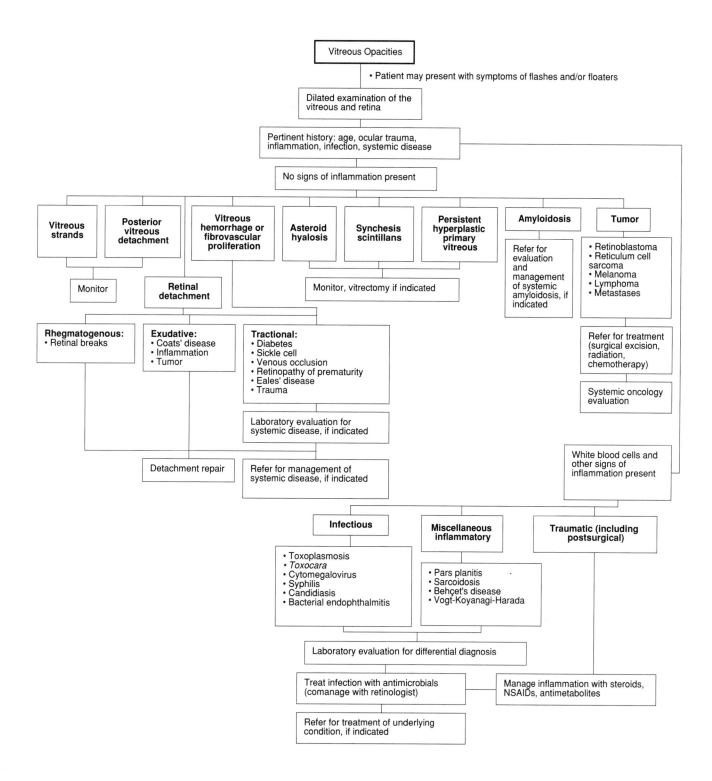

43

Posterior Segment Hemorrhages

DEBRA J. BEZAN

POSTERIOR SEGMENT HEMORRHAGES AT A GLANCE

Vitreous hemorrhages (intravitreous and
  retrovitreous)
  Diabetic retinopathy
  Vitreous detachment
  Retinal detachment
  Venous occlusions
  Hematologic disorders
  Retinopathy of prematurity
  Eales' disease
  Trauma
  Valsalva retinopathy
  Pars planitis
Retinal hemorrhages (nerve fiber layer—flame)
  Hypertensive retinopathy
  Diabetic retinopathy
  Venous occlusive disease
  Acquired immunodeficiency syndrome retinopathy
  Hematologic disorders
  Optic neuritis
  Ischemic optic neuropathy
  Papillophlebitis
  Papilledema
  Glaucoma
  Optic nerve head drusen
  Bacterial endocarditis
  Oral contraceptive use
Retinal hemorrhages (middle and deep sensory retina—
  dot-and-blot)
  Diabetic retinopathy
  Hypertensive retinopathy
  Venous occlusions
  Hematologic disorders
  Posterior vitreous detachment

Acquired immunodeficiency syndrome and cytomegalo-
  virus retinopathy
  Retinal telangiectasias
  Retinal vascular tumors
  Oral contraceptive use
Retinal hemorrhages (subsensory retina)
  Age-related macular degeneration
  Presumed ocular histoplasmosis syndrome
  Degenerative myopia
  Posterior uveitis
  Trauma
  Angioid streaks
  Hematologic disorders
  Coats' disease
  Retinopathy of prematurity
  Diabetic retinopathy
Choroidal hemorrhages
  Age-related macular degeneration
  Presumed ocular histoplasmosis
  Degenerative myopia
  Posterior uveitis
  Trauma
  Surgery, photocoagulation
  Angioid streaks
  Serpiginous (geographic helicoid) peripapillary
    choroidopathy
  Optic nerve head drusen
  Pars planitis
  Osseous choroidoma
  Retinal hamartoma
  Vitelliform dystrophy
  Harada's disease

Most patients with posterior segment hemorrhages are
not symptomatic unless the hemorrhage is sufficiently
large, involves the visual axis, or is associated with mac-

ular edema or scarring. Many hemorrhages are detected in the course of a routine dilated fundus examination.

The location of a posterior segment hemorrhage is fairly easy to determine based on the depth, shape, and color of the hemorrhage. Fresh intravitreous hemorrhages tend to be bright red and diffuse. Long-standing vitreous hemorrhages have a yellow hue. Those that are secondary to proliferative retinopathy may be associated with white vitreoretinal traction bands. Blood trapped between the hyaloid face and the retina or between the inner limiting membrane and the nerve fiber layer tends to become boat shaped as a result of gravitational forces. It is initially bright red but becomes yellowish with time. Retinal hemorrhages located in the nerve fiber layer are bright red and flame shaped, whereas those located in the middle or deeper sensory retinal layers are round (dot-and-blot hemorrhages). Hemorrhages trapped between the sensory retina and retinal pigment epithelium are dark red and somewhat diffuse. Sub–retinal pigment epithelial or choroidal hemorrhages are greenish gray and diffuse in shape.

Most posterior segment hemorrhages are caused by underlying systemic or ocular conditions. When posterior segment hemorrhages are noted, the patient should be asked about a history of systemic or ocular disease, headaches, fatigue, weight changes, or vision loss.

RETINOPATHY OF PREMATURITY

Subjective

Retinopathy of prematurity (ROP) is a condition found primarily in premature, low-birth-weight infants. It is thought to be caused by a failure of the peripheral retina to vascularize normally in a high-oxygen environment. When the infant is removed from oxygen supplementation, the retina becomes relatively hypoxic and forms peripheral neovascular vessels. Patients with this condition may experience vision loss because of tractional misalignment of the macular photoreceptors, vitreous hemorrhage, or retinal detachment.

Objective

The objective findings of ROP observable with a dilated fundus examination or fluorescein angiography vary with the severity of the disease. They include a peripheral demarcation line between vascularized and nonvascularized retina, neovascularization, vitreous hemorrhage, ridge of fibrovascular tissue, dragged disc, and partial or complete retinal detachment. The presence of dilated tortuous vessels in the posterior pole in ROP is called *plus disease*.

Plan

Infants at risk for ROP should be evaluated before leaving the hospital and should be examined frequently during the first 6 months. If ROP is detected, laser photocoagulation or cryotherapy can be used to halt its progression. Vitrectomy or detachment repair may be indicated in more advanced forms of the disease.

TRAUMA

Subjective

Intraocular foreign bodies and retinal breaks are the most common causes of vitreous hemorrhage secondary to trauma; however, blunt trauma to the eye or head can also cause this type of hemorrhage. Vitreous hemorrhages have even been reported in association with subarachnoid hemorrhaging. The patient may complain of floaters, blur, or a red haze over vision. The vision loss may be more profound, depending on the location and extent of the injury.

Objective

Vitreous hemorrhage appears as a red patch or diffuse red cells within the vitreous body. It often obscures the underlying structures so that retinal evaluation is difficult. B-scan ultrasonography, orbital radiography, or computed tomography (CT) can assist in the diagnosis of a penetrating foreign body if the posterior segment cannot be adequately visualized.

Plan

It is important to determine the exact nature of the trauma to manage these cases appropriately. Metallic penetrating foreign bodies should be surgically removed. Vitreous hemorrhages typically resolve spontaneously over time; however, vitrectomy may be indicated for a poorly resolving hemorrhage that impairs visual function. These patients should also be monitored at least annually for other sequelae of trauma, such as retinal detachment or angle-recession glaucoma.

VITREOUS DETACHMENT

Subjective

Posterior vitreous detachments (PVDs) are associated with degenerative changes in the aging vitreous and thus are found primarily in patients over the age of 45. However, certain conditions—including trauma, inflammation, diabetic retinopathy, degenerative myopia, and inherited vitreoretinal degenerations—can cause an earlier onset of PVD.

The isolated floaters noted by patients with PVD typically have a sudden onset and appear as well-defined shapes that shift with fixation. A shower of floaters often indicates a retinal break or torn retinal vessel, which can cause a vitreous hemorrhage. Flashes are phosphenes that occur when movements of the vitreous cause traction on the retina at areas of firm vitreoretinal attachment, such as the vitreous base. Cessation of the flashes usually indicates progression of the PVD and release of traction on the retina.

Objective

Centrally located PVDs can often be observed with a direct ophthalmoscope. Fundus biomicroscopy and binocular indirect ophthalmoscopy are two other techniques for viewing a PVD through a dilated pupil. A PVD often appears as a ring or crescent-shaped opacity just anterior to the optic nerve head (Weis' ring). Large PVDs may appear as a wispy or corrugated veil suspended in the vitreous cavity. A vitreous hemorrhage that is secondary to a PVD gives the vitreous a characteristic red appearance. A PVD can also cause one or more dot-and-blot hemorrhages located near the vitreous base.

Plan

When a patient presents with a recent onset of PVD, the practitioner should carefully evaluate the peripheral retina for the presence of breaks using scleral indentation or a three-mirror contact fundus lens. Retinal breaks occur in 15–30% of symptomatic PVD cases. PVD patients should be counseled about their condition and the symptoms of retinal detachment. They should be monitored closely for the first 1–2 months after the onset of symptoms and then routinely thereafter.

RETINAL DETACHMENT

Subjective

Three basic types of retinal detachment exist: rhegmatogenous, tractional, and exudative. Rhegmatogenous detachments are caused by breaks in the retina and are often associated with trauma, degenerations, or high myopia. Tractional detachments are usually associated with proliferative vasculopathies or trauma. Exudative detachments are associated with conditions causing massive exudation (such as Coats' disease), inflammation (such as Vogt-Koyanagi-Harada syndrome), or tumors (such as choroidal melanoma). Tractional detachments associated with proliferative retinopathies are the most likely to cause vitreous hemorrhaging.

Symptoms of retinal detachment include flashes, floaters, and vision loss. The lightning streak-like flashes caused by vitreoretinal traction are similar to those experienced in PVD. The floaters associated with a retinal break, however, are often multiple and resemble a swarm of gnats.

Objective

Peripheral breaks in the retina, either round holes or linear tears, and rhegmatogenous retinal detachments are often associated with small tobacco dust-like pigment particles in the anterior vitreous (Shafer's sign). Retinal holes are round, and tears are linear or horseshoe shaped. There may be an adjacent vitreoretinal adhesion forming a flap tear. A white cuff surrounding a retinal break indicates the accumulation of fluid under the sensory retina, forming a retinal detachment. Larger retinal detachments have a milky appearance that obscures underlying details and often have an elevated, corrugated surface. They tend to undulate slightly with movements of the eye.

In proliferative retinopathies, exudation from neovascular vessels forms opaque fibrovascular adhesion strands between the vitreous and retina. Tractional forces on these strands can cause hemorrhaging and tractional detachment. Inflammatory cells, exudative debris, or tumor seeds can cause vitreous opacities associated with exudative detachments.

All proliferative retinopathies require a thorough evaluation for underlying systemic disease. A specific health history should be taken that includes questions about any history of premature birth, trauma, and systemic diseases in the patient or family members. Laboratory tests can provide additional diagnostic information. Useful tests include fasting blood sugar for diabetes; Sickledex for sickle-cell disease; purified protein derivative (PPD) test for Eales' disease; and complete blood count (CBC), lipid profile, and blood pressure assessment for occlusive vascular disease.

Plan

Retinal breaks should be carefully monitored or treated prophylactically with a laser procedure when appropriate. Surgical repair of detached retinas is performed through scleral buckling, pneumatic retinopexy and laser photocoagulation, or cryotherapy procedures.

Patients with retinal detachment secondary to systemic disease should be referred for management of the underlying systemic condition.

SICKLE CELL RETINOPATHY

Subjective

Sickle cell retinopathy is associated with sickling hemoglobinopathies, which are found in approximately 10% of African-Americans. The ocular lesions of sickle cell retinopathy are usually asymptomatic unless they are associated with retinal detachment. Nonocular signs and symptoms of sickle-cell disease include pain, fatigue, frequent infections, dehydration, hypoxia, congestive heart failure, organ infarction, gallstones, and skin ulcers.

Objective

Sickle cell retinopathy can be subdivided into nonproliferative and proliferative. Signs of nonproliferative retinopathy include salmon-patch intraretinal hemorrhages, refractile spots, black sunbursts, venous tortuosity, and angioid streaks. Signs of proliferative retinopathy include arteriovenous anastomoses, neovascular sea fans, fibrovascular bands, vitreous hemorrhage, and retinal detachment.

Sickledex and hemoglobin electrophoresis tests are useful in the diagnosis of sickle cell retinopathy.

Plan

Patients with nonproliferative signs of sickle cell retinopathy should be monitored for the development of proliferative retinopathy. If this should occur, photocoagulation or cryotherapy may be used to manage the proliferation. Vitrectomy may be indicated for poorly resolving vitreous hemorrhages. If retinal detachment occurs, scleral buckling procedures may be used for reattachment; however, patients with sickle-cell disease are at high risk for developing anterior segment necrosis secondary to buckling procedures. Patients with sickle cell retinopathy should also be referred for management of the systemic manifestations of sickle-cell disease.

DIABETES MELLITUS

Subjective

Diabetes mellitus affects approximately 6% of the general population. Patients with diabetes may be asymptomatic or may complain of blurred or fluctuating vision. They may also report other symptoms associated with systemic diabetes, including polyuria, polydipsia, polyphagia, weight changes, neuropathy fatigue, and frequent infections.

Objective

Diabetic retinopathy can be subdivided into nonproliferative diabetic retinopathy (NPDR) and proliferative diabetic retinopathy (PDR). The signs of NPDR include dot-and-blot hemorrhages, microaneurysms, exudates, intraretinal microvascular anomalies, cotton-wool spots, venous beading, and capillary nonperfusion. PDR has all of these signs plus neovascularization, which may lead to fibrovascular proliferation, vitreous hemorrhage, and retinal detachment. Macular edema can be associated with either NPDR or PDR.

The fasting blood sugar, 2-hour postprandial glucose, and oral glucose tolerance tests are helpful in the diagnosis of diabetes. Fluorescein angiography is useful in delineating microaneurysms, capillary nonperfusion, macular edema, and neovascularization.

Plan

Patients with NPDR should be examined at least yearly and more frequently if they show signs of increased retinal hypoxia. Patients with high-risk PDR usually benefit from panretinal photocoagulation, and those with clinically significant macular edema usually benefit from focal or grid photocoagulation. Vitrectomy can be used to prevent further neovascularization or to treat poorly resolving vitreous hemorrhages. Diabetic patients should also be referred for management of their systemic disease.

BLOOD DYSCRASIAS (HEMATOLOGIC DISORDERS)

Subjective

Posterior segment hemorrhages can be caused by a number of hematologic disorders, including anemias, leukemia, polycythemia, dysproteinemias, and clotting disorders. Visual symptoms range from none to severe vision loss. Systemic symptoms vary according to the type of disorder, but fatigue, weakness, and malaise are common to most types.

Objective

Many different types of posterior segment hemorrhage—including vitreous, retrovitreous, flame, dot-and-blot, and subsensory retinal hemorrhages—can be found in association with hematologic disorders. Flame hemorrhages are the most commonly observed type. A white-centered flame hemorrhage, or Roth's spot, is another sign seen in many of these disorders. Other posterior segment signs include exudates, cotton-wool spots, venous tortuosity, and disc edema. Ordering a CBC and differential is a useful initial step in the diagnosis of hematologic disorders.

Plan

Management of these cases consists of referral to a hematologist for the treatment of the underlying systemic condition and frequent monitoring of the ocular manifestations.

VALSALVA RETINOPATHY

Subjective

Valsalva retinopathy is caused by any activity that results in a sudden increase in intrathoracic pressure, such as coughing, sneezing, vomiting, straining, or lifting of heavy weights. Patients are usually asymptomatic unless a significant hemorrhage involving the visual axis is produced.

Objective

Posterior segment signs include preretinal and flame hemorrhages, exudates, and edema. The patient may also exhibit subconjunctival hemorrhages.

Plan

Valsalva retinopathy tends to resolve spontaneously, so no treatment is necessary other than routine monitoring.

HYPERTENSIVE RETINOPATHY

Subjective

Hypertension is a very common systemic disease with an increased incidence among blacks and the elderly. Patients with hypertensive retinopathy are usually asymptomatic unless the macula or optic nerve is involved. The underlying systemic hypertension also is typically a "silent" disease, although a few patients experience headaches.

Objective

Signs of hypertensive retinopathy include flame hemorrhages, exudates that occasionally form a macular star,

vessel-crossing changes, arterial constriction, macroaneurysms, and occasional cotton-wool spots. Disc edema is a sign of malignant hypertension.

Systemic blood pressure assessment is an important test in the diagnosis of retinopathy due to hypertension.

Plan

Patients with hypertensive retinopathy should be monitored annually. They should also be referred to their family practitioners or internists for management of the systemic disease.

ACQUIRED IMMUNODEFICIENCY SYNDROME RETINOPATHY

Subjective

Acquired immunodeficiency syndrome (AIDS) is a condition secondary to infection by the human immunodeficiency virus (HIV). It is contracted through direct contact with the blood, semen, vaginal secretions, or breast milk of an infected person. In addition to being affected by the HIV infection itself, the eyes of a person with AIDS can also be affected by a number of opportunistic infections, including cytomegalovirus infections, herpes zoster, herpes simplex, toxoplasmosis, candidiasis, and infection by *Mycobacterium tuberculosis*. Patients infected by HIV may remain asymptomatic for years. Later systemic symptoms include weight loss, fatigue, night sweats, lymphadenopathy, and frequent infections. Ocular symptoms range from none to severe vision loss.

Objective

The signs of HIV retinopathy include cotton-wool spots, flame and blot hemorrhages, and macular edema. Posterior segment signs of opportunistic infections include hemorrhages, retinal necrosis, retinal detachment, pigmentary retinopathy, vitritis, granulomatous posterior uveitis, and papilledema.

The enzyme-linked immunosorbent assay (ELISA) for HIV and the Western blot test are the two main laboratory tests used to screen for HIV infection. CD4 (T lymphocyte) counts are useful in monitoring the progression of AIDS.

Plan

Currently, there is no cure for HIV infection or AIDS, although the symptoms can be diminished with combination therapy. Management consists of careful monitoring and control of both the HIV virus and opportunistic infections. Retinal detachment repair should also be performed when indicated.

GLAUCOMA

Subjective

Occasionally a flame-shaped hemorrhage (Drance hemorrhage) can be found at the edge of a glaucomatous optic nerve head. Such a hemorrhage is most often associated with low-tension glaucoma. Although glaucoma can occur at any age, its incidence increases with age. In its early stages, primary open-angle glaucoma is an asymptomatic disease; as it progresses, however, the patient loses peripheral vision and ultimately central vision. Poor night vision and changes in color perception are less common complaints.

Objective

In addition to the occasional Drance hemorrhage, signs of low-tension glaucoma include optic nerve cupping, nerve fiber defects, and visual field defects. The intraocular pressure is usually within the normal range; this finding differentiates it from typical primary open-angle glaucoma, in which the pressure is elevated. Pressure spikes may be revealed with serial tonometry in cases of low-tension glaucoma.

Plan

The primary therapeutic goal for the glaucoma patient is to maintain intraocular pressure at a level at which no further nerve damage occurs. This goal is attempted through the use of topical or oral antiglaucoma agents, or laser or other surgical procedures.

PAPILLEDEMA

Subjective

True papilledema is a bilateral edema of the optic discs secondary to increased intracranial pressure. Increased intracranial pressure has a number of causes, including tumor, hemorrhage, inflammation, infection, trauma, drug toxicity, and benign intracranial hypertension. Initially, patients with papilledema note no visual symptoms or have brief obscurations of vision. Headache and nausea are common systemic symptoms.

Objective

Papilledema is characterized by an elevated optic nerve head with blurred disc margins. The elevated nerve head is best viewed stereoscopically using fundus biomicroscopy. Paton's folds may also be observed temporal to the disc. Adjacent flame hemorrhages and cotton-wool spots indicate an acute, noncompensated rise in intracranial pressure. Disappearance of a previously noted spontaneous venous pulse is a helpful diagnostic sign. In the acute stages, perimetry reveals an enlarged blind spot. Other field defects occur with increased nerve damage. Another common ocular manifestation is impaired extraocular motility and diplopia secondary to sixth nerve palsy.

The differential diagnosis of papilledema includes evaluation for inflammatory papillitis, ischemic optic neuropathy, demyelinating optic neuropathy, pseudotumor, malignant hypertension, optic nerve head drusen, and other forms of pseudopapilledema. CT, magnetic resonance imaging (MRI), and lumbar puncture are used in the diagnostic evaluation of papilledema.

Plan

Management consists of referral to a neurologist or neurosurgeon to determine and treat the underlying cause.

OPTIC NEURITIS

Subjective

Inflammatory optic neuritis (papillitis) is most commonly found in children and is secondary to a number of systemic infections or inflammatory conditions. Demyelinating optic neuritis (usually in the form of retrobulbar neuritis) is more common in young adulthood and is often associated with multiple sclerosis. During the acute stages, the patient may experience pain on eye movement. The vision loss associated with optic neuropathy runs a typical course in which vision declines rapidly during the first week, stabilizes, then slowly recovers. The ultimate degree of recovery is variable.

Objective

Papillitis typically manifests as a unilateral swollen optic nerve head with blurred margins and adjacent flame hemorrhages. Some forms show a stellate pattern of exudation in the papillomacular area and cells in the vitreous. In contrast, retrobulbar neuritis has few ophthalmoscopically observable features. A central scotoma or other field defects may be revealed with perimetry. Patients also have an afferent pupillary defect and perceive color desaturation with the red cap test.

Laboratory testing to screen for underlying causes of inflammatory papillitis includes fluorescent treponemal antibody absorption (FTA-ABS) test, chest radiography, collagen vascular screening panel, and antibody titers for specific suspected diseases. An increased latency in the visual evoked potential is a useful diagnostic test for demyelinating optic neuritis; however, an MRI scan is needed for definitive diagnosis.

Plan

The management of optic neuritis is currently controversial. Administration of steroids and corticotropin, in addition to treatment of the underlying disease, has been used in managing inflammatory papillitis. Initial use of intravenous steroids followed by oral steroids may hasten visual recovery in demyelinating optic neuritis, but this regimen appears to have no effect on the ultimate level of visual recovery. Oral steroids used alone may increase the incidence of subsequent attacks of optic neuritis.

ISCHEMIC OPTIC NEUROPATHY

Subjective

Ischemic optic neuropathy (ION) can be associated with diabetes, temporal arteritis, and other inflammatory diseases. Fluctuations in blood pressure or intraocular pressure have also been implicated. Many cases, however, are idiopathic and are classified as nonarteritic. ION is primarily found in people over the age of 50; however, it can also occur in younger patients with diabetes. Before an acute episode of ION, the patient may experience transient flashes or obscurations of vision. During the attack, vision decreases suddenly, then stabilizes. Patients with arteritic ION often have a tender, palpable temporal artery and may experience pain on chewing. They may also complain of malaise as well as muscle and joint aches (polymyalgia rheumatica).

Objective

ION usually begins unilaterally but may become bilateral over time. Sectors of the optic disc or the entire disc become edematous, and flame-shaped hemorrhages are observable adjacent to the disc margin. The patient exhibits an afferent pupillary defect and color desaturation with the red cap test. The most common visual field defect demonstrated with perimetry is an altitudinal loss; however,

arcuate scotomas, central scotomas, and other defects are possible. The optic nerve ultimately becomes atrophied.

The initial diagnostic evaluation of ION includes pressure assessment, auscultation for carotid bruits, measurement of fasting blood sugar level, CBC with differential and platelets, and erythrocyte sedimentation rate (ESR). An ESR greater than 50 is suggestive of arteritic ION. In many cases, temporal artery biopsy is needed to confirm the diagnosis.

Plan

Management of ION involves treatment of the underlying disease whenever possible. In the case of arteritic ION, oral steroid therapy should be initiated immediately in an attempt to improve or maintain vision in the affected eye and preserve vision in the other eye.

OPTIC NERVE HEAD DRUSEN (DISC DRUSEN)

Subjective

Drusen of the optic nerve head are a congenital condition with an irregular autosomal dominant mode of inheritance. Disc drusen are not typically associated with symptoms but may occasionally cause peripheral vision loss.

Objective

Disc drusen are classified as a form of pseudopapilledema based on their clinical appearance. The optic nerve is elevated with no cupping. In some cases, splinter or flame hemorrhages occur adjacent to the disc and further confound the clinical picture. Some patients show anomalous vessel patterns such as trifurcations. On rare occasions, neovascular membranes develop adjacent to the disc and may subsequently hemorrhage.

As the patient ages, the drusen begin to surface and appear as yellow, translucent, or refractile bodies. These bodies show autofluorescence when a camera with fluorescein angiography exciter and barrier filters is used. The density of the bodies can be readily demonstrated with B-scan ultrasonography at a low-gain setting. Nerve damage caused by the drusen can lead to a wide variety of field defects.

Plan

No treatment is currently available for disc drusen. Management consists of routine monitoring.

OCCLUSIVE RETINAL VASCULAR DISEASE

Subjective

Occlusive retinal vascular disease is commonly associated with systemic conditions, including carotid artery disease, hypertension, diabetes, hyperlipidemia, chronic lung disease, blood dyscrasias, and certain autoimmune disorders. The patient with a branch retinal vein occlusion (BRVO) often complains of vision loss corresponding to the area of hemorrhage or macular edema. The patient with a central retinal vein occlusion (CRVO) has a more generalized vision loss.

Objective

A BRVO presents as a wedge-shaped area of dot-and-blot hemorrhages and exudates. The apex of the wedge points to the site of occlusion. Flame hemorrhages and cotton-wool spots are more commonly found in the ischemic form, as opposed to the nonischemic form, of BRVO. If the occlusion involves the superior temporal retina, macular edema is likely to result. The manifestation of a CRVO is similar to that of a BRVO except that it involves the entire retina.

Patients who present with a BRVO or CRVO should be evaluated for underlying systemic disease. Useful tests in the initial evaluation include blood pressure assessment, carotid bruit auscultation, measurement of fasting blood sugar level, lipid profile, ESR, and CBC with differential and platelets. Fluorescein angiography is useful in differentiating nonischemic from ischemic occlusive disease and for pinpointing areas of leakage.

Plan

Patients with macular edema should be monitored monthly after the initial presentation. If the edema does not resolve within 4–6 months, grid photocoagulation may be indicated. This procedure tends to be more effective in BRVO than in CRVO. Patients with ischemic venous occlusive disease should be monitored closely for the development of neovascularization and, particularly in the case of ischemic CRVO, for neovascular glaucoma.

COATS' DISEASE (RETINAL TELANGIECTASIA)

Subjective

Coats' disease is typically a unilateral condition found in young boys. It is usually diagnosed between the ages of 2 and 10. It can cause vision loss, particularly if the macula is affected.

Objective

Massive exudation from retinal telangiectasias and aneurysms is the hallmark of Coats' disease. Either the exudate alone or an exudative retinal detachment can cause leukocoria. Subsensory retinal hemorrhages can also occur. Fluorescein angiography is helpful in highlighting the vascular abnormalities characteristic of this disease.

Plan

The treatment of Coats' disease consists of photocoagulation or cryotherapy to seal leaking vessels. Retinal reattachment surgery may be necessary in some cases.

PRESUMED OCULAR HISTOPLASMOSIS SYNDROME

Subjective

Presumed ocular histoplasmosis syndrome (POHS) is thought to be an ocular immune reaction to a previous systemic infection by the fungus *Histoplasma capsulatum*. This organism thrives on soil enriched by bird and bat droppings. In the United States, the disease is found primarily among whites who have resided in the Ohio River/Mississippi River valley complex. During the initial infection, the patient may experience self-limiting flulike symptoms. The ocular disease is usually asymptomatic; however, macular and peripapillary involvement can cause severe vision loss.

Objective

The classic triad of signs of POHS includes peripapillary atrophy, white "histo" spots, and maculopathy. The macular and peripapillary lesions can progress to subretinal neovascularization, hemorrhaging, and ultimately disciform scar formation. The absence of an overlying vitritis is helpful in distinguishing POHS from other forms of posterior segment inflammation. Fluorescein or indocyanine green angiography can be used to define the subretinal neovascular membranes. Chest radiography and the histoplasmin skin test may be useful in diagnosing the primary disease; however, the latter is not recommended in ocular disease because it can promote reactivation of the infection and stimulate the progression of maculopathy. It is important to note that AIDS can also promote the reactivation of histoplasmosis.

Plan

The management of POHS involves close monitoring for the development of neovascularization, both by the clinician in the office and by the patient with an Amsler grid at home. If subretinal neovascularization does form, it is treated with laser photocoagulation or submacular surgical removal of the membrane when possible. If significant vision loss cannot be prevented, the patient may benefit from the prescription of low vision aids.

AGE-RELATED MACULAR DEGENERATION

Subjective

In the United States, age-related macular degeneration (ARMD) is the leading cause of legal blindness among the elderly. In addition to age, other proposed risk factors include positive family history of ARMD, light-colored irides, smoking, hyperopia, certain dietary deficiencies, and prolonged exposure to UV or blue light. The dry, or atrophic, form of the disease is more common than the wet, or exudative, form. Both forms can cause significant loss of central vision; however, loss from the wet form is generally more rapid and devastating.

Objective

Dry ARMD begins as pigmentary changes and drusen formation in the macula. This form may progress until the area of atrophy involves a large portion of the macula. Dry ARMD develops into wet ARMD in 10–20% of cases. Soft, confluent macular drusen are suggestive of a progression toward wet ARMD. In the wet form, subretinal neovascular membranes develop; these can leak, forming macular edema and exudates. Hemorrhage from these membranes has a gray-green appearance. Ultimately, disciform degenerative changes occur. Fluorescein or indocyanine green angiography is useful in distinguishing between wet and dry ARMD.

Plan

Patients with ARMD should be examined regularly and should be instructed in the use of an Amsler grid or similar technique for home monitoring. Subretinal neovascularization, if detected early enough, sometimes can be treated with laser photocoagulation to prevent hemorrhaging and further vision loss. Those patients who have already experienced vision loss may benefit from low vision aids. Currently, a number of therapies are being investigated that are designed to prevent ARMD or improve the prognosis once it does occur. These include the use of oral micronutrients or other pharmaceutical agents, photocoagulation of drusen, photodynamic therapy, radiotherapy, subretinal surgery, retinal pigment epithelium transplantation, and macular translocation.

DEGENERATIVE MYOPIA

Subjective

Degenerative myopia begins in childhood and is a progressive bilateral disease. It is far less common than typical refractive myopia. Permanent vision loss can result from degenerative myopia, particularly if macular hemorrhaging or retinal detachment occurs.

Objective

High refractive error is one of the signs of degenerative myopia. Long axial length as measured by ultrasonography provides additional useful information. The dilated fundus examination often reveals myopic conus, staphyloma, and generalized retinal pigment thinning and degeneration in these elongated eyes. Lacquer cracks and Fuchs' spot signify breaks in Bruch's membrane and indicate increased risk for choroidal neovascularization with hemorrhaging.

Plan

Correction of refractive error and monitoring at least annually for the development of retinal breaks, detachments, and subretinal neovascularization are indicated in the management of patients with degenerative myopia. Neovascular nets sometimes can be treated successfully with photocoagulation or submacular surgery. Retinal detachments usually require surgical repair.

POSTERIOR UVEITIS (CHORIORETINITIS)

Subjective

Infectious posterior uveitis, particularly toxoplasmosis, can set the stage for the development of subretinal neovascular membranes and subsequent hemorrhaging. Many patients with posterior uveitis are asymptomatic; however, those with significant vitritis associated with acute inflammation may complain of blurred vision. In addition, subretinal hemorrhages and chorioretinal scars in the macula can cause significant vision loss.

Objective

The scars in most forms of inactive chorioretinitis have a central white zone of chorioretinal atrophy surrounded by a dark rim of retinal pigment epithelial hyperplasia. The lesions may be single or multiple depending on the nature of the inflammation. In some cases of posterior uveitis, such as in toxoplasmosis, active lesions may form adjacent to inactive chorioretinal scars. There may also be an associated overlying vitritis indicating activity.

A number of laboratory and radiologic tests are available to aid in the differential diagnosis of posterior uveitis. These include the FTA-ABS test or microhemagglutination assay–*Treponema pallidum* test for syphilis, PPD test and chest radiography for tuberculosis, angiotensin-converting enzyme test and chest radiography for sarcoidosis, anti-*Toxoplasma* antigen titer for toxoplasmosis, *Toxocara* ELISA for toxocariasis, serum rubella titer for rubella, and HLA-B5 for Behçet's disease.

Plan

In patients with posterior uveitis, the underlying disease should be treated whenever possible. Inactive chorioretinal scars should be monitored for evidence of reactivation or the development of subretinal neovascularization. Some cases of subretinal neovascularization can be managed with laser photocoagulation or surgical removal of the vascular membrane.

ANGIOID STREAKS

Subjective

Angioid streaks are breaks in Bruch's membrane that are most commonly found in patients with pseudoxanthoma elasticum. They are also associated with a number of other systemic conditions, including Paget's disease, Ehlers-Danlos syndrome, and sickle-cell disease. Severe vision loss can occur with angioid streaks if they result in subretinal neovascularization, hemorrhaging, and scar formation.

Objective

The name *angioid streaks* is derived from the somewhat vessel-like appearance of these brownish-red streaks, which typically radiate outward from the disc. They are usually found in both eyes, although they may not be symmetric in the two eyes. Other ocular signs that may be found in association with angioid streaks include disc drusen, an orange peel–like appearance temporal to the macula, and peripheral retinal degeneration. Fluorescein or indocyanine green angiography is particularly useful in determining the presence of neovascular nets.

It is also important to determine whether an underlying systemic condition is associated with the angioid streaks. Gross observation for skin and joint abnormalities can be useful in the diagnosis of pseudoxanthoma elasticum and Ehlers-Danlos syndrome. Radiographic studies can highlight bone abnormalities in Paget's disease. The Sickledex test can be used to screen for sickle-cell disease.

Plan

The patient with angioid streaks should be referred for further evaluation and management of the underlying systemic condition. Protective eyewear should be prescribed, and the patient should avoid contact sports. The patient should be monitored closely for the development of neovascular membranes so that treatment can be initiated promptly should they occur.

TRAUMATIC DISRUPTION OF BRUCH'S MEMBRANE

Subjective

Blunt trauma to the globe can cause linear choroidal ruptures; sharp trauma, photocoagulation, or cryopexy can cause focal choroidal damage. If the barrier created by Bruch's membrane is disrupted, the eye is at increased risk for developing subretinal neovascularization, hemorrhaging, and scarring. The amount of vision loss resulting depends on the location and extent of the damage.

Objective

Choroidal ruptures secondary to blunt trauma tend to be banana shaped and concentric to the disc. Photocoagulation creates a round area of damage, whereas sharp trauma can cause damage in any shape. Fresh injuries may have retinal or vitreous hemorrhages associated with them; old injuries usually have a surrounding area of pigment epithelium hyperplasia.

Plan

Patients who develop neovascularization secondary to trauma should be monitored closely. In many cases a conservative approach is best, and treatment should be initiated only if the lesion constitutes a significant threat to vision because of its location.

SUGGESTED READING

Alexander LA. Primary Care of the Posterior Segment (2nd ed). Norwalk, CT: Appleton & Lange, 1994.

Beck RW, Cleary PA, Trobe JD, et al. The effect of corticosteroids for acute optic neuritis on the subsequent development of multiple sclerosis. N Engl J Med 1993;329:1764–1769.

Bloch RS. Hematologic Disorders. In W Tasman, EA Jaeger (eds), Duane's Clinical Ophthalmology. Philadelphia: Lippincott, 1990;5:1–13.

Central Vein Occlusion Study Group. Evaluation of grid pattern photocoagulation for macular edema in central vein occlusion. Group M report. Ophthalmology 1995;102:1425–1433.

Roy, FH. Ocular Differential Diagnosis (5th ed). Philadelphia: Lea & Febiger, 1993.

Sternberg P, Lim JI (eds). Macular Disease. Boston: Little, Brown, 1995.

van Heuven WAJ, Zwaan JT. Decision Making in Ophthalmology. St. Louis: Mosby–Year Book, 1992.

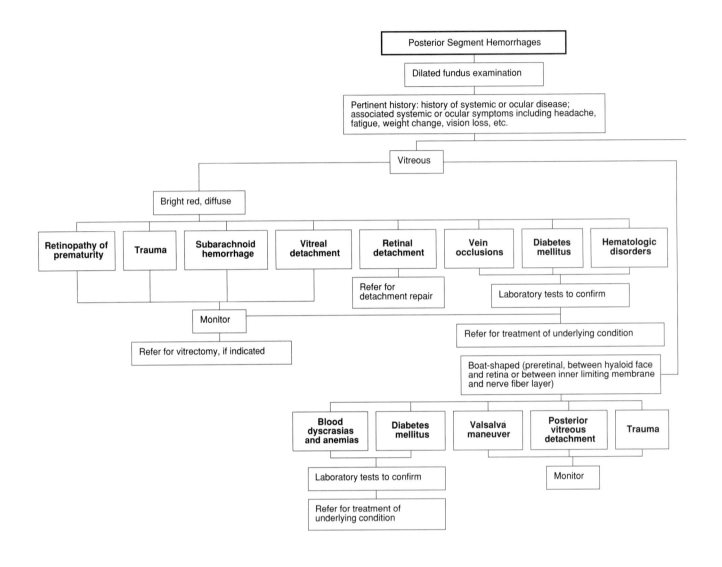

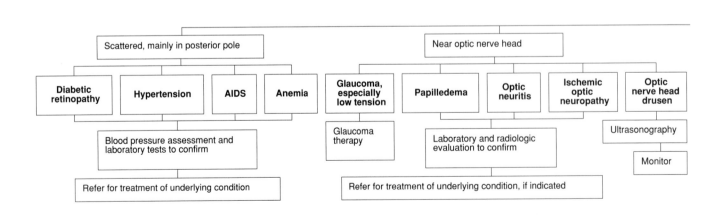

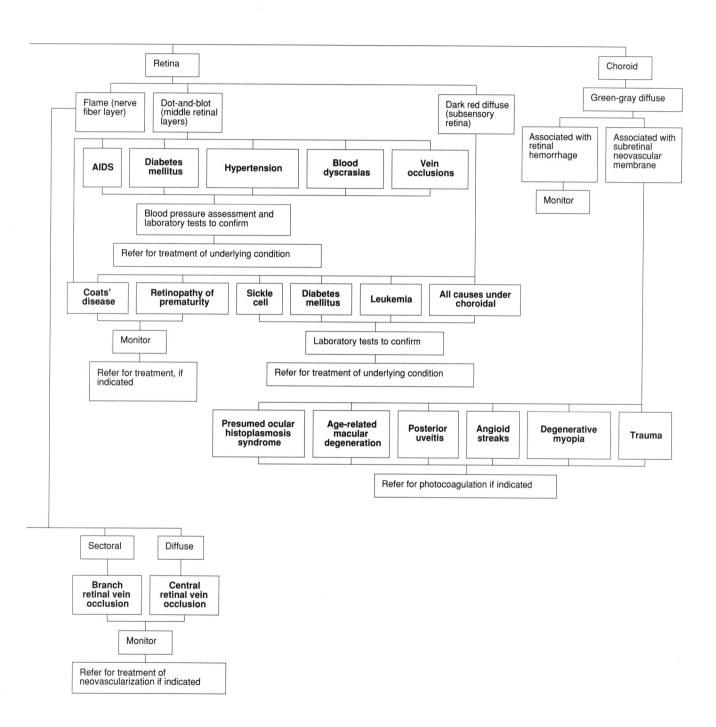

44

Macular Edema

Debra J. Bezan

MACULAR EDEMA AT A GLANCE

Diabetic retinopathy
Occlusive vascular disease
  Branch retinal vein occlusion
  Central retinal vein occlusion
  Carotid artery obstruction
Uveitis
  Behçet's disease
  Pars planitis
  Presumed ocular histoplasmosis syndrome
  Toxoplasmosis
  Toxocariasis
  Lyme disease
Retinitis pigmentosa
Central serous maculopathy
  Idiopathic
  Associated with optic pit
Traumatic maculopathy
  Irvine-Gass syndrome
  Post–laser therapy
  Berlin's edema
  Solar maculopathy
  Radiation maculopathy
Secondary to subretinal neovascularization
  Age-related macular degeneration
  Presumed ocular histoplasmosis syndrome
  Toxoplasmosis
  Other inflammatory chorioretinopathies
  Degenerative myopia
  Angioid streaks
  Choroidal rupture
  Post-photocoagulation or cryosurgery
  Optic nerve head drusen
  Acute multifocal posterior placoid pigment epitheliopathy
  Geographic helicoid peripapillary choroidopathy
  Idiopathic
Dominant macular dystrophy
Coats' disease (retinal telangiectasia)
Eales' disease
Goldmann-Favre syndrome
Mucopolysaccharidoses (MPS II, MPS I-H)
Tumor
  Hemangioma
  Angiomatosis retinae
  Melanoma
Drug toxicity

A patient with macular edema may present complaining of blurred vision, metamorphopsia, or central scotoma. A careful history of systemic disease, ocular disease, trauma, surgery, and medications should be taken when a patient presents with these complaints. In addition to testing of best-corrected visual acuity, a detailed stereoscopic evaluation of the macula and surrounding retina, and central visual field testing (Amsler or static threshold) are useful in the initial diagnostic evaluation of the patient. Some patients, although asymptomatic, may show subtle clinical signs of edema.

DIABETES MELLITUS

Subjective

Patients with diabetic macular edema often present with the symptoms noted above. They may also report systemic symptoms associated with diabetes, such as frequent eating, drinking, and urination; fluctuating vision; neuropathy; fatigue; and recurrent infections.

Objective

Diabetic macular edema may be found in association with either nonproliferative or proliferative diabetic retinopathy. Diabetic macular edema may be classified as clinically significant or non–clinically significant according to the guidelines of the Early Treatment Diabetic Retinopathy Study. Clinically significant macular edema includes

1. Retinal thickening within one-third disc diameter of the center of the macula
2. Hard exudates within one-third disc diameter of the center of the macula if associated with adjacent retinal thickening
3. Retinal thickening of at least one disc diameter in size, any portion of which is within one disc diameter of the center of the macula

Fluorescein angiography is an important adjunct test to help identify subtle areas of edema and sources of leakage.

Plan

Patients with non–clinically significant macular edema should be closely monitored. Those with clinically significant edema are usually treated with focal or grid photocoagulation.

OCCLUSIVE RETINAL VASCULAR DISEASE

Subjective

Occlusive retinal vascular disease is commonly associated with underlying systemic disease, including carotid artery disease, hypertension, diabetes, hyperlipidemia, chronic pulmonary disease, blood dyscrasias, and certain autoimmune disorders. The patient with macular edema secondary to a branch retinal vein occlusion (BRVO) often complains of vision loss corresponding to the area of hemorrhage, in addition to complaining of the symptoms typically associated with the macular edema. The patient with a central retinal vein occlusion (CRVO) has a more generalized vision loss.

Objective

A BRVO presents as a wedge-shaped area of hemorrhages, exudates, and, particularly in the ischemic form, cotton-wool spots. The apex of the wedge points to the occlusion. If the occlusion involves the superior temporal retina, macular edema is likely to result.

The manifestation of a CRVO is similar to that of a BRVO except that the entire retina is involved. Hemi–central vein occlusion (HCVO) involves either the superior or inferior portion of the retina.

Patients who present with a BRVO, HCVO, or CRVO should be evaluated for underlying systemic disease. Useful tests in the initial evaluation include blood pressure assessment, carotid bruit auscultation, fasting blood sugar level, lipid profile, and complete blood count with differential and platelets. Fluorescein angiography is useful in differentiating nonischemic from ischemic occlusive disease and in pinpointing areas of leakage.

Plan

Patients with macular edema should be monitored monthly after the initial presentation. If the edema does not resolve within 4–6 months, grid photocoagulation may be indicated. This procedure is more effective in BRVO than CRVO. Patients should also be monitored closely for the development of neovascularization and, particularly in the case of ischemic CRVO, for neovascular glaucoma.

MACULAR EDEMA SECONDARY TO UVEITIS

Subjective

Macular edema may be one of the manifestations of an intermediate uveitis, such as in pars planitis; a posterior uveitis, such as in histoplasmosis; or uveitis affecting the eye front to back, such as in Behçet's disease. Inflammation of the anterior uveal tissues tends to be painful, whereas inflammation of the posterior uvea typically is not. The only symptoms of these conditions may be those associated with the edema itself. The presence of significant amounts of inflammatory debris in the vitreous can also cause reduced vision.

Objective

In addition to the retinal thickening in the macular area, other signs of uveitis may be noted, including cells and flare in the anterior chamber or vitreous, chorioretinal scar formation, and choroidal neovascularization.

Laboratory and radiologic studies may be helpful in the differential diagnosis of posterior uveitis. These include anti-*Toxoplasma* antibody titer for toxoplasmosis; fluorescent treponemal antibody absorption test and microhemagglutination assay-*Treponema pallidum* for syphilis; purified protein derivative (PPD) test and chest radiography for tuberculosis; angiotensin-converting enzyme test and chest radiography for sarcoidosis; HLA-B5 test for Behçet's disease; *Toxocara* enzyme-linked immunosorbent assay for toxocariasis; and Western blot test for human immunodeficiency virus.

Plan

Oral or injected corticosteroids may be used to control inflammation in intermediate and posterior uveitis. In the case of infectious uveitis such as in toxoplasmosis, antimicrobials (e.g., triple sulfa with pyrimethamine) are used in conjunction with anti-inflammatory agents.

RETINITIS PIGMENTOSA

Subjective

Retinitis pigmentosa is cone-rod dystrophy that has autosomal dominant, recessive, X-linked, and sporadic modes of inheritance. It is characterized by night blindness and progressive peripheral field loss; however, central vision may also be affected by cataracts or macular edema.

Objective

In addition to occasional macular edema, signs include "bone-spicule" pigment clumping, waxy pallor of the optic nerve, vessel attenuation, and sometimes posterior subcapsular cataracts.

Electroretinography, perimetry, and dark adaptometry are all useful adjunct tests in diagnosing and monitoring the progression of retinitis pigmentosa.

Plan

Patients with retinitis pigmentosa should be monitored routinely. Those patients with vision loss often benefit from low vision aids. Vitamin A therapy may have some benefit in slowing the progression of the disease. Genetic counseling is also indicated when the mode of inheritance can be determined.

IDIOPATHIC CENTRAL SEROUS CHOROIDOPATHY (CENTRAL SEROUS MACULOPATHY)

Subjective

Idiopathic central serous choroidopathy (ICSC) is a detachment of the sensory retina or retinal pigment epithelium in the macula. It is most commonly found in young white men. These patients typically complain of metamorphopsia and slightly decreased acuity, and may note some changes in color perception.

Objective

ICSC presents as a smooth, dome-shaped area of elevated tissue in the macula. It may have a central yellow "lemon-drop" appearance. Evaluation of the optic nerve head for the appearance of a grayish optic pit is also important.

A delayed photostress recovery time is a useful clinical finding. Fluorescein angiography is helpful in localizing the area of leakage and determining whether an optic pit is contributing to the edema.

Plan

Most cases of ICSC resolve spontaneously within a few months, although the recurrence rate is approximately 25%. Nonresolving cases may be treated with focal photocoagulation.

TRAUMA

Subjective

Many types of trauma, including surgery, can cause macular edema. Postoperative patients who complain that their vision is getting worse rather than better should be evaluated carefully for macular edema, as well as for other causes of vision loss.

Objective

Cystoid macular edema after cataract surgery is termed *Irvine-Gass syndrome.* Its characteristic flower-petal pattern of edema is highlighted with fluorescein angiography. A similar type of macular edema can also be a sequela of laser procedures such as Nd:YAG capsulotomy.

Solar maculopathy initially presents as a tiny focal area of swelling in the fovea. Later a small, red, slightly depressed area appears.

Berlin's macular edema is a variation on commotio retinae. It is a transient milky opacification of the retina caused by blunt trauma.

Plan

In many cases, traumatic macular edema resolves spontaneously over time. Prostaglandin inhibitors such as topical and oral steroids and nonsteroidal anti-inflammatory agents are of some aid in reducing edema. In cases in which mechanical traction on the vitreous appears to play a role, vitrectomy may be indicated.

PRESUMED OCULAR HISTOPLASMOSIS SYNDROME

Subjective

Presumed ocular histoplasmosis syndrome (POHS) is thought to be an ocular immune reaction to a previous systemic infection by the fungus *Histoplasma capsulatum*. This organism thrives on soil enriched by bird and bat droppings. In the United States, the disease is primarily found among whites who have resided in the Ohio River/Mississippi River valley complex. During the initial infection, the patient may experience self-limiting flulike symptoms. The ocular disease is usually asymptomatic; however, macular and peripapillary involvement can cause symptoms ranging from metamorphopsia to severe vision loss.

Objective

The classic triad of signs of POHS includes peripapillary atrophy, peripheral white "histo spots," and maculopathy. The macular and peripapillary lesions can progress to subretinal neovascularization. Early signs of neovascularization include macular edema and exudates. Subretinal neovascular membranes can hemorrhage and ultimately lead to disciform scar formation. The absence of an overlying vitritis is helpful in distinguishing POHS from other forms of posterior segment inflammation. Fluorescein or indocyanine green angiography can be used to define the subretinal neovascular membranes. Chest radiography and the histoplasmin skin test may be useful in diagnosing the primary disease; however, the latter is not recommended in ocular disease because it can promote reactivation of the infection and stimulate the progression of maculopathy. It is important to note that acquired immunodeficiency syndrome can also promote the reactivation of histoplasmosis.

Plan

The management of POHS involves close monitoring for the development of neovascularization, both by the clinician in the office and by the patient at home. If neovascularization occurs, it is treated with laser photocoagulation or with submacular surgical removal of the membrane

when possible. If significant vision loss cannot be prevented, the patient can benefit from the prescription of low vision aids.

AGE-RELATED MACULAR DEGENERATION

Subjective

In the United States, age-related macular degeneration (ARMD) is the leading cause of legal blindness among the elderly. In addition to age, other proposed risk factors include positive family history of ARMD, light-colored irides, smoking, hyperopia, certain dietary deficiencies, and chronic exposure to UV or visible blue light. The dry, or atrophic, form of the disease is more common than the wet, or exudative, form. Both forms can cause significant loss of central vision; however, the wet form is generally more rapid and devastating.

Objective

Dry ARMD begins as pigmentary changes and drusen formation in the macula. This form may progress until the area of atrophy involves a large portion of the macula. Dry ARMD develops into wet ARMD in approximately 10–20% of cases. Soft, confluent macular drusen or focal detachments of the retinal pigment epithelium are suggestive of a progression toward wet ARMD. In the wet form, subretinal neovascular membranes develop; these can leak, forming macular edema and exudates. Hemorrhage from these membranes has a gray-green appearance. Ultimately, disciform degenerative changes occur. Fluorescein or indocyanine green angiography is useful in distinguishing between wet and dry ARMD.

Plan

Patients with ARMD should be examined regularly and should be instructed in the use of an Amsler grid or similar technique for home monitoring. Subretinal neovascularization, if detected early enough, sometimes can be treated with laser photocoagulation to prevent hemorrhaging and further vision loss. Those patients who have already experienced vision loss may benefit from low vision aids. Currently, a number of therapies are being investigated that are designed to prevent ARMD or improve the prognosis once it has occurred. These include the use of oral micronutrients or other pharmaceutical agents, photocoagulation of drusen, photodynamic therapy, radiotherapy, subretinal surgery, retinal pigment epithelium transplantation, and macular relocation.

DEGENERATIVE MYOPIA

Subjective

Degenerative myopia begins in childhood and is a progressive bilateral disease. It is far less common than typical refractive myopia. Permanent vision loss can result from degenerative myopia, particularly if macular hemorrhaging or retinal detachment occurs.

Objective

High refractive error is one of the signs of degenerative myopia. Myopic conus, staphyloma, and generalized retinal pigment epithelium thinning and degeneration are also found in these elongated eyes. Lacquer cracks and Fuchs' spots signify breaks in Bruch's membrane and indicate increased risk for choroidal neovascularization with edema and hemorrhaging.

Plan

Correction of refractive error and frequent monitoring for the development of retinal breaks, detachments, and subretinal neovascularization are indicated for the management of the patient with degenerative myopia. Neovascular nets can sometimes be treated successfully with photocoagulation or submacular surgery. Retinal detachments usually require surgical repair.

ANGIOID STREAKS

Subjective

Angioid streaks are breaks in Bruch's membrane that are most commonly found in patients with pseudoxanthoma elasticum. They are also associated with a number of other systemic conditions, including Paget's disease, Ehlers-Danlos syndrome, and sickle-cell disease. Severe vision loss can occur with angioid streaks if they result in subretinal neovascularization, macular edema, hemorrhaging, and scar formation.

Objective

The name *angioid streaks* is derived from the somewhat vessel-like appearance of these brownish-red streaks, which typically radiate out from the disc. They are usually found in both eyes, although they may not be symmetric in the two eyes. Other ocular signs that may be found in association with angioid streaks include disc drusen, an orange peel–like appearance temporal to the macula, and peripheral retinal degeneration. Fluores-

cein or indocyanine green angiography is particularly useful in determining the presence of neovascular nets.

It is also important to determine whether an underlying systemic condition is associated with the angioid streaks. Gross observation for skin and joint abnormalities can be useful in the diagnosis of pseudoxanthoma elasticum and Ehlers-Danlos syndrome. Radiographic studies can highlight bone abnormalities in Paget's disease. The Sickledex test can be used to screen for sickle-cell disease.

Plan

The patient with angioid streaks should be referred for further evaluation and management of the underlying systemic condition. Protective eyewear should be prescribed. In addition, the patient should be closely monitored for the development of neovascular membranes so that treatment can be initiated promptly should they occur.

COATS' DISEASE (RETINAL TELANGIECTASIA)

Subjective

Coats' disease is a type of exudative retinopathy associated with congenital telangiectasias. It is most commonly seen in young males. Vision loss in this disease can be due to macular edema, exudates, or retinal detachment.

Objective

This condition is usually unilateral and is variable in its presentation. It can range from small areas of telangiectatic vessels with a surrounding zone of hemorrhages and exudates to large areas of exudation extensive enough to cause leukocoria and retinal detachment.

Fluorescein angiography is a useful adjunct test to localize areas of vascular leakage in Coats' disease.

Plan

Patients with Coats' disease should be monitored frequently. Photocoagulation is occasionally used to treat selected lesions. Retinal detachment repair is performed when indicated.

EALES' DISEASE (RETINAL PERIPHLEBITIS)

Subjective

Eales' disease is most commonly found in young men. In some cases, it may be the result of a tubercular hypersensitivity reaction. Patients with this disease may complain of floaters and blurred vision.

Objective

Eales' disease is characterized by inflammatory perivascular sheathing and vitritis. Peripheral neovascularization can develop in areas of nonperfusion and lead to vitreous hemorrhage. Edema from perimacular telangiectasia can also cause reduced vision.

The PPD test and chest radiography are useful adjunct tests in determining exposure to or active infection with tuberculosis. Fluorescein angiography is also helpful in determining areas of nonperfusion and leakage.

Plan

Patients with Eales' disease should be monitored carefully. Areas of nonperfusion or edema may be treated with laser photocoagulation. These patients should also be referred for management of tuberculosis if indicated.

TUMORS

Subjective

Retinal or choroidal tumors can have an overlying serous retinal detachment, but only rarely cause macular edema.

Objective

Tumors in the posterior pole are elevated and range in color from white to red to dark gray. The overlying edema or detached area may obscure the lesion's detail. The presence of feeder vessels supplying the lesion is a helpful diagnostic sign.

Ultrasonography, fluorescein angiography, and radioisotope uptake studies are useful adjunct tests in the differential diagnosis of posterior pole tumors.

Plan

A number of therapeutic options are available for treating retinal or choroidal tumors, including photocoagulation, radioactive plaque therapy, external beam radiation,

photodynamic therapy, excision, and enucleation. The selection of therapeutic mode often depends on the size and extent of the lesion, and whether the involvement is unilateral or bilateral. Metastatic carcinomas are often left untreated because of the poor survival rate after they are detected. In any case, patients with malignant retinal or choroidal tumors should be evaluated for systemic metastasis. Genetic counseling is also indicated for patients with retinoblastoma and their parents.

DRUG TOXICITY

Subjective

Many drugs have been implicated in the development of macular edema, including acetazolamide, timolol maleate, prednisolone, prednisone, hydroxychloroquine sulfate, hydrochlorothiazide, and aspirin, to name just a few.

Objective

The signs of drug-induced macular edema are similar to those of other forms of macular edema. Some drugs have additional ocular manifestations, such as the bull's-eye pigmentary changes caused by chloroquine and hydroxychloroquine sulfate.

Plan

Patients taking drugs that may cause macular edema should be monitored routinely. If macular edema does appear, the drug regimen should be modified appropriately.

SUGGESTED READING

Alexander LA. Primary Care of the Posterior Segment (2nd ed). Norwalk, CT: Appleton & Lange, 1994.

Roy FH. Ocular Differential Diagnosis (5th ed). Philadelphia: Lea & Febiger, 1993.

Smith RE, Nozik RA. Uveitis: A Clinical Approach to Diagnosis and Management (2nd ed). Baltimore: Williams & Wilkins, 1989.

Weingiest TA, Sneed SR. Laser Surgery in Ophthalmology. Norwalk, CT: Appleton & Lange, 1992.

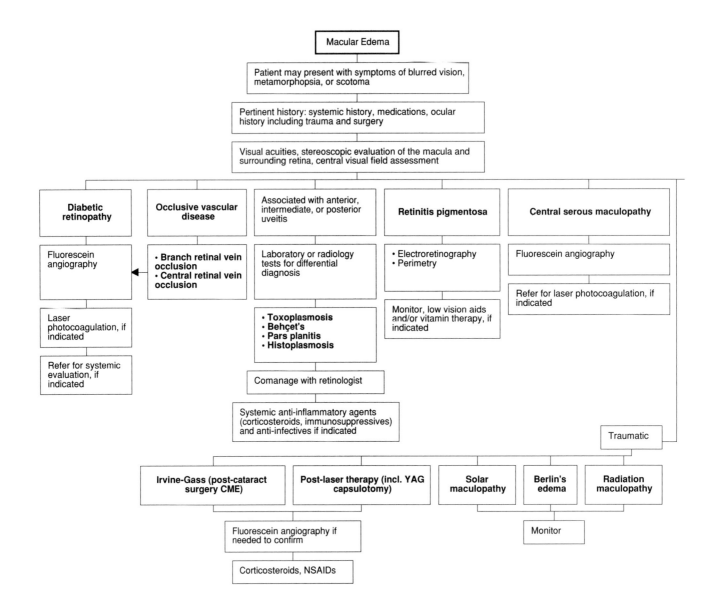

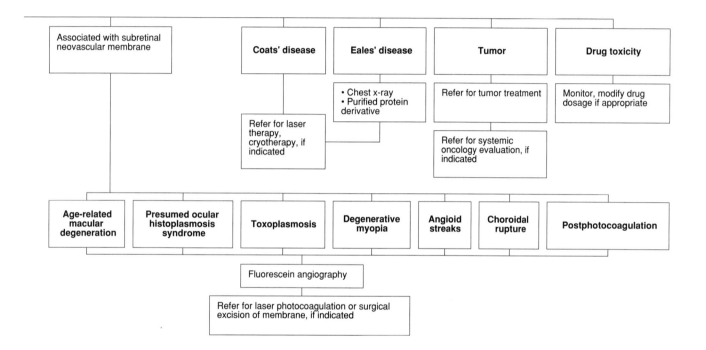

45

Nonhemorrhagic Retinal Vascular Anomalies

DEBRA J. BEZAN

NONHEMORRHAGIC RETINAL VASCULAR ANOMALIES AT A GLANCE

Telangiectasia
  Coats' disease
  Leber's miliary aneurysms
  Idiopathic juxtafoveal retinal telangiectasis
  Venous occlusive disease
  Radiation retinopathy
Microaneurysms
  Diabetes mellitus
  Hypertension
  Venous occlusion
  Aging
  Coats' disease
  Eales' disease
  Systemic lupus erythematosus
  Hematopoietic disease
  Radiation retinopathy
Macroaneurysms
  Hypertension
  Arteriosclerosis
  Congenital
  Idiopathic
Vessel caliber changes (focal)
  Hypertension
  Arteriosclerosis
  Diabetes mellitus
  Branch artery occlusion
  Branch vein occlusion
  Arteriovenous malformation
  Capillary hemangioma
  Cavernous hemangioma
  Trauma
Vessel caliber changes (diffuse)
  Hypertension
  Arteriosclerosis

Diabetes mellitus
Central artery occlusion
Central vein occlusion
Congenital heart disease
Emphysema
Hematologic disorders
Collagen vascular disease
Renal disease
Migraine
Retinopathy of prematurity
Retinitis pigmentosa
Cavernous sinus thrombosis
Carotid cavernous fistula
Trauma
Collaterals (shunt vessels)
  Diabetes mellitus (intraretinal microvascular anomalies)
  Branch vein occlusion
  Central vein occlusion
  Branch artery occlusion
  Sickle-cell disease
Neovascularization
  Diabetes mellitus
  Venous occlusion
  Sickle-cell disease
  Eales' disease
  Inflammatory disorders
  Ocular ischemic syndrome
  Aortic arch syndrome
  Carotid cavernous fistula
  Retinopathy of prematurity
  Familial exudative vitreoretinopathy
  Neoplasms
Tortuosity
  Diabetes mellitus
  Sickle-cell disease
  Congenital heart disease
  Leukemia

Dysproteinemia
Polycythemia
Retinopathy of prematurity (plus disease)
Familial dysautonomia
Mucopolysaccharidoses
Fabry's disease
Congenital arterial tortuosity
Prepapillary loop
Color changes
   Congenital
   Occlusive vascular disease
   Arteriosclerosis
   Lipemia retinalis
   Collagen vascular diseases
   Inflammatory sheathing
   Acute frosted retinal periphlebitis

In most cases, nonhemorrhagic retinal vascular anomalies are asymptomatic unless they involve the macula. They are usually detected during a dilated fundus examination. Because many of these anomalies are ocular manifestations of underlying systemic disease, blood pressure assessment and adjunct laboratory and radiologic tests are often helpful in the differential diagnosis.

RETINAL TELANGIECTASIA

Subjective

Coats' disease, Leber's miliary aneurysms, and idiopathic juxtafoveal retinal telangiectasis are variants of retinal telangiectasia. Coats' disease is typically a unilateral condition. It is most commonly diagnosed in boys between the ages of 2 and 10. It can cause vision loss, particularly if the macula is affected.

Objective

Whitish yellow exudation from retinal telangiectasias and aneurysms are the hallmarks of these diseases. Either the exudate alone, if it is massive, or an exudative retinal detachment can cause leukocoria. Fluorescein angiography is helpful in highlighting the vascular abnormalities characteristic of these conditions.

Plan

Retinal telangiectasia is treated with photocoagulation or cryotherapy to seal leaking vessels. Retinal reattachment surgery may also be indicated in some cases.

DIABETES MELLITUS

Subjective

Diabetes mellitus affects approximately 6% of the general population. Patients with diabetes may be asymptomatic or may complain of blurred or fluctuating vision. They may also report other symptoms associated with systemic diabetes, including polyuria, polydipsia, polyphagia, weight loss, fatigue, neuropathies, and frequent infections.

Objective

Diabetic retinopathy can be subdivided into nonproliferative diabetic retinopathy (NPDR) and proliferative diabetic retinopathy (PDR). The signs of NPDR include dot-and-blot hemorrhages, microaneurysms, exudates, intraretinal microvascular anomalies, cotton-wool spots, venous beading, and capillary nonperfusion. PDR has all of these signs plus neovascularization, which may lead to fibrovascular proliferation, vitreous hemorrhage, and retinal detachment. Macular edema may be associated with either NPDR or PDR and may or may not affect visual acuity.

The fasting blood sugar, 2-hour postprandial glucose, and oral glucose tolerance tests are helpful in the diagnosis of diabetes. Fluorescein angiography is useful in delineating microaneurysms, capillary nonperfusion, macular edema, and neovascularization.

Plan

Patients with NPDR should be examined at least yearly and more frequently if they show signs of increased retinal hypoxia. Patients with high-risk PDR usually benefit from panretinal photocoagulation, and those with clinically significant macular edema that causes a reduction in acuity usually benefit from focal or grid photocoagulation. Diabetic patients should also be referred for management of their systemic disease.

HYPERTENSION

Subjective

Hypertension is a very common systemic disease with an increased incidence among blacks and the elderly. Patients with hypertensive retinopathy are usually asymptomatic unless the macula or optic nerve is involved. Systemic hypertension is typically an asymptomatic, "silent" disease, although some patients experience headaches.

Objective

Signs of hypertensive retinopathy include flame hemorrhages, exudates that occasionally form a macular star, vessel-crossing changes, arterial constriction, macroaneurysms, and occasionally cotton-wool spots. Disc edema is a sign of malignant hypertension.

Systemic blood pressure assessment is an important test in the differential diagnosis of retinopathy due to hypertension.

Plan

Patients with hypertensive retinopathy should be monitored at least annually. They should also be referred for management of their systemic disease.

ARTERIOSCLEROSIS

Subjective

Arteriosclerotic vessel changes may be found to some degree in virtually all adults. Arteriosclerotic retinopathy is an asymptomatic condition.

Objective

Signs of arteriosclerotic retinopathy include arterial constriction, changes in the arterial light reflex (copper to silver to white), vessel-crossing changes, and macroaneurysms. Arteriosclerotic retinopathy often accompanies hypertensive retinopathy.

Plan

Patients with arteriosclerotic retinopathy should be monitored routinely and should be evaluated for systemic hypertension.

VENOUS OCCLUSIVE DISEASE

Subjective

Occlusive retinal vascular disease is commonly associated with underlying systemic disease, including carotid artery disease, hypertension, diabetes, hyperlipidemia, chronic lung disease, hematologic disorders, and certain autoimmune disorders. It can also be associated with glaucoma. The patient with a branch retinal vein occlusion (BRVO) often complains of vision loss corresponding to the area of hemorrhage or macular edema. The patient with a cen-

tral retinal vein occlusion (CRVO) has a more generalized vision loss.

Objective

Increased dilation of the retinal veins is sometimes an indication of impending venous occlusion. Both BRVO and CRVO have a nonischemic and an ischemic form. A BRVO presents as a wedge-shaped area of hemorrhages, microaneurysms, exudates, and, particularly in the ischemic form, cotton-wool spots. The apex of the wedge points to the occlusion. If the occlusion involves the superior temporal retina, macular edema is likely to result. In some cases, collateral or shunt vessels form to bypass the occluded area.

The presentation of a CRVO is similar to that of a BRVO except that the entire retina is involved. Hemi-CRVO involves either the top or bottom half of the retina.

Patients who present with a BRVO or CRVO should be evaluated for underlying systemic disease. Useful tests in the initial evaluation include blood pressure assessment, carotid bruit auscultation, fasting blood sugar, lipid profile, erythrocyte sedimentation rate (ESR), and complete blood count (CBC) with differential and platelets. Fluorescein angiography is useful in differentiating nonischemic from ischemic occlusive disease and in pinpointing areas of leakage.

Plan

Patients with venous occlusive disease should be monitored monthly for the first 6 months after the initial presentation. Grid photocoagulation may be indicated if there is nonresolving macular edema that causes reduced vision. This procedure is more effective in BRVO than in CRVO. Patients should also be monitored closely for the development of neovascularization and, particularly in the case of ischemic CRVO, neovascular glaucoma.

ARTERIAL OCCLUSIVE DISEASE

Subjective

Arterial occlusive disease is usually caused by the lodging of an embolus in the central retinal artery or at a bifurcation of one of its branches. These emboli can originate from a number of sources, including carotid atheromas, diseased cardiac valves, subacute bacterial endocarditis, thrombi associated with inflammatory disease or oral contraceptive use, or exogenous materials such as talc or cornstarch injected intravenously. A central retinal artery occlusion (CRAO) presents as a sudden, painless, unilateral loss of vision. Acuity often declines to the level of finger counting or light perception. Patients with a branch retinal artery occlusion (BRAO) usually note an area of vision loss corresponding to the zone of nonperfusion.

Objective

An acute CRAO presents as a diffuse milky whitening of the retina; the macula appears as the characteristic "cherry-red spot." The arterioles are thinned, and the venules have an irregular caliber. Later, the milky appearance of the retina disappears, and optic atrophy can occur. In acute BRAO, the milky retinal appearance occurs only in the nonperfused area.

A number of tests can be used in the differential diagnosis of the underlying diseases associated with arterial occlusive disease. An initial workup might include blood pressure and pulse assessment, auscultation for carotid bruits, duplex ultrasonography, CBC with differential and platelets, prothrombin and partial thromboplastin times, ESR, and a lipid profile.

Plan

An acute CRAO is considered a true ocular emergency. Attempts should be made to dislodge the embolus by massaging the eye or rapidly lowering the intraocular pressure. Similar procedures or breathing into a bag (elevated CO_2) may be used to move an embolus causing a BRAO if it is affecting central vision. Due to the high incidence of associated systemic disease and the increased risk for stroke, these patients should be referred promptly for a systemic evaluation.

BLOOD DYSCRASIAS (HEMATOLOGIC DISORDERS)

Subjective

Posterior segment hemorrhages can be caused by a number of hematologic disorders, including anemias, leukemia, polycythemia, dysproteinemias, and clotting disorders. Visual symptoms range from none to severe vision loss. Systemic symptoms vary according to the type of disorder, but fatigue, weakness, and malaise are common to most types.

Objective

Many different types of posterior segment hemorrhage—including vitreous, retrovitreous, flame, dot-and-blot, and subsensory retinal hemorrhages—can be found in

association with hematologic disorders. Flame hemorrhages are the most commonly observed type. A white-centered flame hemorrhage, or Roth's spot, is also seen in many of these disorders. Other posterior segment signs include exudates, cotton-wool spots, venous tortuosity, and disc edema. Laboratory testing, including CBC and differential, is a useful initial step in the differential diagnosis of hematologic disorders.

Plan

Management consists of referral for the treatment of the underlying systemic condition and frequent monitoring of the ocular manifestations.

LIPEMIA RETINALIS

Subjective

Lipemia retinalis is associated with hyperlipoproteinemia. Patients with this condition are typically asymptomatic.

Objective

In lipemia retinalis, both the retinal arteries and retinal veins have a creamy or salmon-hued coloration. A lipid profile, including serum triglyceride levels, is an important test in the differential diagnosis of this condition. A fasting blood sugar or similar test should also be performed because of the association of lipemia retinalis with diabetes.

Plan

Patients with lipemia retinalis should be monitored at least annually and should be referred for evaluation of their systemic disease.

SICKLE CELL RETINOPATHY

Subjective

Sickle cell retinopathy is associated with sickling hemoglobinopathies. These are found in approximately 10% of blacks. The ocular lesions of sickle cell retinopathy are usually asymptomatic unless they are associated with retinal detachment.

Objective

Sickle cell retinopathy can be subdivided into nonproliferative and proliferative. Signs of nonproliferative retinopathy include salmon-patch intraretinal hemorrhages, refractile spots, black sunbursts, venous tortuosity, and angioid streaks. Signs of proliferative retinopathy include arteriovenous anastomoses, neovascular sea fans, fibrovascular bands, vitreous hemorrhage, and retinal detachment.

Sickledex and hemoglobin electrophoresis are useful tests in the differential diagnosis of the sickle cell retinopathy.

Plan

Patients with signs of nonproliferative sickle cell retinopathy should be monitored for the development of proliferative retinopathy. If this should occur, photocoagulation or cryotherapy may be used to manage the proliferation. If retinal detachment occurs, scleral buckling procedures may be used for reattachment. However, patients with sickle-cell disease are at high risk for developing anterior segment necrosis secondary to buckling procedures. Patients with sickle cell retinopathy should also be referred for management of the systemic manifestations of sickle-cell disease.

RETINOPATHY OF PREMATURITY

Subjective

Retinopathy of prematurity (ROP) is an iatrogenic condition induced primarily in premature, low-birth-weight infants who undergo oxygen supplementation therapy. Vision loss can be variable and depends on the degree of traction on the macula or the presence of retinal detachment.

Objective

In the early stages, ROP presents as a demarcation line or ridge in the peripheral retina. Later, neovascularization and fibrovascular bands can develop. Tractional forces created by these bands cause macular distortion and the classic dragged-disc appearance. The presence of dilated, tortuous vessels in the posterior pole is called *plus disease*. Partial or total retinal detachments are a possible consequence of the cicatricial stage of ROP.

Plan

Low-birth-weight or premature infants who were on oxygen supplementation therapy should be evaluated before hospital release and should be examined at regular intervals during the first 6 months. Those who appear to be developing vasoproliferative retinopathy may benefit from cryotherapy or photocoagulation.

EALES' DISEASE (RETINAL PERIPHLEBITIS)

Subjective

Eales' disease is most commonly found in young men. In some cases, it may be the result of a tubercular hypersensitivity reaction. Patients with this disease may complain of floaters and blurred vision.

Objective

Eales' disease is characterized by inflammatory perivascular sheathing and vitritis. Peripheral neovascularization can develop in areas of nonperfusion and lead to vitreous hemorrhage. Edema from perimacular telangiectasia can also cause reduced vision.

The purified protein derivative (PPD) test and chest radiography are useful adjunct tests in determining exposure to or active infection with tuberculosis. Fluorescein angiography is also helpful in determining areas of nonperfusion and leakage.

Plan

Patients with Eales' disease should be monitored carefully. Areas of nonperfusion or edema may be treated with laser photocoagulation. These patients should also be referred for management of tuberculosis if indicated.

SYSTEMIC LUPUS ERYTHEMATOSUS

Subjective

Systemic lupus erythematosus (SLE) is an autoimmune disease that may affect any organ system. It is more common among females than males. The manifestations of this disease vary according to which organ systems are affected in a particular individual. Ocular symptoms range from dry-eye irritation to loss of vision. Systemic symptoms include joint ache and malaise.

Objective

SLE can affect both the anterior and posterior eye. Anterior segment manifestations include keratoconjunctivitis sicca, marginal corneal ulcer, lid rash, conjunctivitis, episcleritis, scleritis, and iritis. Posterior segment signs include cotton-wool spots, microaneurysms, hemorrhages, secondary hypertensive retinopathy, vasculitis, vascular occlusions, and optic neuritis.

Systemic signs include malar rash, discoid skin lesions, oral ulcers, arthritis, pleuritis, pericarditis, glomerulonephritis, hematologic disorders, and central nervous system disorders.

Tests used to help confirm the diagnosis include antinuclear antibody (ANA) test, anti-DNA antibody test, and lupus erythematosus cell preparation.

Plan

Patients with SLE should be referred for management of the systemic disease. These patients are treated with corticosteroids, other immunosuppressives, and antimalarials to help control their symptoms. Eye care providers treat the dry-eye symptoms and monitor ocular changes associated with the disease or the systemic therapy.

PERIVASCULAR INFLAMMATORY SHEATHING

Subjective

Inflammatory sheathing is most commonly associated with infectious posterior uveitis. It is typically asymptomatic.

Objective

The clinical appearance is of a white, yellow, or gray cuff encircling a portion of a vessel. It is sometimes accompanied by hemorrhages and exudates.

Laboratory and radiologic studies may be helpful in determining an underlying systemic cause of the perivascular sheathing. These include fluorescent treponemal antibody absorption test for syphilis, PPD and chest radiography for tuberculosis and Eales' disease, chest radiography and angiotensin-converting enzyme for sarcoidosis, ESR for temporal arteritis, and HLA-B5 for Behçet's disease.

Plan

Patients with perivascular sheathing should be examined on a regular basis and should be referred for management of the underlying systemic disease when indicated.

RETINITIS PIGMENTOSA

Subjective

Retinitis pigmentosa is rod-cone dystrophy that has autosomal dominant, recessive, X-linked, and sporadic modes of inheritance. It is characterized by night blindness and progressive peripheral field loss; however, the central vision may also be affected by cataracts or macular edema.

Objective

Signs of retinitis pigmentosa include "bone-spicule" pigment clumping, waxy pallor of the optic nerve, vessel constriction or attenuation, and occasionally macular edema and posterior subcapsular cataracts.

Electroretinography, perimetry, and dark adaptometry are all useful adjunct tests in diagnosing and monitoring the progression of retinitis pigmentosa.

Plan

Patients with retinitis pigmentosa should be monitored routinely. Those patients with vision loss often benefit from low vision aids. Vitamin A therapy may also have some benefit in slowing the progression of this disease. Genetic counseling is indicated when the mode of inheritance can be determined.

CONGENITAL ARTERIAL TORTUOSITY

Subjective

This uncommon condition has an autosomal dominant mode of inheritance. Most of these patients are asymptomatic; however, on rare occasions a patient with congenital arterial tortuosity may complain of vision loss secondary to a macular hemorrhage.

Objective

The primary sign of this condition is tortuous retinal arteries with normal-appearing veins.

Plan

No treatment other than routine monitoring is required for congenital arterial tortuosity.

PREPAPILLARY LOOP

Subjective

Prepapillary loops are congenital malformations of retinal vessels (usually arteries) or cilioretinal vessels. Patients with these loops are usually asymptomatic unless an arterial obstruction occurs that results in vision loss.

Objective

Vessels in prepapillary loops have a twisted, corkscrew-like appearance extending from the disc. Approximately one-third of these loops are surrounded by a glial sheath or have a visible associated Bergmeister's papilla.

Plan

Patients who have prepapillary loops have a higher than normal risk of developing a retinal artery obstruction; therefore, they should be counseled regarding the risk factors and monitored routinely.

CAPILLARY HEMANGIOMA (ANGIOMATOSIS RETINAE, VON HIPPEL–LINDAU DISEASE)

Subjective

Capillary hemangioma of the retina is a condition that has an autosomal dominant mode of inheritance with variable expression. Capillary hemangiomas may be unilateral or bilateral and usually become apparent in young adulthood. When capillary hemangiomas are found in association with angiomas, cysts, or other tumors elsewhere in the body—including the spinal cord, adrenal glands, kidney, liver, pancreas, ovaries, or epididymis—the syndrome is termed *von Hippel–Lindau disease*. This disorder is one of the phakomatoses. Capillary hemangiomas are usually asymptomatic; however, they may cause vision loss due to hemorrhage, exudation, or edema involving the macula, or exudative retinal detachment.

Objective

Capillary hemangiomas are most commonly found in the temporal periphery of the retina, but they may be found elsewhere, including at the optic disc. Small peripheral lesions have a reddish gray color. Larger lesions appear as reddish pink, balloonlike structures with enlarged feeder vessels. Retinal hemorrhages, exudates, and cystoid edema may be associated with these hemangiomas. Significant amounts of exudation may lead to retinal detachment. Fluorescein angiography is helpful in highlighting the vascular anomaly and associated leakage.

Plan

Patients with suspected von Hippel–Lindau disease should be referred to a neurologist or internist for further evaluation. Capillary hemangiomas should be monitored closely and can be treated with photocoagulation in some cases to prevent vision loss. Genetic counseling is also indicated.

RETINAL ARTERIOVENOUS MALFORMATION (RACEMOSE ANGIOMA, WYBURN-MASON SYNDROME)

Subjective

Wyburn-Mason syndrome, one of the phakomatoses, is characterized by intracranial and retinal angiomas. Ocular symptoms are rare, but occasionally leakage from the affected vessels can cause vision loss.

Objective

The hallmark retinal sign of Wyburn-Mason syndrome is a dilated, tortuous vessel that leaves and re-enters the optic disc. It can be small or very prominent and can take on a "bag-of-worms" appearance. Systemic signs include occasional hemiparesis, seizures, psychological disturbances, and facial angiomas (Klippel-Trenaunay-Weber syndrome).

Plan

The ocular manifestations of Wyburn-Mason syndrome should be monitored on a routine basis. The patient may also be referred for a neurologic evaluation. In addition, the patient should be counseled about the increased risk of hemorrhage during dental procedures if maxillary or mandibular angiomas are present.

CAVERNOUS HEMANGIOMA

Subjective

Cavernous hemangioma of the retina is thought to have an autosomal dominant pattern of inheritance with variable expression. The condition is typically unilateral and manifests by young adulthood. It is occasionally associated with hemangiomas elsewhere in the nervous system. Cavernous hemangioma is usually asymptomatic, but occasionally an associated epiretinal membrane can cause blurred or distorted vision.

Objective

Cavernous hemangioma presents as a cluster of red saccular dilatations along a retinal vessel ("cluster-of-grapes" appearance). There is frequently an epiretinal membrane lying on the surface of the hemangioma. Fluorescein angiography is useful in differentiating this condition from other retinal vascular anomalies.

Plan

Cavernous hemangiomas are benign and should simply be monitored during routine examinations. If hemangiomas elsewhere in the nervous system are suspected, a referral to a neurologist is indicated.

CAVERNOUS SINUS THROMBOSIS

Subjective

Cavernous sinus thrombosis can be either septic or aseptic. The clinician should take a careful history to determine whether the patient has had a recent infection of the throat, mouth, ears, sinuses, or other regions of the face. Factors that may contribute to aseptic cavernous sinus thrombosis include head trauma; surgery for tic douloureux or carotid cavernous fistula; and phlebothrombosis of the orbital veins secondary to dysproteinemia, collagen vascular disease, or the use of oral contraceptives. Symptoms of cavernous sinus thrombosis include dry-eye sensation due to exposure keratitis and diplopia if the extraocular muscles are involved. Vision loss may occur due to ischemic optic neuritis or secondary glaucoma.

Objective

External signs of cavernous sinus thrombosis include engorged episcleral veins and proptosis with secondary exposure keratopathy. There may be an afferent pupillary defect and extraocular motility restrictions secondary to internal ophthalmoplegia. Internal signs include dilated retinal veins, hemorrhages, cotton-wool spots, and occasionally disc edema or ischemic optic neuritis. The disc may show glaucomatous cupping if secondary open-angle glaucoma is present. Cavernous sinus thrombosis can be easily confused with carotid cavernous fistula; however, cavernous sinus thrombosis does not have an audible orbital bruit associated with it.

A carotid angiogram or orbital venogram can be used to help confirm the diagnosis. Other useful diagnostic tests include radiography, computed tomographic or magnetic resonance imaging scans of the skull and sinuses, blood or sinus cultures, and ESR.

Plan

Patients with cavernous sinus thrombosis should be referred to an internist for further evaluation and management. Septic cavernous sinus thrombosis is treated with an intravenous broad-spectrum antibiotic, with appropriate modification of the therapy once the infecting organism has been identified. Aseptic cavernous sinus thrombosis is usually treated with systemic anticoagulants and anti-inflammatory agents when indicated. Bed rest with elevation of the head also helps to relieve symptoms. The primary eye care provider can treat the exposure keratopathy with lubricants, punctal occlusion, and lid taping. The secondary glaucoma associated with cavernous sinus thrombosis is often difficult to manage medically.

SUGGESTED READING

Alexander LA. Primary Care of the Posterior Segment (2nd ed). Norwalk, CT: Appleton & Lange, 1994.

Berkow R, Fletcher AJ. The Merck Manual of Diagnosis and Therapy (16th ed). Rahway, NJ: Merck, 1992.

Duker JS, Brown GC. Vascular Anomalies of the Fundus. In Tasman W, Jaeger EA (eds), Duane's Clinical Ophthalmology. Philadelphia: Lippincott, 1990.

Loeb S (ed). Clinical Laboratory Tests: Values and Interpretation. Springhouse, PA: Springhouse, 1991.

Margo CE, Hamed LM, Mames RN. Diagnostic Problems in Clinical Ophthalmology. Philadelphia: Saunders, 1994.

Roy FH. Ocular Differential Diagnosis (5th ed). Philadelphia: Lea & Febiger, 1993.

Spalton DJ, Hitchings RA, Hunter PA. Atlas of Clinical Ophthalmology (2nd ed). London: Wolfe, 1994.

van Heuven WAJ, Zwaan JT. Decision Making in Ophthalmology. St. Louis: Mosby–Year Book, 1992.

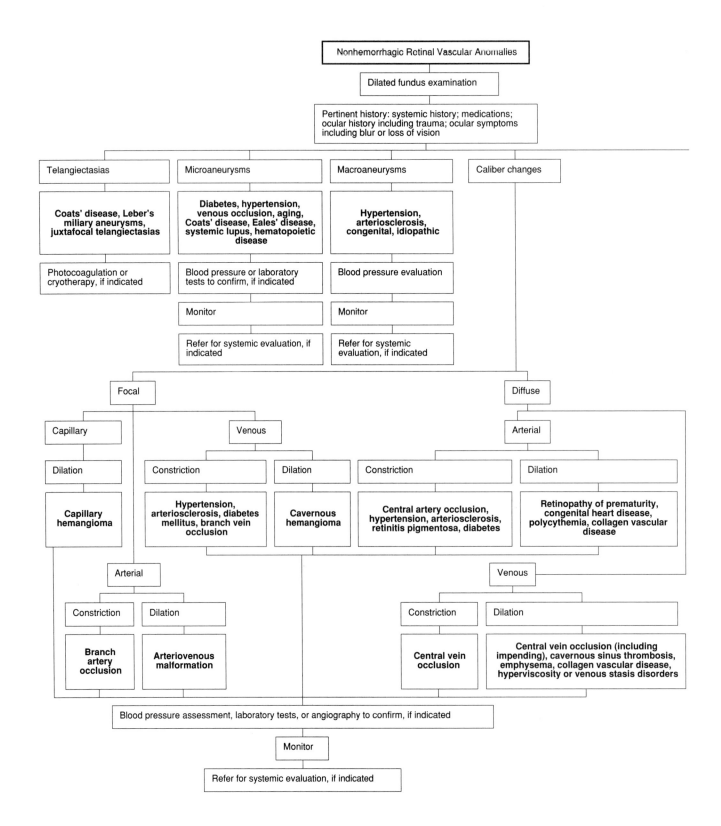

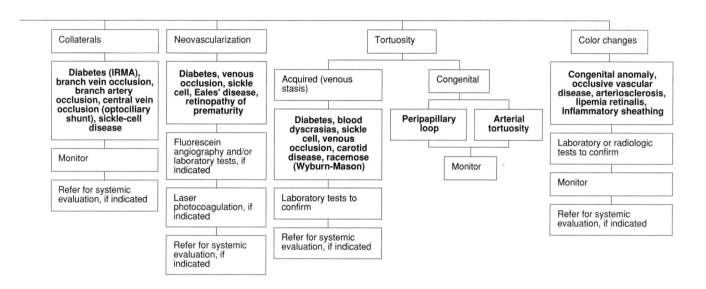

46

Yellow or White Fundus Lesions

DEBRA J. BEZAN

YELLOW OR WHITE FUNDUS LESIONS AT A GLANCE

Exudates
  Diabetes mellitus
  Hypertension
  Occlusive vascular disease
  Subretinal neovascularization
  Optic neuropathy (papillitis)
  Papilledema
  Macroaneurysm
  Coats' disease
Cotton-wool spots
  Diabetes mellitus
  Occlusive vascular disease
  Hypertension
  Collagen vascular disorders
    Systemic lupus erythematosus
    Giant cell arteritis
    Dermatomyositis
    Polyarteritis nodosa
    Scleroderma
    Wegener's granulomatosis
  Hematologic disorders
    Anemia
    Leukemia
    Dysproteinemia
  Papillitis
  Papilledema
  Toxemia of pregnancy
  Subacute bacterial endocarditis
  Human immunodeficiency retinopathy
  Lyme disease
  Acute pancreatitis
  Purtscher's retinopathy

Retinal necrosis
  Cytomegalovirus retinopathy
  Acute retinal necrosis
Drusen
Coloboma
Medullated nerve fibers
Retinal pigment epithelial window defect
Retinal embolus
Presumed ocular histoplasmosis syndrome
Other types of posterior uveitis
Trauma, including panretinal photocoagulation
Central serous choroidopathy
Best's disease
Stargardt's disease
Fundus flavimaculatus
Dominant drusen
Fundus albipunctatus
Birdshot chorioretinopathy
Acute multifocal posterior placoid pigment epitheliopathy
Multiple evanescent white dot syndrome
Serpiginous (geographic helicoid) peripapillary choroidopathy
Acute retinal pigment epithelitis
Radiation retinopathy
Tumors
  Retinoblastoma
  Metastatic choroidal tumor
  Astrocytic hamartoma
  Amelanotic melanoma

Many lesions of the retina or choroid are asymptomatic and therefore are first noted on dilated fundus examination. Aspects of the fundus lesion to be assessed include whether the lesion is single or multiple, whether multiple lesions are focal or diffuse, and whether the condition is unilateral or bilateral. The size, shape, color, and depth of the lesion and the presence of other ocular signs should also be noted.

Once a posterior segment lesion is noted, aspects to review or explore in more depth include a patient history of systemic disease, ocular disease, or ocular trauma, and medications the patient is taking. With some conditions, patients complain of blurred or reduced vision, photophobia, or changes in color perception. Patients who are symptomatic should be questioned about the onset, duration, and stability of their symptoms.

COLOBOMA

Subjective

Coloboma is a congenital condition caused by incomplete closure of the fetal fissure. Vision loss can range from mild to severe depending on the extent of the coloboma.

Objective

Colobomas can be unilateral or bilateral, and can involve the iris, retina, choroid, or optic nerve head. They usually appear as well-demarcated, rounded areas of white bare sclera in the inferior fundus. Morning-glory syndrome, a condition characterized by an enlarged optic nerve head covered by whitish glial tissue, is considered by some to be a variation of optic nerve coloboma. B-scan ultrasonography can be helpful in the diagnosis of these conditions.

Plan

Patients with coloboma should be educated about the symptoms of retinal detachment and should be monitored at least yearly.

TUMORS

Subjective

Tumors can be primary ocular tumors, including retinoblastoma, amelanotic choroidal melanoma, or astrocytoma, or tumors that have metastasized from other sites. Vision loss and strabismus can result depending on the location and extent of the tumor.

Objective

The ocular tumors mentioned above usually have a white or creamy yellow appearance and may have single or multiple foci. They are usually elevated and may have an overlying retinal detachment that complicates the clinical picture. Ultrasonography, computed tomographic (CT) scan, and fluorescein angiography are useful procedures in the differential diagnosis of retinal tumors. For example, the calcific nature of a retinoblastoma is highlighted with ultrasonography or CT, whereas the characteristic late staining pattern of a melanoma is quite evident with fluorescein angiography.

Plan

Primary ocular tumors such as retinoblastoma and choroidal melanoma can metastasize and become life-threatening. Enucleation or radiation are generally used to manage these tumors. A referral for a systemic oncology evaluation is also indicated. Benign retinal tumors should be monitored on a regular basis, and surgical excision should be considered when appropriate.

MEDULLATED (MYELINATED) NERVE FIBERS

Subjective

This condition is a congenital anomaly caused by myelination of the retinal nerve fibers extending beyond the lamina cribrosa. It is usually asymptomatic but can occasionally cause a relative scotoma.

Objective

Medullated nerve fibers manifest as a feathery white patch that follows the pattern of the nerve fiber layer.

Plan

Medullated nerve fibers require no treatment other than routine observation.

RETINAL PIGMENT EPITHELIAL WINDOW DEFECT

Subjective

Retinal pigment epithelial window defects are focal areas where there is an absence of melanin within the retinal pigment epithelial cells. These defects are quite common in the general population and are asymptomatic.

Objective

Retinal pigment epithelial window defects are whitish yellow, well-defined areas most commonly located in the equatorial region of the retina. Their borders are rounded or slightly scalloped, and typically do not have retinal pigment epithelial hyperplasia surrounding them.

Plan

Retinal pigment epithelial window defects have no significant consequences and merely should be noted on routine examination.

BEST'S DISEASE (VITELLIFORM DYSTROPHY)

Subjective

Best's disease is a macular disorder with an autosomal dominant mode of inheritance. It is thought to be caused by an abnormal accumulation of lipofuscin in the retinal pigment epithelium. It typically manifests between the ages of 4 and 10. Early in the disease visual acuity is mildly reduced (20/30 to 20/50), but acuity may drop to 20/100 or worse in some cases as the condition progresses.

Objective

A yellow lesion 0.5–5.0 disc diameters in size that looks like an egg yolk is characteristic of early Best's disease. The lesion sometimes has a pseudohypopyon appearance. Later in the disease, the lesion ruptures, giving a "scrambled egg" appearance. Electrodiagnostic testing is helpful in the diagnosis of Best's disease because the electro-oculogram (EOG) becomes abnormal even before vision loss occurs, whereas the electroretinogram (ERG) remains normal. The abnormal EOG is helpful in differentiating this condition from pseudovitelliform macular dystrophy (adult-type foveomacular vitelliform dystrophy), which has a similar clinical presentation.

Plan

Although no specific treatment is available for Best's disease, the prescription of tinted lenses and low vision aids may be of benefit. Genetic counseling is also indicated.

CHORIORETINITIS

Subjective

Chorioretinal scarring is a response to mechanical trauma (including surgery), infection, or other inflammation of the retina or underlying choroid. Although most patients report no symptoms, some patients may complain of blurred vision in the active phase of the inflammation. In addition, some patients with larger inactive chorioretinal scars may note a corresponding scotoma, particularly if the scars are located in the posterior pole.

Objective

Most chorioretinal scars have a central white zone of chorioretinal atrophy surrounded by a dark rim of retinal pigment epithelial hyperplasia. Histoplasmosis lesions tend to have less surrounding pigmentation than the lesions associated with most other types of posterior uveitis. Chorioretinal scars may be single or multiple depending on the nature of the inflammation. In some cases of posterior uveitis, such as toxoplasmosis, active lesions may form adjacent to inactive chorioretinal scars. There may also be an associated overlying vitritis.

A number of laboratory and radiologic tests are available to aid in the differential diagnosis of posterior uveitis. These include fluorescent treponemal antibody absorption test (FTA-ABS) or microhemagglutination assay–*Treponema pallidum* for syphilis; purified protein derivative test and chest radiography for tuberculosis; angiotensin-converting enzyme test and chest radiography for sarcoidosis; anti-*Toxoplasma* antigen titer for toxoplasmosis; *Toxocara* enzyme-linked immunosorbent assay (ELISA) for toxocariasis; serum rubella titer for rubella; and HLA-B5 for Behçet's disease.

Plan

Inactive chorioretinal scars should be monitored during routine examination for evidence of reactivation or the development of subretinal neovascularization. Some cases of subretinal neovascularization can be managed with laser photocoagulation or surgical removal of the vascular membrane. In the case of a lesion caused by posterior uveitis, the underlying disease, ocular or systemic, should be treated.

RETINAL EMBOLUS

Subjective

A number of different substances can cause endogenous retinal emboli, including cholesterol, calcium, fibrin, platelets, microorganisms, and fat. Substances introduced exogenously that can cause retinal emboli include talc, cornstarch, and silicone. Symptoms associated with retinal emboli range from transient episodes of vision loss (amaurosis fugax) to total monocular blindness, depending on the location and nature of the occlusion. Systemic symptoms of transient ischemic attacks or stroke also may be found in association with the presence of retinal emboli.

Objective

Cholesterol emboli are yellow and highly refractile. They tend to lodge in arterial bifurcations. Calcium emboli are white or slightly gray. Fibrin-platelet emboli are elongated and dull white. Talc or cornstarch emboli are shiny and variable in color. They tend to lodge in the perimacular capillaries. Extensive white peripapillary patches are associated with fat embolization (Purtscher's retinopathy).

Plan

Patients with emboli should be referred to an internist or cardiovascular specialist for further evaluation and management of the underlying systemic condition. They should also be closely monitored by the primary eye care provider for the development of retinal occlusive vascular disease.

IDIOPATHIC CENTRAL SEROUS CHOROIDOPATHY (CENTRAL SEROUS MACULOPATHY)

Subjective

Idiopathic central serous choroidopathy (ICSC) is a detachment of the sensory retina or retinal pigment epithelium in the macula. It is found most commonly in young adult white males. These patients typically complain of metamorphopsia and slightly decreased acuity, and may note some changes in color perception.

Objective

ICSC presents as a smooth, dome-shaped area of elevated tissue in the macular area. It may have a central yellow "lemon-drop" appearance. Evaluation of the optic nerve head for the appearance of a grayish optic pit is also important. Fluorescein angiography is helpful in localizing the area of leakage and in determining whether an optic pit is contributing to the edema.

Plan

Most cases of ICSC resolve spontaneously within a few months, although the recurrence rate is approximately 25%. Nonresolving and recurring cases may be treated with focal photocoagulation.

PHOTOCOAGULATION SCARS

Subjective

Laser photocoagulation is used to treat a variety of retinal vascular conditions or retinal breaks. The symptoms patients experience after laser photocoagulation depend on the location and the extent of the treatment. Many patients are asymptomatic, but some complain of blurred vision, peripheral field loss, or reduced night vision.

Objective

Immediately after treatment, photocoagulation burns appear as small, round, whitish yellow lesions that may have a surrounding gray ring. In the months after treatment, the lesions develop a pigmented rim. The burns may be isolated, clustered together in a grid pattern, or scattered throughout the midperipheral retina, depending on the desired treatment effect.

Plan

Patients who have had photocoagulation should be monitored at least annually for recurrence of their original condition or for the development of subretinal neovascularization.

STARGARDT'S DYSTROPHY AND FUNDUS FLAVIMACULATUS

Subjective

Once considered separate entities, Stargardt's dystrophy and fundus flavimaculatus are now thought to be variants of the same condition. Some forms of this condition have an autosomal dominant pattern of inheritance. The primary symptom is reduced central vision that becomes apparent during the adolescent years or early adulthood and worsens progressively. Color vision defects can also occur later in the disease.

Objective

One of the first signs of this condition is a pigment stippling of the macula in a bull's-eye pattern. Later the macula and midperiphery develop yellow pisciform (fish-shaped) flecks. As this condition progresses, there is further atrophy of the macula in an oval "beaten-bronze" pattern and degeneration of the surrounding retina. The macular changes are more pronounced in the Stargardt's variant than in the fundus flavimaculatus variant. The finding of an abnormal EOG with a normal or slightly abnormal ERG can be helpful in confirming the diagnosis.

Plan

Little can be done to prevent the progressive vision loss associated with Stargardt's dystrophy and fundus flavimaculatus; however, some practitioners advocate the use of spectacle tints that block short-wavelength light. Low vision aids can be very helpful in allowing patients to maximize their existing vision. Genetic counseling may also be beneficial. In addition, patients should be monitored on a regular basis for the development of subretinal neovascularization. Should it occur, prompt treatment should be initiated if possible.

DRUSEN

Subjective

Drusen are deposits of lipids and mucopolysaccharides on Bruch's membrane. They are associated with a malfunction of the retinal pigment epithelium. The condition is sometimes inherited as an autosomal dominant trait. Hereditary drusen become apparent in early adulthood. Degenerative drusen are more common in old age. The vision changes associated with drusen range from very mild to severe. Metamorphopsia can signal the development of an associated subretinal neovascular membrane.

Objective

Drusen have a variety of forms. Typical drusen are small, discrete yellow dots. Calcified drusen tend to be whiter and more refractile. Confluent "soft" drusen are larger and have less distinct borders. The lesions found in the hereditary form are scattered throughout the posterior pole, while those associated with degenerative changes (age-related macular degeneration) are found primarily in the macula. Drusen can also occur in the peripheral retina.

Plan

Patients with drusen should be monitored on a routine basis. Patients, particularly those with confluent drusen, should be educated to perform home vision monitoring with an Amsler grid or similar technique. Those who develop subretinal neovascular membranes (wet age-related macular degeneration) should be treated promptly with laser photocoagulation whenever possible. The prescription of low vision aids can be quite beneficial to patients who have already lost significant vision. Currently, a number of therapies are being investigated that are designed to prevent macular degeneration or improve the prognosis once it does occur. These include the prescription of vitamins and other micronutrients, laser photocoagulation of drusen, photodynamic therapy, radiotherapy, subretinal surgery, and retinal pigment epithelium transplantation and macular relocation.

BIRDSHOT CHORIORETINOPATHY

Subjective

Birdshot chorioretinopathy is a rare condition that occurs primarily in middle-aged whites. Patients with this condition may complain of floaters and vision loss due to macular edema.

Objective

Birdshot chorioretinopathy is typically a bilateral condition that presents as small, discrete whitish yellow spots scattered throughout the posterior pole and midperipheral retina. As the name implies, the retina looks as if it has received a shotgun blast. Other signs include vitritis, vasculitis, cystoid macular edema, and disc edema.

Fluorescein angiography can be helpful in highlighting vascular leakage and ruling out subretinal neovascularization. The HLA-A29 test is another useful diagnostic test, because 80–95% of patients with birdshot chorioretinopathy have this genetic marker.

Plan

Local or oral corticosteroid therapy is sometimes beneficial in managing birdshot chorioretinopathy. In other cases, immunosuppressive drugs or vitrectomy are more effective. Patients with birdshot chorioretinopathy should also be monitored carefully for the development of subretinal neovascularization so that prompt laser treatment can be initiated when appropriate. Patients who have sustained significant vision loss may benefit from the prescription of low vision aids.

MULTIPLE EVANESCENT WHITE DOT SYNDROME

Subjective

Multiple evanescent white dot syndrome (MEWDS) is found most commonly among young adult females. Some patients with this syndrome report a recent episode of a flulike condition. During the acute phase of the disease, the central acuity may drop to between 20/50 and 20/200, and the patient may complain of paracentral scotomas. As the condition resolves over a course of several weeks, the acuity usually returns to 20/30 or better.

Objective

MEWDS tends to be a unilateral condition that presents as several small white or salmon-colored dots clustered in the posterior pole. The macula may have a granular pigment appearance. A mild vitritis may occasionally be present. Perimetry often demonstrates an enlarged blind spot or paracentral scotomas. The clinical signs of MEWDS tend to disappear as the condition resolves.

Plan

The management of MEWDS consists of monitoring the condition during the active phase and providing reassurance to the patient.

ACUTE MULTIFOCAL POSTERIOR PLACOID PIGMENT EPITHELIOPATHY

Subjective

Acute multifocal posterior placoid pigment epitheliopathy (AMPPPE) is a disease of the pigment epithelium most commonly found in young adults. Patients with this condition often report a recent history of a viral illness. Vaccinations or ingestion of antibiotics or certain other oral medications have also been implicated as triggers for the development of AMPPPE. Patients with this condition complain of a rapid bilateral loss of vision that usually recovers to 20/40 or better in a few weeks to months.

Objective

AMPPPE is characterized by the sudden appearance of multiple dull-yellow or cream-colored plaquelike lesions clustered in the posterior poles. Fluorescein angiography is useful in defining these lesions. Approximately half of patients with active AMPPPE also have iridocyclitis or vitritis. As AMPPPE resolves, pigment mottling—indicating disruption of the retinal pigment epithelium—remains.

Plan

Topical corticosteroids and cycloplegic agents should be used to treat anterior uveitis if it occurs in association with

AMPPPE. Otherwise, frequent monitoring and patient reassurance are indicated in the management of active AMPPPE. Once the patient has recovered, the patient still should be monitored on a regular basis for recurrence or development of secondary retinal vascular disease such as subretinal neovascularization.

PRESUMED OCULAR HISTOPLASMOSIS SYNDROME

Subjective

Presumed ocular histoplasmosis syndrome (POHS) is thought to be an ocular immune reaction to a previous systemic infection by the fungus *Histoplasma capsulatum*. This organism thrives on soil enriched by bird and bat droppings. In the United States, the disease is found primarily among whites who have resided in the Ohio River/Mississippi River valley complex. During the initial infection, the patient may experience self-limiting flulike symptoms. The ocular disease is usually asymptomatic; however, macular and peripapillary involvement can cause severe vision loss.

Objective

The classic triad of signs of POHS includes peripapillary atrophy, white "histo spots," and maculopathy. The macular and peripapillary lesions can be the sites of subsequent subretinal neovascularization, hemorrhaging, and ultimately disciform scar formation. The absence of an overlying vitritis is helpful in distinguishing POHS from other forms of posterior segment inflammation. Macular edema and a circinate ring of exudates can herald the presence of a subretinal neovascular membrane. Fluorescein or indocyanine green angiography can be used to confirm and define the neovascular membrane. Chest radiography and the histoplasmin skin test may be useful in diagnosing the primary disease; however, the latter is not recommended in ocular disease because it can promote reactivation of the infection and stimulate the progression of maculopathy. It is important to note that acquired immunodeficiency syndrome (AIDS) can also promote the reactivation of histoplasmosis.

Plan

The management of POHS involves close monitoring for the development of neovascularization, both by the clinician in the office and by the patient with an Amsler grid at home. If neovascularization occurs, it is treated with laser photocoagulation or with submacular surgical removal of the membrane when possible. If significant vision loss cannot be prevented, the patient can benefit from the prescription of low vision aids.

INFLAMMATORY OPTIC NEURITIS

Subjective

Inflammatory optic neuritis (papillitis) is found most commonly in children and is secondary to a number of systemic infections or inflammatory conditions. These include bacterial, viral, and fungal infections, as well as collagen-vascular diseases. Demyelinating optic neuritis (usually in the form of retrobulbar neuritis) is more common in young adulthood and is often associated with multiple sclerosis.

The changes in visual acuity associated with optic neuropathy run a typical course in which vision declines rapidly during the first week, stabilizes, then slowly recovers. The ultimate degree of recovery is variable. During the acute stages, the patient may also experience pain on eye movement.

Objective

Papillitis typically manifests as a unilateral swollen optic nerve head with blurred margins and adjacent flame hemorrhages. Some forms show a stellate pattern of exudation in the papillomacular area. In contrast, retrobulbar neuritis has few ophthalmoscopically observable features. A central scotoma or other defects may be revealed with perimetry. Patients also have an afferent pupillary defect and perceive color desaturation with the red cap test.

Laboratory testing to screen for underlying causes of inflammatory papillitis includes FTA-ABS test, chest radiography, collagen vascular screening panel, and antibody titers for specific suspected diseases. An increased latency in the visual evoked potential is a useful diagnostic test for demyelinating optic neuritis; however, magnetic resonance imaging (MRI) is needed for definitive diagnosis.

Plan

The management of optic neuritis is still controversial. Administration of steroids and corticotropin, in addition to treatment of the underlying disease, has been used in managing inflammatory papillitis. Initial intravenous steroids followed by oral steroids may hasten visual recovery in demyelinating optic neuritis, but this regimen appears to have no effect on the ultimate visual recovery. Oral steroids used alone may increase the rate of subsequent attacks of optic neuritis.

PAPILLEDEMA

Subjective

True papilledema is a bilateral edema of the optic discs secondary to increased intracranial pressure. Increased intracranial pressure has a number of causes, including tumor, hemorrhage, inflammation, infection, trauma, drug toxicity, and benign intracranial hypertension. Initially, patients with papilledema note no visual symptoms or have brief obscurations of vision. Headache and nausea are common systemic symptoms.

Objective

Papilledema is characterized by elevated optic nerve heads with blurred disc margins. The elevated nerve head is best viewed stereoscopically using fundus biomicroscopy. Paton's folds may also be observed temporal to the disc. Adjacent flame hemorrhages and cotton-wool spots indicate an acute, noncompensated rise in intracranial pressure. Occasionally, exudates are noted in a macular star pattern. Disappearance of a previously noted spontaneous venous pulse is a helpful diagnostic sign. In the acute stages, perimetry reveals an enlarged blind spot. Other field defects occur with increased nerve damage. Another common ocular manifestation is impaired extraocular motility and diplopia secondary to sixth nerve palsy.

The differential diagnosis of papilledema includes evaluation for inflammatory papillitis, ischemic optic neuropathy, demyelinating optic neuropathy, pseudotumor, malignant hypertension, optic nerve head drusen, and other forms of pseudopapilledema. CT, MRI, and lumbar puncture are used in the diagnostic evaluation of papilledema.

Plan

Management consists of referral to a neurologist or neurosurgeon for determination and treatment of the underlying cause.

SUBRETINAL (CHOROIDAL) NEOVASCULARIZATION

Subjective

Any condition that causes a break in Bruch's membrane can set the stage for the development of subretinal neovascularization. Among the more common of these conditions are age-related macular degeneration, presumed ocular histoplasmosis, other inflammatory chorioretinopathies, and degenerative myopia. Symptoms of subretinal neovascularization involving the macula include metamorphopsia and vision loss, which may become severe.

Objective

Signs of early subretinal neovascularization include macular edema and an associated ring of yellow exudates. A grayish green spot in this area usually indicates that the subretinal neovascular membrane has begun to hemorrhage. The end stage of subretinal neovascularization is the formation of a disciform scar. Fluorescein angiography is a good way to confirm the presence of a suspected subretinal neovascular membrane. If there is a significant amount of overlying hemorrhage, angiography with indocyanine green dye may be of greater benefit than angiography with fluorescein dye.

Plan

Some subretinal neovascular membranes can be treated with laser photocoagulation. Extrafoveal membranes (i.e., those that extend no closer than 200 μm from the center of the foveal avascular zone) have the best prognosis. In a few cases, subfoveal neovascular membranes can be surgically excised. This procedure appears to have a greater success rate when the membranes are a result of presumed ocular histoplasmosis than when they are associated with age-related macular degeneration or degenerative myopia.

HYPERTENSION

Subjective

Hypertension is a very common systemic disease with an increased incidence among blacks and the elderly. Although the majority of cases of hypertension are classified as essential, some are secondary to other conditions such as renal disease, pheochromocytoma, or toxemia of pregnancy (pre-eclampsia or eclampsia). Patients with hypertensive retinopathy are usually asymptomatic unless the macula or optic nerve is involved. Systemic hypertension also is typically a "silent" disease, although some patients may experience headaches.

Objective

Signs of hypertensive retinopathy include flame hemorrhages, exudates that occasionally form a macular star, vessel-crossing changes, arterial constriction, macroaneurysms, and occasionally cotton-wool spots. Disc edema is a sign of malignant hypertension.

Systemic blood pressure assessment is an important test in the differential diagnosis of retinopathy due to hypertension.

Plan

Patients with hypertensive retinopathy should be monitored at least annually. They should also be referred for management of the systemic disease.

OCCLUSIVE RETINAL VASCULAR DISEASE

Subjective

Occlusive retinal vascular disease is commonly associated with underlying systemic disease, including carotid artery disease, hypertension, diabetes, hyperlipidemia, chronic lung disease, blood dyscrasias, and certain autoimmune disorders. The patient with macular edema secondary to a branch retinal vein occlusion (BRVO) often complains of vision loss corresponding to the area of hemorrhage, in addition to complaining of the symptoms typically associated with the macular edema. The patient with a central retinal vein occlusion (CRVO) has a more generalized vision loss.

Objective

A BRVO presents as a wedge-shaped area of hemorrhages, exudates, and, particularly in the ischemic form, cotton-wool spots. The apex of the wedge points to the occlusion. If the occlusion involves the superior temporal retina, macular edema is likely to result.

The manifestation of a CRVO is similar to that of a BRVO except that the entire retina is involved. Hemi–central vein occlusion (HCVO) involves either the superior or inferior portion of the retina.

Patients who present with a BRVO, HCVO, or CRVO should be evaluated for underlying systemic disease. Useful tests in the initial evaluation include blood pressure assessment, carotid bruit auscultation, fasting blood sugar level, lipid profile, erythrocyte sedimentation rate, and complete blood count (CBC) with differential and platelets. Fluorescein angiography is useful in differentiating non-ischemic from ischemic occlusive disease and in pinpointing areas of leakage.

Plan

Patients with macular edema should be monitored monthly after the initial presentation. If the edema does not resolve within 4–6 months, grid photocoagulation may be indicated. This procedure is more effective in BRVO than in CRVO. Patients should also be monitored closely for the development of neovascularization and, particularly in the case of ischemic CRVO, neovascular glaucoma.

DIABETES MELLITUS

Subjective

Diabetes mellitus affects approximately 6% of the general population. Patients with diabetes may be asymptomatic or may complain of blurred or fluctuating vision. They may also report other symptoms associated with systemic diabetes, including polyuria, polydipsia, polyphagia, weight loss, fatigue, neuropathies, and frequent infections.

Objective

Diabetic retinopathy can be subdivided into nonproliferative diabetic retinopathy (NPDR) and proliferative diabetic retinopathy (PDR). The signs of NPDR include dot-and-blot hemorrhages, microaneurysms, exudates, intraretinal microvascular anomalies, cotton-wool spots, venous beading, and capillary nonperfusion. Proliferative retinopathy has all of these signs plus neovascularization, which may lead to fibrovascular proliferation, vitreous hemorrhage, and retinal detachment. Macular edema may be associated with either NPDR or PDR.

The fasting blood sugar, 2-hour postprandial glucose, and oral glucose tolerance tests are helpful in the diagnosis of diabetes. Fluorescein angiography is useful in defining microaneurysms, capillary nonperfusion, macular edema, and neovascularization.

Plan

Patients with NPDR should be examined at least yearly and more frequently if they show signs of increased retinal hypoxia. Patients with high-risk PDR usually benefit from panretinal photocoagulation, and those with clinically significant macular edema usually benefit from focal or grid photocoagulation. Diabetic patients should also be referred for management of the systemic disease.

MACROANEURYSM

Subjective

Retinal macroaneurysms are focal dilatations of a major retinal vessel. They are most often associated with systemic hypertension, arteriosclerosis, or atherosclerosis;

however, they are occasionally congenital or idiopathic. They are found most commonly in older women. Peripheral macroaneurysms are usually asymptomatic, whereas more central lesions can cause vision loss.

Objective

A retinal macroaneurysm initially manifests as an area of bulging or ballooning in the retinal vessel. As the vessel begins to leak, the area becomes edematous and is usually surrounded by a ring of exudates. Subretinal or intraretinal hemorrhaging may occur. Once the macroaneurysm hemorrhages, it often self-seals and becomes sclerotic.

Fluorescein angiography may be helpful in confirming the diagnosis of a macroaneurysm and in determining where to treat if photocoagulation is indicated.

Plan

Many macroaneurysms can be managed by close monitoring. Those that fail to self-seal, cause persistent edema, or otherwise threaten vision may be treated with laser photocoagulation. In all cases, the patient should be referred for an evaluation for underlying cardiovascular disease.

COATS' DISEASE

Subjective

Coats' disease, Leber's miliary aneurysms, and idiopathic juxtafoveal retinal telangiectasis are variants of retinal telangiectasia. Coats' disease is typically a unilateral condition. It is most commonly diagnosed in boys between the ages of 2 and 10. It can cause vision loss, particularly if the macula is affected.

Objective

Whitish yellow exudation from retinal telangiectasias and aneurysms are the hallmarks of these diseases. Either the exudate alone, if it is massive, or an exudative retinal detachment can cause leukocoria. Fluorescein angiography is helpful in highlighting the vascular abnormalities characteristic of these conditions and determining where to treat.

Plan

Retinal telangiectasia is treated with photocoagulation or cryotherapy to seal leaking vessels. If an associated retinal detachment is found, reattachment surgery is usually indicated.

COLLAGEN VASCULAR DISORDERS

Subjective

A number of collagen vascular disorders can cause retinopathy, including systemic lupus erythematosus, dermatomyositis, polyarteritis nodosa, scleroderma, Wegener's granulomatosis, and giant cell arteritis. The ocular symptoms vary, and the amount of vision loss is related to the location and extent of retinopathy.

Objective

Many of the collagen vascular disorders affect both the anterior and posterior eye. Posterior segment signs often resemble those of hypertensive retinopathy; indeed, the patient may concurrently have systemic hypertension. Cotton-wool spots, exudates, and hemorrhages are common. Roth's spots may also be present. Disc edema or optic atrophy may be seen in some cases.

The systemic signs and symptoms vary with the specific condition. Joint pain, facial rash, or other characteristic dermatologic disorders should alert the practitioner to the possibility of a collagen vascular disorder.

Plan

Patients with suspected collagen vascular disorders should be referred for further evaluation and treatment of the underlying condition.

BLOOD DYSCRASIAS (HEMATOLOGIC DISORDERS)

Subjective

Posterior segment manifestations can occur from a number of hematologic disorders, including anemias, leukemia, polycythemia, dysproteinemias, and clotting disorders. Visual symptoms range from none to severe vision loss. Systemic symptoms vary according to the type of disorder, but fatigue, weakness, and malaise are common to most types.

Objective

Exudates and cotton-wool spots are seen in association with a number of hematologic disorders. Many different types of posterior segment hemorrhage—including vitreous, retrovitreous, flame, dot-and-blot, and subsensory

retinal hemorrhages—can be found in association with hematologic disorders. Flame hemorrhages are the most commonly observed type. A white-centered flame hemorrhage, or Roth's spot, is also seen in many hematologic disorders. It should be noted that Roth's spots are not pathognomonic of hematologic disorders; the spots can be found in other conditions such as subacute bacterial endocarditis. Other posterior segment signs of hematologic disorders include venous tortuosity and disc edema. Laboratory testing, including CBC and differential, is a useful initial step in the differential diagnosis of hematologic disorders.

Plan

Management consists of referral to a hematologist for the treatment of the underlying systemic condition and frequent monitoring of the ocular manifestations.

PURTSCHER'S RETINOPATHY

Subjective

Purtscher's retinopathy occurs after crushing injuries such as thoracic compression. It is thought to be a result of the embolization of fat from bone marrow or a disseminated intravascular coagulation. The primary symptom associated with this condition is vision loss.

Objective

The clinical manifestation of acute Purtscher's retinopathy typically consists of numerous cotton-wool spots in the posterior pole. Exudates and retinal or vitreous hemorrhages may also be present. Later, the cotton-wool spots disappear, but attenuated arterioles, nerve fiber loss, and disc pallor may remain.

Plan

There is no specific treatment for Purtscher's retinopathy. These patients should be monitored on a regular basis, because they are at increased risk for retinal detachment. Those who sustain permanent vision loss may benefit from the prescription of low vision aids.

CYTOMEGALOVIRUS RETINOPATHY

Subjective

Cytomegalovirus (CMV) is an opportunistic organism that typically infects an immunocompromised host, for example, one with AIDS. The symptoms of CMV retinopathy vary according to the location and extent of the tissue damage. Some patients may be totally asymptomatic, while others may complain of floaters and central or peripheral vision loss.

Objective

CMV retinopathy begins as a focal area of necrosis, often at the site of a cotton-wool spot representing human immunodeficiency virus (HIV) retinopathy. The necrosis spreads over a period of weeks to months, usually in a "brush fire" pattern. Other signs of ocular CMV infection include vitreous opacities, microaneurysms, hemorrhages, perivascular sheathing, and ischemic areas due to capillary nonperfusion. This condition has been called the "mustard and catsup fundus" or the "pizza fundus" because of the large yellow and red patches caused by hemorrhaging and necrosis. CMV retinopathy can lead to retinal detachment.

A laboratory evaluation for HIV infection (ELISA for HIV or Western blot test) should be performed on patients with suspected CMV retinopathy. A serum CMV antibody screener can be used to confirm the diagnosis of CMV. A CD4 lymphocyte count may also be useful in monitoring the progression of AIDS. CMV retinopathy is usually associated with a low CD4 count.

Plan

The primary drugs currently available to treat CMV retinopathy are ganciclovir, foscarnet sodium, cidofovir, and fomiversen. These drugs do not cure the condition but can cause it to stabilize or regress. Patients who develop retinal detachments may require reattachment surgery.

ACUTE RETINAL NECROSIS

Subjective

Acute retinal necrosis (ARN) occurs primarily in patients aged 20–60. Patients may otherwise be healthy or may be immunocompromised. Viral infection with varicella zoster,

herpes simplex, or cytomegalovirus has been suggested as the cause of ARN. Symptoms of ARN include pain on eye movement, photophobia, floaters, and reduced central or peripheral vision.

Objective

ARN is an acute severe occlusive vasculitis that predominantly affects the peripheral retinal and choroidal arteries. It may be either unilateral or bilateral. It is characterized by peripheral whitish patches of necrotizing retina. These areas of necrosis may be mistaken for CMV retinitis. Other signs of ARN include retinal detachment, perivasculitis, optic neuritis, vitritis, neovascularization, vitreous hemorrhage, anterior uveitis, episcleritis, and conjunctival injection.

Plan

Intravenous followed by oral acyclovir is used to treat active ARN. Oral steroids may be used once antiviral treatment is under way to help decrease inflammation. Prophylactic laser photocoagulation may be used in some cases to prevent retinal detachment. If detachment occurs, a vitrectomy and gas or oil tamponade are typically used in the repair. If the patient is not known to have an immunosuppressive condition, further testing should be done to rule out AIDS.

SUGGESTED READING

Alexander LA. Primary Care of the Posterior Segment (2nd ed). Norwalk, CT: Appleton & Lange, 1994.
Margo CE, Hamed LM, Mames RN. Diagnostic Problems in Clinical Ophthalmology. Philadelphia: Saunders, 1994.
Marks ES, Adamczyk DT, Thomann KH (eds). Primary Eyecare in Systemic Disease. Norwalk, CT: Appleton & Lange, 1995.
Roy FH. Ocular Differential Diagnosis (5th ed). Philadelphia: Lea & Febiger, 1993.
Spalton DJ, Hitchings RA, Hunter PA. Atlas of Clinical Ophthalmology (2nd ed). London: Wolfe, 1994.
van Heuven WAJ, Zwaan JT. Decision Making in Ophthalmology. St. Louis: Mosby–Year Book, 1992.

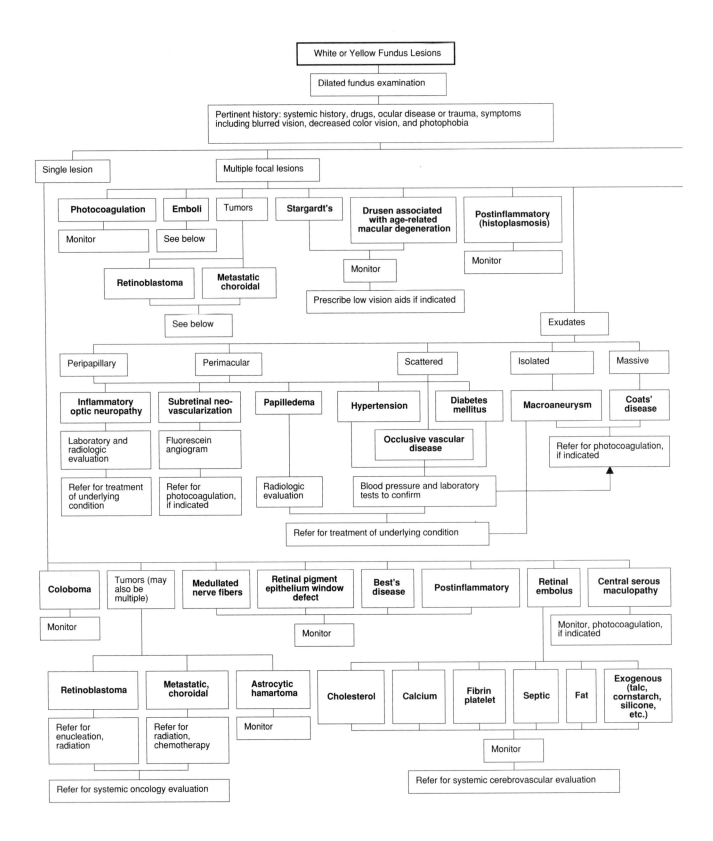

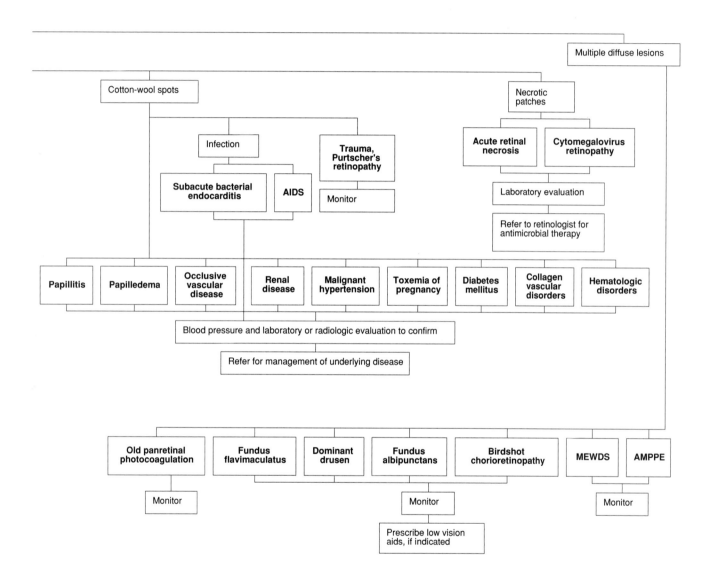

47

Black or Gray Fundus Lesions

Debra J. Bezan

Most darkly colored fundus lesions are asymptomatic and are discovered during routine fundus examination. Once a dark fundus lesion is noted, the clinician may wish to review pertinent aspects of the case history, including history of systemic or ocular disease in the patient or family members, use of medications, and ocular symptoms such as loss of peripheral or central vision or night blindness.

LATTICE DEGENERATION

Subjective

Lattice degeneration is found in 6–10% of the general population. The patient with lattice degeneration may be asymptomatic or may experience flashes.

Objective

Lattice degeneration may be unilateral or bilateral. It presents as a dark, linear lesion usually concentric to the ora, which may be interspersed with a white lattice of sclerosed vessels. Degenerated vitreous usually overlies areas of lattice degeneration. Atrophic holes within the lesion are common and usually insignificant. Breaks at the edge of the lattice lesion are of more concern.

Plan

Patients with lattice degeneration should be monitored at least annually because of the increased risk of developing retinal breaks and detachments. High-risk, symptomatic lesions are occasionally treated prophylactically with laser photocoagulation.

CONGENITAL HYPERTROPHY OF THE RETINAL PIGMENT EPITHELIUM

Subjective

Most patients with lesions representing congenital hypertrophy of the retinal pigment epithelium (CHRPE) are asymptomatic. Those with large lesions may note a corresponding scotoma in their peripheral field.

Objective

CHRPE may occur as a single large, dark lesion with a surrounding zone of retinal pigment epithelial (RPE) hypoplasia. This appearance gives rise to the name *haloed nevus*. These lesions occasionally have depigmented zones of chorioretinal atrophy within them called lacunae. Another form of CHRPE occurs as a localized cluster of small, dark lesions called *bear tracks*.

Plan

CHRPE lesions are benign and should be monitored on routine examination. Persons who have a family history of familial adenomatous polyposis and who have four or more CHRPE lesions should be referred for an evaluation for this disease.

RETINAL PIGMENT EPITHELIAL HYPERPLASIA

Subjective

RPE hyperplasia is a response to mechanical trauma (including surgery) or inflammation of the retina or underlying choroid. Although most patients report no symptoms, some with larger lesions may note a corresponding scotoma.

Objective

RPE hyperplasia appears as a black lesion and may have adjacent depigmented zones of chorioretinal atrophy. In some cases of posterior uveitis, such as in toxoplasmosis, active lesions may form adjacent to inactive chorioretinal scars. There may also be an associated overlying vitritis. Linear bands of RPE hyperplasia may indicate an area in which a detached retina became reattached either spontaneously or post-treatment.

A number of laboratory and radiologic tests are available to aid in the differential diagnosis of posterior uveitis. These include fluorescent treponemal antibody absorption test for syphilis, purified protein derivative test and chest radiography for tuberculosis, angiotensin-converting enzyme and chest radiography for sarcoidosis, anti-*Toxoplasma* antigen titer for toxoplasmosis, *Toxocara* enzyme-linked immunosorbent assay for toxocariasis, serum rubella titer for rubella, HLA-B5 test for Behçet's disease, and Western blot test for human immunodeficiency virus.

Plan

Inactive areas of RPE hyperplasia should be monitored during routine examination. When a lesion caused by posterior uveitis is found, the underlying disease, either ocular or systemic, should be treated.

VOGT-KOYANAGI-HARADA SYNDROME OR HARADA SYNDROME

Subjective

Vogt-Koyanagi-Harada (VKH) syndrome is a syndrome with both ocular and dermal manifestations; Harada syndrome affects primarily the posterior segment of the eye. VKH syndrome is more common among darkly pigmented people than among whites. Patients with VKH syndrome may be asymptomatic or may have vision loss due to cataract, uveitis, glaucoma, or retinal detachment. They may also experience central nervous system symptoms such as headache, stiff neck, paralysis, seizures, tinnitus, or deafness.

Objective

The dermal manifestations of VKH syndrome include vitiligo (depigmentation), poliosis (whitening of the cilia), and alopecia (baldness). Ocular signs include anterior uveitis, cataract, secondary glaucoma, chorioretinitis, Dalen-Fuchs nodules, retinal hemorrhages, and exudative retinal detachment. Pigment clumping may be due to the chorioretinitis or may be due to spontaneous retinal reattachment ("watermarks"). Although VKH syndrome is usually diagnosed based on the clinical appearance, testing for the presence of HLA-B22 is occasionally performed to help confirm the diagnosis.

Plan

Patients with VKH syndrome need to be monitored closely. Topical corticosteroids and cycloplegic agents are used to treat anterior uveitis associated with VKH syndrome. Oral corticosteroids or other immunosuppressive agents are used to manage posterior inflammation. Retinal detachment repair is performed when indicated.

CHOROIDAL NEVUS

Subjective

Choroidal nevi are benign tumors present in approximately one-third of the general population. They are asymptomatic.

Objective

Choroidal nevi present as rounded, gray lesions with slightly indistinct borders. They occasionally have yellowish drusen on the surface. The size of the lesions varies but is usually less than three disc diameters.

The relative disappearance of this lesion when it is viewed through a red-free filter is a finding that is helpful in differentiating it from RPE hyperplasia or hypertrophy or a subretinal hemorrhage.

Plan

Nevi should be monitored routinely for changes in size or shape, which may indicate malignant transformation.

CHOROIDAL MELANOMA

Subjective

Choroidal melanoma is the most common primary ocular tumor. It is more prevalent in whites than in darkly pigmented populations, and its incidence increases with age. Most melanomas are asymptomatic until they are large enough to involve the central retina or cause an overlying retinal detachment.

Objective

Choroidal melanomas range in color from dark to pale (amelanotic) and may have surface drusen, lipofuscin, or

RPE hyperplasia. Occasionally they have an overlying retinal detachment that obscures the view of the surface details. Melanomas commonly develop a mushroom or collar-stud morphology after they break through Bruch's membrane.

A-scan and B-scan ultrasonography, fluorescein angiography, and radioactive isotope uptake procedures are useful adjunct tests in the differential diagnosis of choroidal and retinal tumors.

Plan

A number of therapeutic options are available for treating choroidal melanomas, including photocoagulation, radioactive plaque therapy, external beam radiation, excision, enucleation, and no therapy at all. The selection of therapy often depends on the size and extent of the lesion. Regardless of the treatment selected, patients with malignant melanomas should be evaluated for systemic metastasis.

CHOROIDAL HEMORRHAGE SECONDARY TO SUBRETINAL NEOVASCULAR MEMBRANES

Subjective

Choroidal hemorrhages secondary to subretinal neovascular membranes are a result of breaks in Bruch's membrane and are associated with a number of ocular conditions. These include age-related macular degeneration (ARMD), presumed ocular histoplasmosis and other types of posterior uveitis, degenerative myopia, angioid streaks, choroidal rupture, and post–laser photocoagulation. Symptoms of subretinal neovascular membranes are reduced visual acuity, metamorphopsia, or central scotoma.

Objective

Subretinal hemorrhages present as diffuse gray-green lesions. They are often accompanied by edema and exudates. Fluorescein angiography is an important test in diagnosing and localizing subretinal neovascular membranes, but a dense choroidal hemorrhage may make this test difficult to interpret. In these cases, indocyanine green angiography may be of more benefit. The presence of other clinical signs such as drusen, "histo" spots, peripapillary atrophy, toxoplasmosis scars, high refractive error, angioid streaks, choroidal rupture, or photocoagulation scars can aid in the differential diagnosis of the underlying cause of the choroidal hemorrhage.

Plan

Patients with conditions that could cause subretinal neo-vascular membranes should be examined regularly and should be instructed in the use of an Amsler grid or similar technique for home monitoring. Extrafoveal subretinal neovascular membranes, if detected early enough, can be treated with laser photocoagulation to prevent hemorrhaging and further vision loss. Subfoveal membranes may be irradiated or surgically removed in some cases. Those patients who have already experienced vision loss may benefit from low vision aids.

SIEGRIST STREAKS AND ELSCHNIG SPOTS

Subjective

Siegrist streaks and Elschnig spots are caused by regional infarction of the choriocapillaris. They are most commonly associated with hypertensive retinopathy and cause no symptoms.

Objective

Elschnig spots are focal areas of mottled pigmentation due to retinal pigment epithelium degeneration. They tend to occur in the posterior pole. Siegrist streaks are linear areas of mottling that most commonly occur in the peripheral retina.

Plan

Patients with either of these lesions should be evaluated for hypertension and should be monitored on a routine basis.

AGE-RELATED MACULAR DEGENERATION

Subjective

ARMD is found in approximately 10% of the population over the age of 50. Its incidence increases with age. Symptoms of ARMD range from mild central vision loss or metamorphopsia to legal blindness.

Objective

ARMD can be subdivided into the nonexudative or dry form and the exudative or wet form. The more common dry form exhibits pigment mottling of the retinal pigment epithelium and drusen in the macula. It may progress to a geographic RPE atrophy or develop into wet ARMD. The wet form is characterized by subretinal neovascularization, exudates, and hemorrhages, and can ultimately lead to disciform macular scarring.

Fluorescein angiography is helpful in confirming the presence of subretinal neovascular membranes.

Plan

Patients with ARMD should be examined regularly and should be instructed in the use of a home Amsler grid or in a similar technique. Subretinal neovascular membranes, if detected early enough, may sometimes be treated with laser photocoagulation to prevent further vision loss. Low vision aids are often beneficial to those patients who have already experienced vision loss. Currently a number of therapies are being investigated that are designed to prevent ARMD or improve the prognosis once it has occurred. These include prescription of oral micronutrients or other pharmaceutical agents, photocoagulation of drusen, photodynamic therapy, radiotherapy, subretinal surgery, retinal pigment epithelium transplantation, and macular relocation.

PROGRESSIVE CONE DYSTROPHY

Subjective

Progressive cone dystrophy is an inherited condition that usually manifests in childhood. Symptoms include photophobia, progressive vision loss, and changes in color perception.

Objective

Progressive cone dystrophy has a variable presentation. One form shows "bull's-eye" RPE changes in the macula. Color vision testing and electroretinography (ERG), which should show reduction in the photopic response, are useful adjunct tests.

Plan

Patients with this condition often benefit from the use of tinted spectacles and other low vision aids. Genetic counseling is also in order.

DRUG TOXICITY

Subjective

Numerous drugs have been implicated in pigmentary changes in the macula. Of these, the antimalarials chloroquine and hydroxychloroquine sulfate, used in the treatment of rheumatoid arthritis and systemic lupus erythematosus, are the most notorious. Symptoms of antimalarial toxicity include glare sensitivity, mildly reduced central vision or central scotoma, and changes in color perception.

Objective

Antimalarial retinopathy presents as pigmentary changes in the macula that show a bull's-eye pattern. It may be accompanied by corneal deposits.

Plan

Drug-induced maculopathies are often dosage related; therefore, the drug regimen should be modified when appropriate.

RETINITIS PIGMENTOSA

Subjective

Retinitis pigmentosa is cone-rod dystrophy that has autosomal dominant, recessive, X-linked, and sporadic modes of inheritance. It is characterized by night blindness and progressive peripheral field loss; however, central vision may also be affected by cataracts or macular edema.

Objective

Signs of retinitis pigmentosa include peripheral "bone-spicule" pigment clumping, waxy pallor of the optic nerve, vessel attenuation, and occasionally macular edema and posterior subcapsular cataracts. When the patient has deafness associated with retinitis pigmentosa, it is termed *Usher's syndrome.*

ERG, perimetry, and dark adaptometry are all useful adjunct tests in diagnosing and monitoring the progression of retinitis pigmentosa.

Plan

Patients with retinitis pigmentosa should be monitored routinely. Those patients with vision loss often benefit from low vision aids. Vitamin A therapy may have some benefit in slowing the progression of this disease. Genetic counseling is also indicated when the mode of inheritance can be determined.

MUCOPOLYSACCHARIDOSES (MUCOPOLYSACCHARIDE STORAGE DISORDERS)

Subjective

The mucopolysaccharidoses are a group of mucopolysaccharide (MPS) storage disorders. They all have an autosomal recessive mode of inheritance except MPS II-A

(Hunter's syndrome), which is X-linked recessive. The most common ocular symptoms associated with the MPS disorders are night blindness and reduced acuity.

Objective

The posterior segment signs of the MPS disorders resemble those of retinitis pigmentosa. Many of the MPS subtypes also exhibit corneal clouding. The systemic manifestations of the MPS disorders are quite varied. They include skeletal and facial anomalies, cardiac disease, deafness, and mental retardation.

Laboratory tests are available to help differentiate between the MPS subtypes.

Plan

Patients with MPS disorders should be routinely monitored. Some may benefit from keratoplasty. These patients should also be referred for management of their systemic conditions when appropriate.

ABETALIPOPROTEINEMIA (BASSEN-KORNZWEIG SYNDROME)

Subjective

Abetalipoproteinemia is due to an absence of beta-lipoproteins, which in turn causes a lowering of serum levels of fat and fat-soluble vitamins such as A and E. Ocular symptoms are similar to those of retinitis pigmentosa and include progressive peripheral vision loss and nyctalopia. Acuity may also be reduced in some cases secondary to nystagmus or strabismus.

Objective

Ocular signs of this condition include a pigmentary retinopathy resembling retinitis pigmentosa. Some patients have strabismus or nystagmus. Systemic signs include ataxia and fat intolerance. Laboratory testing to determine serum levels of lipids and vitamins and to look for malformed erythrocytes (acanthocytosis) is useful in confirming the diagnosis. Dark adaptometry and ERG can be used to monitor the progression of the disease.

Plan

In cases with known deficiency, vitamin A therapy has been effective in improving dark adaptation and ERG waveforms. This result suggests that some forms of this condition are reversible if treated early in the disease course.

REFSUM'S DISEASE (HEREDOPATHIA ATACTICA POLYNEURITIFORMIS)

Subjective

Refsum's disease is a disorder that affects both the eye and nervous system. The disease has an autosomal recessive mode of inheritance. It is due to a metabolic disorder that results in an abnormally high production of phytanic acid. Ocular symptoms are similar to those of retinitis pigmentosa and include night blindness and peripheral vision loss. Deafness and paresis of the extremities are found in some patients with this condition.

Objective

The ocular signs, including bone-spicule pigmentary changes, are very similar to those found in retinitis pigmentosa. Other signs include dry skin, ataxia, polyneuritis, and skeletal abnormalities. Laboratory testing to determine serum phytanic acid levels and to check for elevated cerebrospinal fluid proteins can be useful in the differential diagnosis.

Plan

Some patients have shown improvement in retinal and neurologic function after they have been put on a low-phytanic-acid diet.

LAURENCE-MOON SYNDROME AND BARDET-BIEDL SYNDROME

Subjective

The Laurence-Moon and Bardet-Biedl syndromes have many common features, although they are usually considered separate conditions. The ocular symptoms of these syndromes are similar to those of retinitis pigmentosa except that central vision is more often affected early in the disease. The mode of inheritance is usually difficult to determine.

Objective

Pigmentary retinopathy that is often more pronounced in the macula than in the periphery is common to both syndromes. Both are also associated with mental retardation and hypogenitalism. Polydactyly (extra fingers) and obesity are associated with Bardet-Biedl syndrome, whereas spastic paraplegia is associated with Laurence-Moon syndrome.

Plan

The management of these syndromes consists of routine monitoring and prescription of low vision aids when indicated.

RETICULAR PIGMENTARY DEGENERATION

Subjective

Reticular pigmentary degeneration is more commonly seen in older adults and is asymptomatic.

Objective

The condition manifests as a reticular or netlike pattern of pigmentary changes in the retinal pigment epithelium of the peripheral retina.

Plan

There are no significant sequelae of these lesions; therefore, they should simply be noted on routine examination.

RETINAL PHOTOCOAGULATION

Subjective

Laser photocoagulation is used to treat a number of retinal vascular conditions and retinal breaks. Laser burns near the macula can cause noticeable scotomas. Panretinal photocoagulation can cause reduced night vision.

Objective

The appearance of the photocoagulation site varies with the duration and intensity of the laser application. Fresh burns appear white or gray, while older burns are pigmented. Depending on the condition to be treated, the laser burns may be single or isolated (focal), clustered in a small pattern (grid), or scattered throughout the midperipheral retina (panretinal).

Plan

Photocoagulation burns can usually be monitored during routine examination. Occasionally subretinal neovascular membranes can develop at a photocoagulation site, and further treatment may be necessary.

SUGGESTED READING

Alexander LA. Primary Care of the Posterior Segment (2nd ed). Norwalk, CT: Appleton & Lange, 1994.

Carr RE, Heckenlively JR. Hereditary pigmentary degenerations of the retina. In W Tasman, EA Jaeger (eds), Duane's Clinical Ophthalmology. Vol 3. Philadelphia: Lippincott, 1990.

Margo CE, Hamed LM, Mames RN. Diagnostic Problems in Clinical Ophthalmology. Philadelphia: Saunders, 1994.

Roy FH. Ocular Differential Diagnosis (5th ed). Philadelphia: Lea & Febiger, 1993.

Smith RE, Nozik RA. Uveitis: A Clinical Approach to Diagnosis and Management (2nd ed). Baltimore: Williams & Wilkins, 1989.

Spalton DJ, Hitchings RA, Hunter PA. Atlas of Clinical Ophthalmology (2nd ed). London: Wolfe, 1994.

van Heuven WAJ, Zwaan JT. Decision Making in Ophthalmology. St. Louis: Mosby–Year Book, 1992.

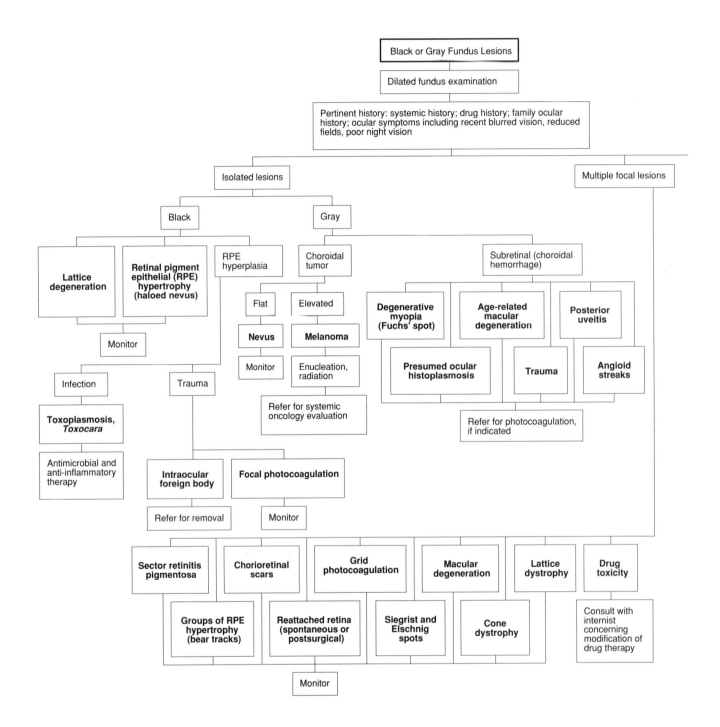

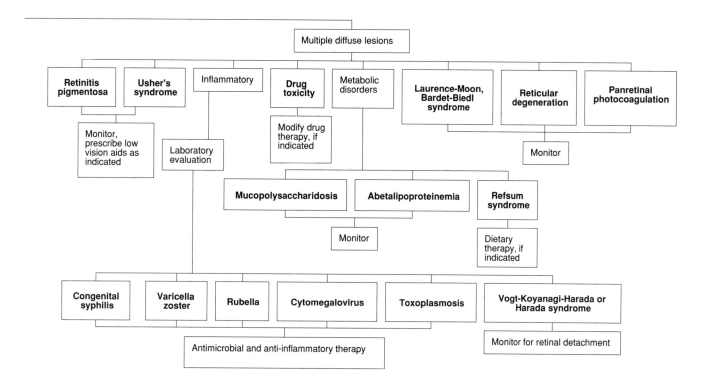

48

Lesions of the Peripheral Retina

DEBRA J. BEZAN

LESIONS OF THE PERIPHERAL RETINA AT A GLANCE

Pale lesions
   Cystoid degeneration
   White without pressure
   White with pressure
   Retinal pigment epithelium window defect
   Presumed ocular histoplasmosis lesion
   Paving-stone degeneration
   Enclosed ora bay
   Ora pearl
   Pars plana cyst
   Drusen
   Vitreoretinal tuft
   Meridional fold or complex
   Retinoschisis
   Snail-track degeneration
   Snowflake degeneration
   Commotio retinae
   Retinopathy of prematurity
   Familial exudative vitreoretinopathy
   Retinal detachment
   Scleral buckle
   Coloboma
   Retinoblastoma
   Amelanotic melanoma
   Gyrate atrophy
   Sickle cell retinopathy
   Pars planitis
   Sarcoidosis
   Behçet's disease
   Toxoplasmosis
   Toxocariasis
   Coats' disease

Dark lesions
   Lattice degeneration
   Age-related pigmentary degeneration
      Reticular degeneration
      Senile pigmentary degeneration
      Tapetochoroidal (honeycomb) degeneration
   Nevus
   Retinal pigment epithelial hypertrophy
   Retinal pigment epithelial hyperplasia
      Infection
      Inflammation
      Trauma, including surgery
   Retinitis pigmentosa
   Pseudo–retinitis pigmentosa
   Choroidal detachment
   Melanoma
   Wagner's hereditary vitreoretinal degeneration
   Goldmann-Favre disease
   Stickler syndrome
Red lesions
   Retinal hole
   Retinal tear
   Hemorrhage
   Neovascularization
   Choroidal hemangioma
   Cavernous hemangioma
   Retinal angioma
   Arteriovenous malformation

Most lesions of the peripheral retina are asymptomatic and are discovered only during a dilated fundus examination. Scleral indentation used in conjunction with binocular indirect ophthalmoscopy or three-mirror fundus biomicroscopy can aid the clinician in performing a complete stereoscopic evaluation of the peripheral retina.

TYPICAL CYSTOID DEGENERATION

Subjective

No symptoms are associated with typical cystoid degeneration. It is found in virtually all patients aged 9 and older.

Objective

Cystoid degeneration appears as a hazy, gray-white area with enclosed reddish dots that usually extends approximately 0.5 disc diameter from the ora serrata. It is most commonly located in the superior and temporal retina.

Plan

Cystoid degeneration should be monitored at routine examinations. In some cases typical cystoid lesions may coalesce and form retinoschisis.

WHITE WITHOUT PRESSURE

Subjective

White without pressure is usually asymptomatic. The condition is more common among myopes and in darkly pigmented populations. Its incidence increases with age.

Objective

It typically appears as a gray area of peripheral retina adjacent to the ora serrata. It is often bounded by a reddish brown line. The borders may be scalloped. The condition is thought to be caused by traction between the vitreous and retina.

Plan

Patients with this condition should be monitored every 6–12 months, because it puts them at higher risk for developing a retinal tear or detachment. They should also be made aware of the symptoms of a detachment to facilitate timely evaluation.

RETINAL PIGMENT EPITHELIAL WINDOW DEFECT

Subjective

Retinal pigment epithelial (RPE) window defects are asymptomatic.

Objective

The defect appears as an isolated, round, yellow lesion with flat, well-defined borders. It may be located any place in the retina. It is thought to be an area of RPE with reduced melanin rather than a region from which RPE is absent.

Plan

RPE window defects simply should be noted at routine examinations.

"HISTO" SPOT (PRESUMED OCULAR HISTOPLASMOSIS)

Subjective

Peripheral lesions associated with presumed ocular histoplasmosis are usually asymptomatic; however, the macular lesions can cause significant vision loss. Presumed ocular histoplasmosis is most commonly found in patients between the ages of 20 and 50 who have a history of living in central North America. They may also report a history of exposure to chickens or bats. (The feces of these animals in the environment created by the Mississippi, Missouri, and Ohio river systems of the central United States promote the growth of the *Histoplasmosis capsulatum* fungus.)

Objective

Histo spots appear as white "punched-out" lesions. They may be located anywhere in the retina. They are usually 0.2–0.7 disc diameter in size, occur in multiples, and are usually found in both eyes. They are occasionally surrounded by a ring of RPE hyperplasia. Other signs of ocular histoplasmosis include peripapillary atrophy and subretinal neovascularization, especially in the macula.

Plan

Peripheral histo spots do not need to be treated; however, the patient should be monitored for the development of subretinal neovascularization, both by the clinician in the office and by the patient with a grid at home. If neovascularization does develop and is detected promptly, it may be treated with laser photocoagulation, irradiation, or membrane surgery in an attempt to prevent further vision loss.

PAVING-STONE DEGENERATION (COBBLESTONE DEGENERATION, PRIMARY CHORIORETINAL ATROPHY)

Subjective

Paving-stone degeneration is asymptomatic. It is found in more than one-fourth of patients aged 20 or older, and the incidence increases with age.

Objective

Paving-stone lesions may occur unilaterally or bilaterally. They typically present as whitish yellow lesions 0.33–1.00 disc diameter in size located between the equator and ora, usually between the 5- and 7-o'clock positions. They are often surrounded by an area of RPE hyperplasia.

Plan

Although paving-stone degeneration is thought to be caused by a focal occlusion of the choriocapillaris, it has no significant consequences. Therefore, it should simply be noted during routine examination.

ENCLOSED ORA BAY

Subjective

Enclosed ora bays are found in approximately 6% of the general population and are usually asymptomatic.

Objective

Enclosed ora bays appear as circular areas of brownish pars plana surrounded by sensory retina at the ora serrata.

Plan

Patients with enclosed ora bays should be monitored at least yearly, because there is a 15–20% chance that a retinal break will develop at the posterior border of these lesions.

GYRATE DYSTROPHY OF THE RETINA AND CHOROID (GYRATE ATROPHY)

Subjective

Gyrate dystrophy is a progressive condition associated with a deficiency in the enzyme ornithine ketoacid aminotransferase. It is inherited as an autosomal recessive trait.

The symptoms usually appear during the adolescent to young adult years and include peripheral field loss and night blindness. Loss of central and color vision appears later in the disease course, and legal blindness usually occurs by middle age.

Objective

The midperipheral choroid and RPE begin to atrophy in the early stages of this disease. As these areas coalesce, they appear as large yellow patches with scalloped, pigmented borders. The lesions spread both peripherally and centrally until the entire retina is involved. Other associated ocular manifestations include myopia, macular edema, and early-onset posterior subcapsular cataracts.

Elevated plasma ornithine and reduced serum lysine levels help to confirm the diagnosis of this disease. Abnormal electroretinogram, electro-oculogram, and dark adaptometry findings, as well as peripheral field losses, are useful in monitoring the progression of gyrate dystrophy.

Plan

In some cases, dietary modification through the use of vitamin B_6 or proline supplementation, or reduction of protein intake has been effective in slowing the progression of gyrate dystrophy. Vision rehabilitation may be very helpful for those patients who have already experienced significant vision loss. Genetic counseling is also indicated due to the autosomal recessive mode of inheritance of this disease.

DRUSEN

Subjective

Equatorial drusen are found primarily among the elderly and are thought to be incompletely digested photoreceptor outer segments. They are not necessarily related to macular drusen or age-related macular degeneration. Equatorial drusen are typically asymptomatic.

Objective

Drusen appear as small, well-defined, whitish yellow bodies. They can occur alone or in clusters and are often found in association with honeycomb pigmentary degeneration.

Plan

Equatorial drusen need no treatment and can simply be monitored during routine examination.

ORA PEARL

Subjective

Ora pearls are asymptomatic lesions that are found in approximately 20% of the general population.

Objective

An ora pearl appears as a small, whitish, spherical body located adjacent to a dentate process of the ora serrata. Ora pearls are similar to large drusen.

Plan

There are no significant consequences associated with ora pearls; thus, they should simply be noted during routine examination.

PARS PLANA CYST

Subjective

Pars plana cysts occur in 3–18% of the general population and are asymptomatic.

Objective

Pars plana cysts are caused by a split between the pigmented and nonpigmented epithelia of the pars plana. The space between these layers fills with hyaluronic acid and forms a smooth cyst approximately 0.25–3.00 disc diameters in size.

Plan

Pars plana cysts have no significant sequelae and merely should be monitored during routine examination.

VITREORETINAL TUFT

Subjective

Vitreoretinal tufts are adhesions between the vitreous and retina. Tugging on a tuft due to movement of the vitreous can cause the patient to experience a phosphene similar to a flash of light. Noncystic retinal tufts occur in more than 70% of the general population, whereas cystic tufts occur in approximately 7%, and zonular traction tufts occur in approximately 15%.

Objective

The tufts appear as triangular, slightly elevated, grayish adhesions between the vitreous and retina. They are located between the equator and ora, and are more common nasally. They may be either unilateral or bilateral.

Plan

Patients with vitreoretinal tufts should be monitored regularly, because they have a slightly elevated risk of developing a retinal break or detachment. These are most likely to occur in association with a posterior vitreous detachment.

MERIDIONAL FOLD AND MERIDIONAL COMPLEX

Subjective

Meridional folds occur in approximately 25% of the general population; meridional complexes occur in about 10%. Both conditions are asymptomatic.

Objective

A meridional fold is an elevated ridge of retinal tissue that runs perpendicular to the ora serrata. A meridional complex is a meridional fold that is aligned with an enlarged dentate and ciliary process. It often has an excavated area adjacent to it that may mimic a retinal hole.

Plan

Patients with meridional folds and complexes should be monitored regularly, because both of these types of lesion put patients at a slightly elevated risk for developing a retinal break.

RETINOSCHISIS (DEGENERATIVE RETINOSCHISIS)

Subjective

Degenerative retinoschisis occurs in 1–7% of the population age 40 and over. Patients with this condition may be asymptomatic or may complain of peripheral visual field loss.

Objective

Degenerative retinoschisis is a splitting of the sensory retina at the outer plexiform layer. There are two types:

flat (typical) and bullous (reticular). The flat type may be an advanced form or coalescing of cystoid degeneration. The bullous type presents as a taut, transparent bulge of retinal tissue that, unlike a retinal detachment, does not undulate with eye movement. The surface may have a snowflake- or honeycomb-like appearance. Visual field testing shows a corresponding area of absolute scotoma; this finding can help differentiate this lesion from a retinal detachment, which often causes a relative scotoma.

Plan

Patients with retinoschisis may develop a corresponding retinal detachment; thus, it is important to monitor these patients at least yearly.

COMMOTIO RETINAE

Subjective

Commotio retinae occurs as a result of blunt trauma to the eye. Patients with this condition may be asymptomatic or may notice visual field loss corresponding to the affected area.

Objective

Commotio retinae appears within a few hours after the trauma and presents as an area of slightly elevated, opaque whitening of the outer retinal layers. It tends to resolve over a period of days to weeks. After resolution is complete, the involved area may show pigmentary changes in the RPE or no changes at all.

Plan

Patients who have had blunt trauma to the eye are at increased risk for developing retinal breaks and detachment; therefore, such patients should be examined soon after the trauma and routinely thereafter. They should also be monitored for the development of angle-recession glaucoma.

RETINAL DETACHMENT

Subjective

Symptoms that often accompany retinal detachments include flashes of light, floaters, and the feeling of having a curtain over a portion of the visual field. Retinal detachments occur in 0.005–0.010% of the general population. Among the risk factors for developing retinal detachments are trauma (including intraocular surgery), high myopia, certain peripheral retinal degenerations, retinal breaks, and exudative or proliferative retinopathies.

Objective

Retinal detachments can be subdivided into rhegmatogenous (associated with retinal break) and nonrhegmatogenous. Nonrhegmatogenous detachments can be further classified into tractional and exudative detachments. Retinal detachments commonly appear as a semitransparent, elevated area of retina that has a corrugated surface and undulates with eye movements. The underlying choroidal detail is obscured. The overlying detached retina becomes more opacified with time. Older retinal detachments may have adjacent rows of pigment ("watermarks") indicating zones of detachment and reattachment.

B-scan ultrasonography is a useful test for diagnosing a retinal detachment behind opaque media.

Plan

Most retinal detachments require surgical repair. Scleral buckling procedures combined with laser photocoagulation or cryotherapy commonly are used to anatomically reattach the retina. The reattachment success rate is greater than 90%. Following this treatment the buckled retina appears elevated, and the site of cryotherapy has areas of depigmentation and hyperpigmentation. The visual recovery success rate is lower than the success rate for anatomic reattachment and depends on the location and extent of the detachment, as well as the timeliness of the repair.

TUMOR

Subjective

Most peripheral retinal or choroidal tumors are asymptomatic until they are large enough to involve the central retina or cause an overlying retinal detachment. Retinoblastomas are primarily found in children, while choroidal melanomas and metastatic carcinomas are more common in adults.

Objective

Retinoblastomas are elevated tumors with white calcified areas within them. They may be single or multiple, unilateral or bilateral, and may seed into the vitreous. Choroidal melanomas range in color from dark to pale (amelanotic) and may show surface drusen, lipofuscin, or RPE hyperplasia. They develop a mushroom or collar-stud morphology after they break through Bruch's membrane. Metastatic carcinomas tend to be pale yellow and occur in multiples.

A-scan and B-scan ultrasonography, serial fundus photography, fluorescein angiography, and radioactive isotope uptake procedures are useful adjunct tests in the diagnosis of choroidal and retinal tumors.

Plan

A number of therapeutic options are available for treating retinal or choroidal tumors, including photocoagulation, radioactive plaque therapy, external beam radiation, excision, and enucleation. The selection of therapy often depends on the size and extent of the lesion and whether the involvement is unilateral or bilateral. Metastatic carcinomas are often left untreated because of the poor survival rate after they are detected. Regardless of the treatment selected, patients with malignant retinal or choroidal tumors should be evaluated for systemic metastasis. Genetic counseling is also indicated for patients or the parents of patients with retinoblastoma.

PARS PLANITIS

Subjective

Pars planitis is an inflammatory disease that commonly has its onset in young adulthood and may run a long course of exacerbations and remissions. Patients often complain of floaters and blurred central vision.

Objective

The condition is often bilateral and appears as whitish "snowbanks" of inflammatory debris on the far peripheral retina. "Snowballs," or clumps of this debris, may also be seen in the anterior vitreous. Cystoid macular edema is a common associated finding and may account for the central vision loss.

Plan

Oral administration or sub-Tenon injections of corticosteroids may be used to minimize the inflammatory response in this disease. Other immunosuppressive agents or cryotherapy may be used in unresponsive cases. The patients should also be monitored closely for the development of associated complications, including cataracts, glaucoma, neovascularization, and retinal hemorrhages and breaks.

COATS' DISEASE

Subjective

Coats' disease is a type of exudative retinopathy associated with congenital telangiectasias. It is most commonly seen in young males. It may be asymptomatic or may result in significant vision loss if the macula is involved.

Objective

The condition is usually unilateral and is variable in its presentation. It can range from small areas of telangiectatic vessels with a surrounding zone of hemorrhages and exudates to large areas of exudation that are extensive enough to cause leukocoria and retinal detachment.

Fluorescein angiography is a useful adjunct test to localize areas of vascular leakage in Coats' disease.

Plan

Patients with Coats' disease should be monitored frequently. Photocoagulation is occasionally used to treat selected lesions. Retinal detachment repair is performed when indicated.

RETINAL BREAKS

Subjective

Retinal breaks (holes or tears) occur in 2–15% of the general population. Patients may be asymptomatic or may complain of flashes or floaters. Trauma, posterior vitreous detachment, high myopia, and certain peripheral degenerations are risk factors for developing retinal breaks.

Objective

Atrophic retinal holes appear as small, round, reddish lesions that often are surrounded by a small white cuff of intraretinal fluid. RPE hyperplasia encircling a hole indicates a long-standing lesion. Some retinal holes have an overlying operculum of retinal tissue, which shrinks in size with time. Horseshoe-shaped breaks often have vitreous adhering to the inner apex of the horseshoe. These are more likely than operculated holes to tear further as a result of vitreous traction and lead to retinal detachment.

Plan

In patients with few risk factors, asymptomatic breaks with a minimal surrounding fluid cuff should be monitored. Higher-risk lesions may be treated with photocoagulation or cryotherapy to prevent retinal detachment.

HEMORRHAGE

Subjective

Hemorrhages are less common in the peripheral retina than in the posterior pole. They may be idiopathic or associated with conditions such as sickle cell retinopathy, retinopathy of prematurity, or posterior vitreous detachment. They are usually asymptomatic, although patients occasionally complain of floaters.

Objective

Peripheral retinal hemorrhages appear as red lesions that vary in size and shape. They may be found associated with neovascular vessels, retinal breaks, or vitreous hemorrhages.

Plan

Peripheral hemorrhages tend to resolve over time. Associated neovascularization or retinal breaks may be treated with photocoagulation or cryotherapy.

NEOVASCULARIZATION

Subjective

Neovascularization of the peripheral retina is a result of ischemia and is associated with diseases such as sickle cell retinopathy, retinopathy of prematurity, Eales' disease, and other inflammatory disorders. Diabetes mellitus and venous occlusive disease are more likely to cause neovascularization near the posterior pole but occasionally may cause peripheral changes. Peripheral neovascularization is usually asymptomatic unless it results in fibrovascular tractional forces that distort the macula or detach the retina.

Objective

Peripheral neovascularization manifests as a network of lacy abnormal vessels. It may take on a "sea-fan" appearance. Whitish fibrovascular traction bands extending into the vitreous are a sequela of peripheral neovascularization. They may lead to photoreceptor misalignment, vitreous hemorrhaging, or retinal detachment.

Fluorescein angiography is a useful test to localize peripheral areas of nonperfusion and leakage. Laboratory and radiologic tests are also helpful in determining an underlying systemic cause of peripheral neovascularization. These include Sickledex, purified protein derivative, chest radiography, fasting blood sugar level, and complete blood count with differential.

Plan

Patients with peripheral neovascularization often benefit from photocoagulation or cryotherapy procedures. They should also be carefully monitored for the development of vitreous hemorrhage or retinal detachment.

RETINAL AND CHOROIDAL VASCULAR TUMORS

Subjective

Vascular tumors of the retina and choroid are usually asymptomatic unless they involve the posterior pole or create significant exudation or retinal detachment. Many vascular tumors are associated with systemic vascular, dermatologic, and neurologic anomalies and are classified as phakomatoses.

Objective

Vascular tumors vary in appearance. Choroidal hemangioma manifests as a reddish, slightly elevated lesion, while the arteriovenous malformations of racemose hemangioma have a dramatic "bag of worms" appearance.

Plan

Choroidal and retinal vascular tumors should be monitored closely. Photocoagulation or cryopexy may be indicated when there is significant exudation and may be combined with buckling procedures to repair retinal detachment. Patients should also be evaluated for systemic manifestations of the phakomatoses if indicated.

LATTICE DEGENERATION

Subjective

Lattice degeneration is found in 6–10% of the general population. The patient with lattice degeneration may be asymptomatic or may experience flashes.

Objective

Lattice degeneration may be unilateral or bilateral. It presents as a dark, linear lesion concentric to the ora, which may be interspersed with a white lattice of sclerosed vessels. Degenerated vitreous usually overlies areas of lattice degeneration. Atrophic holes within the lesion are common and usually insignificant. Breaks at the edge of the lattice lesion are of more concern.

Plan

Patients with lattice degeneration should be monitored at least annually because of the increased risk of developing retinal breaks and detachments. High-risk, symptomatic lesions are occasionally treated prophylactically.

RETICULAR PIGMENTARY DEGENERATION

Subjective

The lesions associated with reticular pigmentary degeneration are seen more commonly in older adults and are asymptomatic.

Objective

The lesions appear as a reticular or netlike pattern of pigment changes in the RPE of the peripheral retina.

Plan

There are no significant sequelae of these lesions; therefore, they should simply be noted on routine examination.

CHOROIDAL NEVUS

Subjective

Choroidal nevi are benign tumors present in approximately one-third of the general population. They are asymptomatic.

Objective

A nevus presents as a rounded, gray lesion with slightly indistinct borders. Nevi occasionally have yellowish drusen on the surface. The size of the lesions varies but is usually less than three disc diameters.

The relative disappearance of this lesion when it is viewed through a red-free filter is a finding that is helpful in differentiating it from RPE hyperplasia or hypertrophy or a subretinal hemorrhage.

Plan

Nevi should be monitored routinely for changes in size or shape, which may indicate malignant transformation.

CONGENITAL HYPERTROPHY OF THE RETINAL PIGMENT EPITHELIUM

Subjective

Most patients with lesions representing congenital hypertrophy of the retinal pigment epithelium (CHRPE) are asymptomatic. Those with large lesions may note a corresponding scotoma in their peripheral field.

Objective

CHRPE may occur as a single large, dark lesion with a surrounding zone of RPE hypoplasia. This appearance gives rise to the name *haloed nevus*. These lesions occasionally have depigmented zones of chorioretinal atrophy within them called *lacunae*. Another form of CHRPE occurs as a localized cluster of small, dark lesions called *bear tracks*.

Plan

CHRPE lesions are benign and should be monitored on routine examination. Persons who have a family history of familial adenomatous polyposis and who have four or more CHRPE lesions should be referred for an evaluation for this disease.

RETINAL PIGMENT EPITHELIAL HYPERPLASIA

Subjective

RPE hyperplasia is a response to mechanical trauma or inflammation of the retina or underlying choroid. The clinician should question the patient carefully about previous ocular infections, trauma, and surgery, including laser procedures. Although most patients report no symptoms, some with larger lesions may note a corresponding scotoma.

Objective

RPE hyperplasia appears as a black lesion and may have adjacent depigmented zones of chorioretinal atrophy. In some cases of posterior uveitis, such as in toxoplasmosis, active lesions may form adjacent to inactive chorioretinal scars. There may also be an associated overlying vitritis.

Plan

Inactive areas of RPE hyperplasia should be monitored routinely. When a lesion caused by posterior uveitis is found, the underlying disease, either ocular or systemic, should be treated when appropriate.

CHOROIDAL DETACHMENT

Subjective

Choroidal detachment is most commonly associated with penetrating ocular trauma, including surgery. It may be either serous or hemorrhagic. The patient may be asymptomatic or may complain of severe eye pain and vision loss.

Objective

A choroidal detachment presents as a reddish brown, bullous elevation of both the retina and choroid. Serous detachments are usually accompanied by a low intraoc-

ular pressure, while hemorrhagic detachments are accompanied by a high intraocular pressure. In both types the anterior chamber is shallow and usually has cells and flare.

B-scan ultrasonography is a helpful adjunct test in the differential diagnosis of choroidal detachment.

Plan

Choroidal detachments often need to be repaired surgically. Topical corticosteroids and cycloplegics may be used to manage the anterior chamber reaction.

SUGGESTED READING

Alexander LA. Primary Care of the Posterior Segment (2nd ed). Norwalk, CT: Appleton & Lange, 1994.

Jones WL. Atlas of the Peripheral Ocular Fundus (2nd ed). Boston: Butterworth–Heinemann, 1998.

Margo CE, Hamed LM, Mames RN. Diagnostic Problems in Clinical Ophthalmology. Philadelphia: Saunders, 1994.

Roy FH. Ocular Differential Diagnosis (5th ed). Philadelphia: Lea & Febiger, 1993.

Zinn KM. Clinical Atlas of Peripheral Retinal Disorders. New York: Springer-Verlag, 1988.

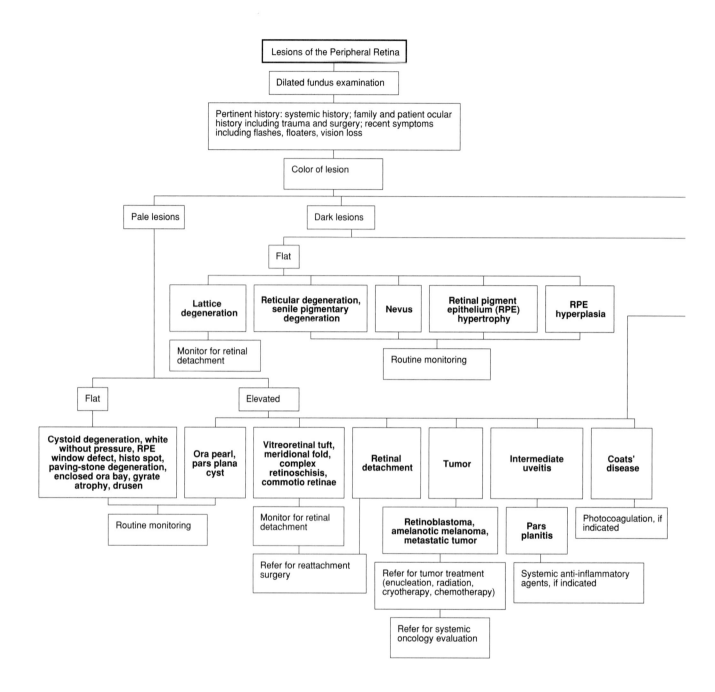

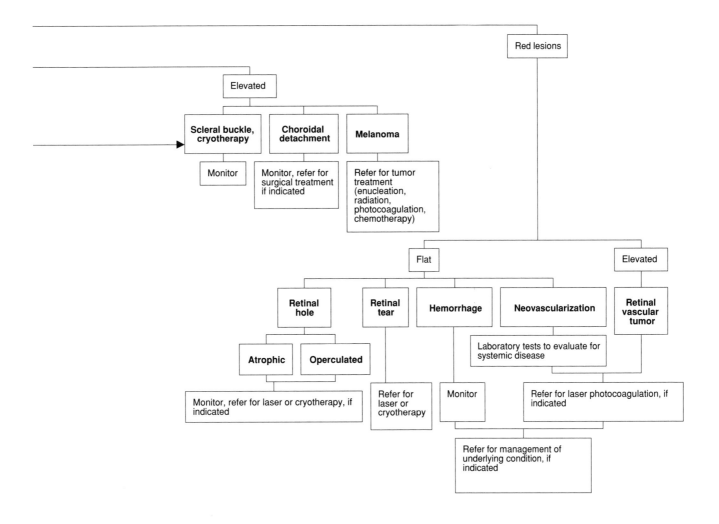

49

Anomalies of Optic Disc Color

John H. Nishimoto

ANOMALIES OF OPTIC DISC COLOR AT A GLANCE

Dark-colored (black or gray) anomalies
  Melanocytoma
  Retinal pigment epithelial or choroidal crescent
Light-colored (yellow or white) anomalies
  Bergmeister's papilla
  Myelination of optic nerve head
  Scleral crescent
  Optic atrophy
    Inherited optic atrophies
      Autosomal dominant congenital
      Autosomal dominant juvenile
      Behr's optic atrophy
      Autosomal recessive congenital
      Autosomal recessive juvenile
      Leber's optic atrophy
    Circulatory optic atrophies
      Central retinal artery occlusion
      Ischemic optic neuropathy
      Carotid artery disease
    Toxic optic atrophies
      Tobacco or alcohol
      Arsenic
      Lead
      Some antimicrobials
    Optic atrophies associated with central nervous
      system disease
      Multiple sclerosis
      Herpes zoster
      Tertiary syphilis
      Charcot-Marie-Tooth atrophy
    Pressure or compressive optic atrophies
      Glaucoma

      Papilledema
      Aneurysm
      Exophthalmos
    Postinflammatory optic atrophies
      Optic neuritis
      Orbital cellulitis
      Choroiditis
    Consecutive optic atrophies
      Pigmentary retinal dystrophies (e.g., retinitis
        pigmentosa)
  Coloboma
  Optic pit
  Morning-glory syndrome
  Optic nerve hypoplasia
  Optic nerve head drusen
  Tumors
    Metastatic carcinoma
    Retinoblastoma
    Malignant melanoma (amelanotic)
    Glioma
    Osteoma
    Meningioma
    Astrocytic hamartoma
Red-colored anomalies
  Neovascularization
  Papilledema
  Papillitis
  Hypertensive papillopathy
  Central retinal vein occlusion
  Hemangioma

In most cases, anomalies of optic disc color are benign variations of normal presentation. However, some color anomalies are pathologic and may be due to infection, vascular disease, or congenital conditions. This chapter

379

discusses several of the many causes of abnormal optic disc color, and their diagnosis and management.

MELANOCYTOMA

Subjective

A melanocytoma is a benign pigmented tumor that typically involves the optic nerve and adjacent nerve fiber layer. Patients with a melanocytoma of the optic nerve head usually have normal vision and are asymptomatic. If the tumor is fairly large, the observant patient may notice slightly blurred vision or a scotoma due to an enlarged blind spot. On rare occasions, progressive but often reversible loss of visual acuity occurs in the involved eye secondary to compression, necrosis of the tumor, obstruction of adjacent blood vessels, or a coincidental optic neuritis.

Objective

In ophthalmoscopic examination, a melanocytoma usually appears as an elevated jet-black mass located eccentrically over the edge of the optic disc. Occasionally, the edges of the lesion have a feathery appearance that follows the pattern of the nerve fiber layer. The uninvolved optic disc is often normal but may occasionally be edematous. In older patients there may be chronic degenerative changes in the retinal pigment epithelium around the melanocytoma. Although most melanocytomas can be recognized by ophthalmoscopy alone, ancillary procedures such as serial fundus photography, fluorescein angiography, and visual field testing are helpful in diagnosis and subsequent follow-up examinations. Typically, the tumor is hypofluorescent throughout the angiogram. The hypofluorescence occurs because the deeply pigmented, densely packed cells block the underlying fluorescence, and the tumor itself is relatively avascular. This finding is in contrast to the patchy hyperfluorescence seen in a choroidal melanoma. Visual field testing most frequently shows enlargement of the blind spot, but nerve fiber bundle defects and nasal steps have also been noted.

Plan

Management of melanocytoma of the optic disc consists of the proper diagnosis and follow-up to ensure that the lesion is not enlarging or progressing. After the initial diagnostic evaluation, the lesion be should re-examined within 3 months to monitor its stability and should be followed at least annually thereafter.

BERGMEISTER'S PAPILLA

Subjective

Bergmeister's papilla is a congenital anomaly of the optic nerve head. Patients with Bergmeister's papilla rarely have symptoms and do not realize that they have such a condition until the practitioner observes it on funduscopic examination. However, if the persistence of the hyaloid system is extensive, the patient may complain of vitreous floaters.

Objective

Bergmeister's papilla is formed from the hyaloid artery, which courses from the optic nerve to the lens near the end of the 4-week stage of embryonic development to form the tunica vasculosa lentis. Regression of the artery usually begins in the third embryonic month and is generally complete by the eighth month. Incomplete regression can leave a tuft of glial tissue, usually on the nasal side of the disc, called *Bergmeister's papilla*.

Plan

Bergmeister's papilla generally is a benign condition and should merely be noted during routine examination. In rare instances in which the hyaloid vessel is still patent or there is an associated prepapillary vascular loop, a vitreous hemorrhage may occur. In this event, the patient should be referred to a retinologist for further diagnosis and management.

MYELINATION OF THE OPTIC NERVE HEAD

Subjective

Myelination (medullation) of the retinal nerve fibers is a common benign congenital condition in which the myelin sheath around the axons extends beyond the lamina cribrosa. This condition typically is asymptomatic, but it can cause a mild relative scotoma if the myelination is particularly dense.

Objective

Myelination often extends outward from the optic nerve in a feathery white pattern. Occasionally, the myelination appears remote from the optic nerve head. Both the distribution and density of the myelinated nerve fibers vary greatly.

Plan

Myelinated nerve fibers are typically benign and stable. Once diagnosed, this condition should be noted during routine examination. Disappearance of the myelination is suggestive of demyelinating disease.

RETINAL PIGMENT EPITHELIAL, SCLERAL, AND CHOROIDAL CRESCENTS

Subjective

Crescents around the optic nerve may be congenital or acquired. Usually patients with crescents are asymptomatic; however, they may experience symptoms caused by underlying conditions such as progressive myopia, retinopathy of prematurity, or proliferative sickle cell retinopathy.

Objective

Crescents are caused by elongation of the globe or peripheral retinal traction. Stretching pulls the more superficial tissues from the disc margin, exposing deeper layers. Retinal pigment epithelial and choroidal crescents are pigmented, while scleral crescents are white. Crescents may extend only a few clock-hour positions or may totally encircle the disc. They are more commonly found on the temporal side of the disc. Large scleral crescents may cause an enlarged blind spot detectable with perimetry. History, refraction, and careful peripheral retinal evaluation are useful in detecting underlying ocular conditions that cause traction on the peripapillary tissues. Other conditions to be considered in the differential diagnosis of crescents include peripapillary atrophy due to presumed ocular histoplasmosis, glaucoma, or aging; circumpapillary choroiditis; and angioid streaks.

Plan

Crescents are benign and require no management other than routine monitoring.

OPTIC ATROPHY

Subjective

Many types of optic atrophy exist, both hereditary and acquired. Depending on the cause, visual acuity, color vision, and visual fields can be mildly to severely affected. Nystagmus is a common finding in congenital or juvenile optic atrophies that cause severe visual impairment.

There are three main classifications of optic atrophy: primary, secondary, and consecutive. Primary optic atrophies present with a pale, flat optic disc. The inherited optic atrophies include autosomal dominant congenital and juvenile, autosomal recessive congenital and juvenile, Behr's optic atrophy, and Leber's hereditary optic atrophy. The dominant type may appear between the ages of 5 and 8 years, and visual acuity is only moderately affected. The recessive type presents at an earlier age with more severe vision loss. Secondary optic atrophy follows long-standing swelling of the optic disc. Etiologic factors include papillitis, ischemic optic neuropathies, and papilledema. Other causes include toxic optic neuropathies, infiltrative optic neuropathies, glaucoma, and radiation of the optic nerve. In consecutive optic atrophy, there may be associated degenerative changes to the retina. Retinitis pigmentosa is a classic example. In this condition impaired night vision and peripheral vision are common symptoms.

Objective

In primary optic atrophy, the ophthalmoscopic appearance is typically of a pale optic disc with clearly defined margins. The pallor generally involves all of the disc but may be more pronounced in the temporal sector. Atrophy of the neural rim causes loss of the physiologic cup and flattening of the disc. In secondary optic atrophy, the optic disc is pale and may be slightly elevated. The physiologic cup is partially or completely filled in, and the disc margins are poorly defined. In consecutive optic atrophy, especially when associated with retinitis pigmentosa, the optic disc has a waxy pallor. It is flat, and the margins are well defined. The central retinal vessels are attenuated, and there are scattered areas of pigmentary degeneration in the midperipheral fundus.

Plan

In primary optic atrophy, the clinician must make the correct diagnosis by ruling out acquired causes. Patient education and genetic counseling are often beneficial. It is important to provide the best possible spectacle prescription and low vision rehabilitation if necessary. In autosomal recessive optic atrophy, because vision loss is usually severe, blindness rehabilitation services may be indicated. In acquired optic atrophy, if the cause is not established, a radiologic evaluation (computed tomography [CT] and magnetic resonance imaging [MRI]), a laboratory workup to rule out vascular disease such as diabetes and temporal arteritis, and a referral to a neuro-ophthalmologist or neurologist for further testing to uncover the cause are indicated. For consecutive optic atrophy, genetic counseling is advisable, especially if the optic atrophy is from retinitis pigmentosa. Low vision devices and other forms of vision rehabilitation are often beneficial in these cases.

PAPILLEDEMA

Subjective

Papilledema is a bilateral swelling of the optic discs secondary to elevated intracranial pressure. Underlying causes include tumor, hypertension, and pseudotumor cerebri (benign intracranial hypertension). Patients presenting with papilledema may complain of transient episodes of vision loss lasting for a few seconds. These episodes can occur with changes in posture. The patient may also complain of headache, nausea, vomiting, or diplopia.

Objective

On fundus examination, the optic nerve head appears swollen and hyperemic, with blurred disc margins. Physiologic cupping may still be present in early stages; however, in chronic or severe cases the cup is obscured. Associated findings include flame hemorrhages along the disc margin and a loss of spontaneous venous pulsation if it was present previously. Due to the swelling of the nerve, venous outflow becomes difficult, and the retinal veins become dilated and tortuous. The nerve fiber layer surrounding the disc develops circular folds called *Paton's folds.* Eventually chronic papilledema leads to optic atrophy, with a resultant loss of color vision and visual acuity.

Plan

Papilledema is considered medically urgent. The initial evaluation includes blood pressure assessment to rule out severe hypertension. A CT or MRI scan is crucial to rule out mass lesions such as intracranial tumors, hamartomas, subarachnoid hemorrhage, brain abscesses, and meningitis that may be causing the problem. Patients with mass lesions should be referred to a neurosurgeon for further diagnosis and management.

If the radiologic studies are negative, a lumbar puncture is indicated. If benign elevated intracranial pressure (pseudotumor cerebri) is the underlying cause, treatment may include a weight-reduction diet and oral acetazolamide. In severe cases, a shunt procedure may be required to reduce the pressure.

NEOVASCULARIZATION

Subjective

Neovascularization of the optic nerve head is most commonly associated with proliferative diabetic retinopathy. Symptoms vary from none to severe vision loss. A patient with uncontrolled diabetes mellitus often notices changes in vision associated with fluctuations in blood glucose level. Associated systemic symptoms include peripheral neuropathies and increased thirst, urination, and appetite.

Objective

Neovascularization of the optic nerve head presents as a fine lacy network of blood vessels that originate from the capillaries of the optic nerve head. Neovascularization may appear in small areas or cover the entire disc. It is usually accompanied by other signs of diabetic retinopathy, including cotton-wool spots, venous beading, intraretinal microvascular anomalies, dot-and-blot hemorrhages, hard exudates, and neovascularization elsewhere. Neovascularization of the disc indicates that the patient is at increased risk for developing vitreous hemorrhages, rubeosis iridis, and neovascular glaucoma.

Plan

If neovascularization of the disc is detected, a retinal specialist should be consulted regarding the feasibility of treatment with panretinal laser photocoagulation. If the neovascularization of the disc covers more than one-third of the disc, the patient is at high risk for significant vision loss, and prompt referral is indicated. Patients should also be referred to their internists or family practitioners for assessment of their blood sugar control.

MALIGNANT HYPERTENSION

Subjective

Patients with hypertensive retinopathy that involves swelling of the disc (malignant hypertension) may have no symptoms or may have symptoms ranging from mild to severe loss of central vision. A common systemic symptom of malignant hypertension is a headache occurring in the occipital region.

Objective

In malignant hypertension, the hallmark ophthalmoscopic finding is a swollen, hyperemic optic nerve head.

The margins of the disc are blurred and indistinct with adjacent flame hemorrhages. Cotton-wool spots and hard exudates that form a star-shaped pattern around the macula may also be present. Blood pressure is typically extremely elevated, and the patient is at risk for kidney failure.

Plan

Immediate referral to an internist or cardiologist is indicated to control the hypertension and evaluate kidney function. Many of the retinal signs clear once the blood pressure is brought under control. If persistent macular edema is present and vision loss has occurred, laser photocoagulation may be beneficial.

CENTRAL RETINAL VEIN OCCLUSION

Subjective

Central retinal vein occlusion (CRVO) is often associated with systemic or ocular diseases, including diabetes, hypertension, hyperlipidemia, autoimmune disorders, chronic lung disease, hyperviscosity syndromes, and glaucoma. Patients with a CRVO usually present complaining of a painless loss of vision that occurred over a 48-hour period. The symptoms are usually unilateral; however, if the condition is due to a blood viscosity disorder, the symptoms may be bilateral.

Objective

The typical presentation of CRVO is diffuse flame hemorrhaging in all quadrants of the retina. The hemorrhaging is particularly dense toward the posterior pole and optic nerve. The veins are dilated and tortuous due to reduced venous drainage. Associated signs include a hyperemic, swollen optic disc and cotton-wool spots.

There are classically two types of CRVO: ischemic and nonischemic. Ischemic CRVO is characterized by numerous cotton-wool spots and extensive capillary nonperfusion visible with fluorescein angiography. Visual acuity is severely reduced (acuity of 20/200 or worse), and, if the CRVO is unilateral, an afferent pupillary defect is often present. Neovascularization of the disc and iris may develop in later phases, particularly in ischemic CRVO. In nonischemic CRVO, fewer signs of ischemia (fewer cotton-wool spots) are found. Flame hemorrhages and disc edema may be minimal, and visual acuity loss is not as pronounced as in ischemic CRVO (acuity is better than 20/200).

Plan

The diagnosis of CRVO calls for an investigation to rule out underlying systemic disease. The initial workup includes fasting blood sugar level, complete blood count with differential, lipid profile, platelet count, and blood pressure assessment. In addition the patient should be evaluated for chronic open-angle glaucoma. The patient must be monitored closely for at least 3 months for the formation of neovascularization, rubeosis iridis, and subsequent neovascular glaucoma. Panretinal laser photocoagulation is helpful in reducing neovascularization and preventing secondary glaucoma. In some cases anticoagulant therapy such as administration of aspirin or warfarin has been used to help decrease the coagulation of blood and facilitate venous drainage.

SUGGESTED READING

Alexander LJ. Primary Care of the Posterior Segment (2nd ed). Norwalk, CT: Appleton & Lange, 1994.

Gurwood AS, Muchnick BG. The Optic Nerve in Clinical Practice. Boston: Butterworth–Heinemann, 1997.

Hess RF, Plant GT. Optic Neuritis. New York: Cambridge University Press, 1986.

Kritzinger EE, Beaumont HM. A Colour Atlas of Optic Disc Abnormalities. Chicago: Wolfe Medical Publications Ltd., 1987.

Spoor TC. Atlas of Optic Nerve Disorders. New York: Raven Press, 1992.

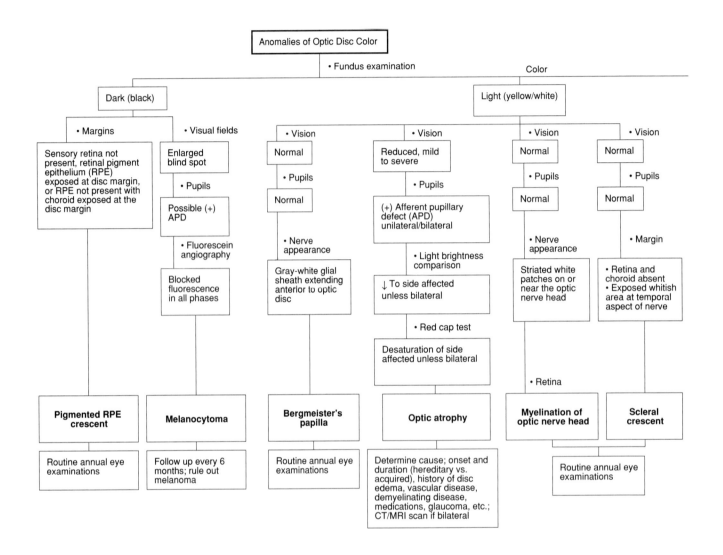

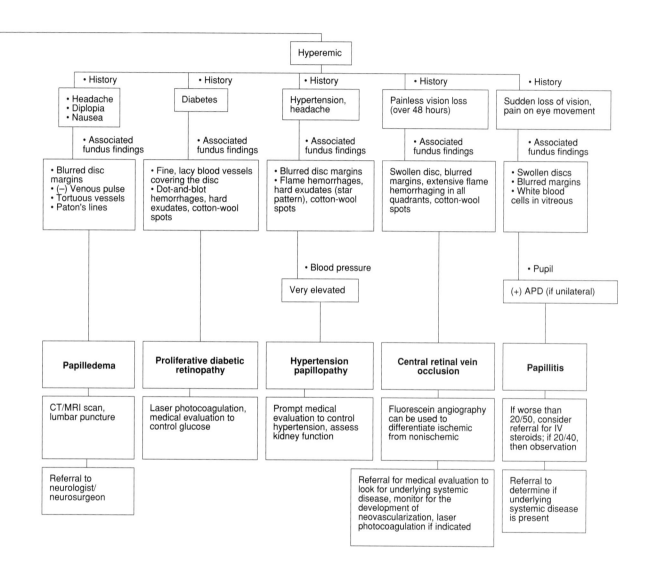

50

Anomalies of Optic Disc Contour
and Position

JOHN H. NISHIMOTO

ANOMALIES OF OPTIC DISC CONTOUR AND POSITION AT A GLANCE

Oblique insertion
Coloboma
Hypoplasia
Drusen of the optic nerve head
Optic pit
Retinopathy of prematurity
Tilted disc syndrome
Megalopapilla
Papilledema
Papillitis
Glaucoma
Optic nerve head tumors

Abnormalities of optic disc contour and position are often associated with congenital conditions, although some are a result of acquired ocular or systemic pathologies. This chapter describes conditions that cause anomalies of the profile and position of the optic nerve head.

OBLIQUE INSERTION

Subjective

Oblique insertion exists when there is an oblique insertion of the optic nerve through the scleral canal. Usually, no symptoms are associated with oblique insertion. However, there appears to be a correlation between this condition and myopia.

Objective

With oblique insertion, the disc is typically raised nasally and depressed temporally. This conformation gives the disc the appearance of a pseudopapilledema when viewed by ophthalmoscopy because the raised portion creates blurred disc margins.

Plan

There are no significant consequences to oblique insertion of the optic disc except that it may confound the differential diagnosis of true tilted discs. Routine eye and vision examinations are the normal protocol for follow-up.

COLOBOMA OF THE OPTIC NERVE HEAD

Subjective

A coloboma is caused by incomplete closure of the embryonic fissure. Patients with coloboma have varying symptoms, depending on the extent of involvement. Vision can range from normal to light perception only. There may be systemic associations, including transphenoidal encephalocele, cardiac defects, and drug-related congenital anomalies. Patients may have peripheral vision loss of which they themselves are unaware but which may be observed by close relatives and friends.

Objective

A coloboma is a depression of the retina, choroid, or optic nerve head due to an absence of tissue. Several types of optic nerve coloboma exist. A coloboma can be confined to the nerve head, can involve portions of the retina and choroid, or can involve all of these areas. Some patients also have an associated iris or lens coloboma. The site of the coloboma is usually the inferior portion of the disc or retina, which coincides with the expected final aspect of closure of the fetal fissure. Some form of unusual vessel arrangement as well as enlargement of the optic disc is present in most cases. Pigmentary anomalies usually surround the coloboma because of the stretching of the retinal tissue and subsequent reactive retinal pigment epithelial hyperplasia. Visual field changes are related to the position at the extent of the coloboma and can involve a large portion of the visual field. Glial tissue may fill the coloboma, giving an unusual appearance that is similar to that of morning-glory syndrome. Morning-glory syndrome is considered by some to be a variant presentation of optic nerve coloboma. B-scan ultrasonography can be of value in the differential diagnosis.

Plan

There is a strong association between optic nerve head coloboma and nonrhegmatogenous retinal detachment, which usually occurs early in life. This detachment is generally due to subretinal fluid leakage in the papillomacular area. Eye protection is necessary, particularly if the patient participates in contact sports. Patient education involves presenting information regarding the possible severe consequences of the condition, informing the patient of the symptoms of retinal detachment, and stressing the importance of immediate evaluation if these symptoms are noted. In most cases, routine yearly eye examinations are sufficient. The health care practitioner must also ensure that the patient has no associated neurologic anomalies such as midline defects or other systemic abnormalities. If these are suspected, referral is indicated to ensure that the systemic manifestations, such as endocrine imbalance, are properly managed.

DISC HYPOPLASIA

Subjective

In patients with disc hypoplasia, the reduction in disc size is the result of a reduction in or absence of retinal nerve fibers and an absence of corresponding ganglion cells. Visual acuity can range from normal to no light perception. Bilateral optic nerve hypoplasia may be associated with a number of systemic conditions, including anencephaly, septo-optic dysplasia, pituitary dysfunction, cerebral palsy, epilepsy, and absence of the septum pellucidum. There is also an association with maternal viral infections or the use of drugs—including alcohol, quinine, diphenylhydantoin (Dilantin), lysergic acid diethylamide, or phencyclidine—during pregnancy. Hypoplasia may occur unilaterally or bilaterally. It occurs in approximately 2 of 100,000 births, with no difference in incidence for males and females.

Objective

The nerve head is typically one-third to one-half the size of a normally developed optic nerve. The nerve head is often more pale than normal and is usually surrounded by a yellow zone. This appearance is termed the *double-ring sign*. In some cases, only a segment of the disc is involved. There is a visual field defect corresponding to the affected area. Another useful test is measurement of the disc-macula to disc-disc ratio. A normal disc-macula to disc-disc ratio is from 2 to 1, to 3 to 2; values greater than 3 to 2 are suggestive of congenital optic nerve hypoplasia.

Other ocular findings may include slow pupillary reaction to bright light, positive afferent pupillary defect in cases of unilateral hypoplastic strabismus, nystagmus, or persistent hyperplastic primary vitreous. Visual field defects vary considerably, depending on the location and extent of the hypoplasia. Particularly when the disc hypoplasia is bilateral, diagnostic imaging and neurologic and endocrine evaluations are indicated if associated systemic anomalies are suspected.

Plan

Congenital optic nerve hypoplasia is a benign, nonprogressive condition that requires no ocular management. The only concern is management of the associated systemic conditions mentioned above, if indicated.

DRUSEN OF THE OPTIC NERVE HEAD

Subjective

Optic nerve drusen are hyaline bodies found in the optic disc. They occur in approximately 1% of the general population and are found more commonly in whites than in other population groups. The clinician may be able to elicit a family history of optic nerve head drusen, since this condition is inherited in an autosomal dominant pattern with incomplete penetrance. In most cases, patients with optic nerve head drusen are asymptomatic unless visual fields are significantly compromised. On rare occasions, disc drusen may have associated symptoms, including migraine headaches, seizures, and other neurologic disorders.

Objective

Optic nerve head drusen present bilaterally in approximately 70% of cases. In childhood, the drusen appear as pseudopapilledema with no physiologic cupping. In the adolescent or early adult years, the discs become yellowed and the round, refractile drusen erupt to the surface and become more visible. The disc margins often have an indistinct or lumpy appearance. These refractile bodies autofluoresce (glow), especially when illuminated with a red-free light. Ultrasonography is very helpful in detecting disc drusen, which have high reflectivity even on low gain settings. Computed tomographic scans also reveal disc drusen in some cases. Optic nerve head drusen occasionally can cause visual field defects and circumpapillary hemorrhages. The field defects can have a variety of manifestations; arcuate, sectorial, and altitudinal scotomas are the most common.

Plan

Although many patients remain asymptomatic, buried drusen of the optic nerve head can be visually devastating in some cases. Vision loss can be secondary to progressive nerve fiber damage, choroidal neovascular membranes, and hemorrhages. No therapy is currently available to prevent either the associated nerve fiber layer loss or hemorrhages.

OPTIC PIT

Subjective

Optic pits are congenital malformations of the optic disc and are thought by some to be a variant form of coloboma. Most patients with optic pits are asymptomatic, but some may complain of metamorphopsia due to serous maculopathy, or of vision loss due to serous retinal detachment.

Objective

Optic pits appear as a focal discolored area within the optic nerve head. They are most commonly located in the inferior temporal quadrant but may occur anywhere on the disc. Centrally located pits may be mistaken for glaucomatous cupping. This picture is further complicated by the fact that many optic pits have an associated arcuate scotoma. Other findings associated with optic pits include enlarged disc, circumpapillary atrophy, cilioretinal artery, serous maculopathy, and serous retinal detachment. Fluorescein angiography is useful in demonstrating the hypofluorescence of the pit and in detecting any serous leakage.

Plan

The management of optic pits consists of regular examination of the patient, home monitoring with an Amsler grid, and education of the patient regarding the symptoms of serous detachment. In addition, protective eyewear should be prescribed. If serous detachment does occur, laser photocoagulation may be of value.

RETINOPATHY OF PREMATURITY (DRAGGED DISC)

Subjective

The patient with retinopathy of prematurity (ROP) typically has a history of premature birth (less than 36 weeks' gestation), low birth weight (under 4 lb 6 oz), and supplemental oxygen therapy. The manifestations of ROP depend on the stage of the condition. Vision loss can be due to tractional displacement of the macula, strabismus, or retinal detachment.

Objective

The clinical manifestations of ROP occur in three stages: primary vaso-obliteration, secondary fibrovascular proliferation, and tertiary scarring. Changes are classified according to location, extent, and severity. In the early phases, there is a demarcation line between the vascular and avascular peripheral retina that develops into a ridge. Later, in the proliferative stage, peripheral fibrovascular bands can cause traction on the retina, which results in macular heterotopia (dragged disc) and retinal detachment. In the advanced cicatricial stage, the detached retina may form a white retrolental mass. It is important to note that, in many patients, ROP does not progress to the more advanced stages.

Plan

Because ROP can progress to blindness during the first 3 months of life and because treatment such as cryopexy and laser photocoagulation has been proved effective in controlling the condition, for very low-birth-weight infants (i.e., less than or equal to 1,500 g), a dilated fundus examination should be performed between 4 and 6 weeks' chronologic age or between 31 and 33 weeks' postconception age. Follow-up examinations depend on the initial examination. According to the International Classification of Retinopathy of Prematurity, follow-up examinations should be planned at approximately 2- to 4-week intervals until evidence is found of normal vascularization of the retina. Other patients at risk for retinal damage (i.e., retinal detachment and tears) from ROP should be evaluated at 3 months of age at a minimum and then regularly thereafter (approximately every 6–12 months).

TILTED DISC SYNDROME

Subjective

Tilted disc syndrome is a congenital anomaly in which the vertical axis of the disc is tilted away from the normal 90-degree orientation. Patients with tilted disc syndrome are usually asymptomatic. In some cases, however, there is a bilateral temporal visual field loss that resembles a chiasmal neurologic defect except that it crosses the vertical midline.

Objective

Tilted disc syndrome can be unilateral or bilateral. In addition to the obliquely oriented disc, other signs include crescents, nasal staphyloma, and situs inversus vessel pattern. Perimetry is useful in determining whether a field defect accompanies the tilted disc.

Plan

Tilted disc syndrome is a nonprogressive condition and should merely be noted during routine examination.

MEGALOPAPILLA

Subjective

Megalopapilla is a congenital, nonprogressive unilateral enlargement of the optic nerve head. Patients with megalopapilla are usually asymptomatic and have normal visual acuity.

Objective

On ophthalmoscopy, the optic nerve appears to be very large and may be almost twice the normal size. Otherwise, the optic nerve characteristics (margins, cup-to-disc ratio, rim tissue) appear normal. It should be noted that, although the cup-to-disc ratio is normal, the cup is larger than in the fellow eye, and this enlargement may be mistaken for glaucomatous enlargement. The visual field shows an enlarged blind spot.

An enlarged optic nerve may be found in isolation or in association with other congenital ocular anomalies such as coloboma, optic pit, morning-glory syndrome, or optic nerve head drusen. It can also be associated with systemic congenital anomalies such as sphenoethmoidal encephalocele and cleft palate. Radiologic imaging is helpful in determining the presence of these abnormalities.

Plan

Since vision is usually normal and the optic nerve head enlargement is nonprogressive, no treatment is necessary. A referral to rule out other congenital anomalies should be considered.

SUGGESTED READING

Acers TE. Congenital Abnormalities of the Optic Nerve and Related Forebrain. Philadelphia: Lea & Febiger, 1983.

Alexander LJ. Primary Care of the Posterior Segment (2nd ed). Norwalk, CT: Appleton & Lange, 1994.

American Academy of Pediatrics. Screening examination of premature infants for retinopathy of prematurity. Pediatrics 1997;100:273.

Gurwood AS, Muchnick BG. The Optic Nerve in Clinical Practice. Boston: Butterworth–Heinemann, 1997.

Kothe AC. Optic nerve pits. Clinical Eye Vision Care 1993;5(3): 101–103.

Kritzinger EE, Beaumont HM. A Colour Atlas of Optic Disc Abnormalities. Chicago: Wolfe Medical Publications Ltd., 1987.

Ryan SJ. Retina. Vol. 2. St. Louis: Mosby, 1994.

Van Dalen JT. Congenital Anomalies of the Eye. 1. Optic Nerve Coloboma, Optic Nerve Hypoplasia, Morning Glory Syndrome. Amersfoort, the Netherlands: Holland Ophthalmic Publishing, 1983.

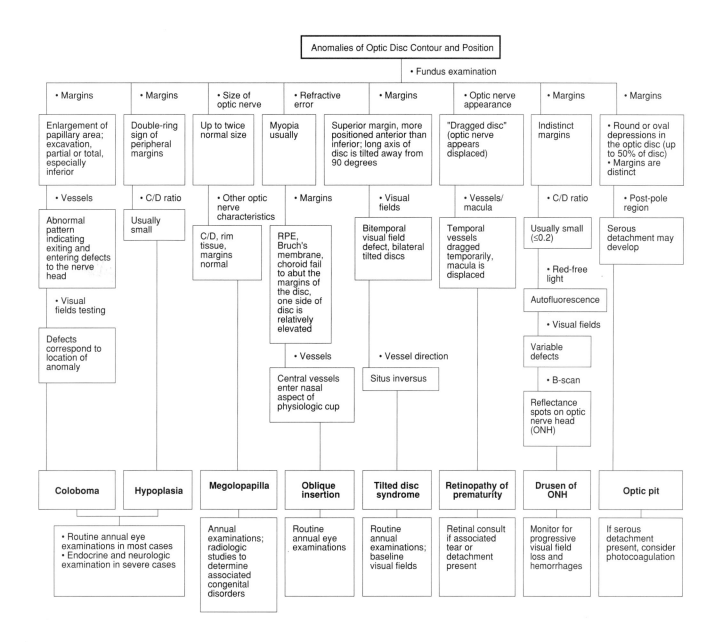

Anomalies of Optic Disc Contour and Position

• Fundus examination

• Margins	• Margins	• Size of optic nerve	• Refractive error	• Margins	• Optic nerve appearance	• Margins	• Margins
Enlargement of papillary area; excavation, partial or total, especially inferior	Double-ring sign of peripheral margins	Up to twice normal size	Myopia usually	Superior margin, more positioned anterior than inferior; long axis of disc is tilted away from 90 degrees	"Dragged disc" (optic nerve appears displaced)	Indistinct margins	• Round or oval depressions in the optic disc (up to 50% of disc) • Margins are distinct

• Vessels | • C/D ratio | • Other optic nerve characteristics | • Margins | • Visual fields | • Vessels/ macula | • C/D ratio | • Post-pole region

Abnormal pattern indicating exiting and entering defects to the nerve head | Usually small | C/D, rim tissue, margins normal | RPE, Bruch's membrane, choroid fail to abut the margins of the disc, one side of disc is relatively elevated | Bitemporal visual field defect, bilateral tilted discs | Temporal vessels dragged temporarily, macula is displaced | Usually small (≤0.2) | Serous detachment may develop

• Visual fields testing

Defects correspond to location of anomaly

• Red-free light

Autofluorescence

• Visual fields

Variable defects

• Vessels | • Vessel direction

Central vessels enter nasal aspect of physiologic cup | Situs inversus

• B-scan

Reflectance spots on optic nerve head (ONH)

Coloboma	**Hypoplasia**	**Megolopapilla**	**Oblique insertion**	**Tilted disc syndrome**	**Retinopathy of prematurity**	**Drusen of ONH**	**Optic pit**
	• Routine annual eye examinations in most cases • Endocrine and neurologic examination in severe cases	Annual examinations; radiologic studies to determine associated congenital disorders	Routine annual eye examinations	Routine annual examinations; baseline visual fields	Retinal consult if associated tear or detachment present	Monitor for progressive visual field loss and hemorrhages	If serous detachment present, consider photocoagulation

51

Vascular Anomalies of the Disc

JOHN H. NISHIMOTO

VASCULAR ANOMALIES OF THE DISC AT A GLANCE

Anterior ischemic optic neuropathy (nonarteritic)
Anterior ischemic optic neuropathy (arteritic)
Optic neuritis from demyelinating disease
Optic neuritis from viral infection
Neuroretinitis
Retrobulbar optic neuritis
Prepapillary vascular loops
Neovascularization of the disc
Optociliary shunt vessels
Hemangioma
Central retinal vein occlusion
Low-tension glaucoma
Optic nerve head drusen

The optic nerve head contains substantial microcirculation and is therefore prone to pathologies caused by inflammation and vascular occlusion. This chapter discusses some of the conditions that cause vascular anomalies of the optic nerve head.

ANTERIOR ISCHEMIC OPTIC NEUROPATHY (NONARTERITIC)

Subjective

Nonarteritic anterior ischemic optic neuropathy (AION) usually occurs in patients over 50 years of age. Men are affected more frequently than women. The patient may have a history of diabetes or hypertension. Patients with this condition may complain of transient blurring, flashing, or flickering of vision, as well as areas of visual field loss similar to the amaurosis found in carotid artery disease. With the onset of attack, vision is decreased, and visual field loss may occur over a period of 24 hours to 4 weeks without remission. The patient often notices a sudden decrease in vision on awakening. Orbital pain that is not associated with eye movement may be present.

Objective

The condition begins unilaterally and may become bilateral over time. The optic disc changes can be variable, ranging from isolated sectorial optic disc edema to full-blown disc swelling. The amount of loss of acuity and peripheral visual field is correlated with the degree of disc involvement. Small peripapillary flame-shaped hemorrhages appear initially then disappear in 3–5 weeks. Eventually, the acute manifestations subside, and optic atrophy appears in about 3 months. A positive afferent pupillary defect is often present, as are other indications of optic nerve conduction defects. The classic visual field defect is an altitudinal loss, but other defect patterns are possible. Visual acuity stabilizes at 20/60 or better in approximately half of the cases of nonarteritic AION and at worse than 20/200 in the rest.

Plan

The current prevailing view is that no therapeutic intervention is of any benefit in the treatment of nonarteritic AION; however, some clinicians believe steroid therapy may be beneficial. It has been postulated that the steroid decreases capillary permeability in the optic nerve, thereby reducing swelling and improving circulation. In most cases of nonarteritic AION, identifying and managing the underlying systemic disease is the primary management goal.

A Westergren erythrocyte sedimentation rate (ESR) should be ordered to rule out arteritic AION. Other useful tests include blood pressure assessment, carotid auscultation, duplex ultrasonography, fasting blood glucose level, complete blood count (CBC) with differential and platelets, and serum protein electrophoresis. A follow-up visit should be scheduled in 1 month if the condition is acute or to assure that there is no associated neurologic disease.

ANTERIOR ISCHEMIC OPTIC NEUROPATHY (ARTERITIC)

Subjective

Arteritic ION is an autoimmune disorder usually affecting patients over the age of 60 years. Females are more often affected than males. Temporal arteritis (giant cell arteritis) causes inflammation of the elastic tissue on the media and adventitia of the arterial walls, which leads to occlusion. Prodromal symptoms such as transient vision loss and flashing or flickering vision occur in approximately 75% of patients with arteritic AION about 1–2 weeks before the acute attack. Systemic symptoms of temporal arteritis include headache, scalp tenderness, palpable temporal artery, weight loss, suboccipital neck pain, malaise, muscle and joint pain, and jaw ache (claudication) associated with chewing. During the attack of arteritic AION, there is acute vision loss that may range from an acuity of 20/60 to no light perception. The second eye frequently becomes involved shortly after the first one.

Objective

Fundus examination usually reveals one of two types of presentation, each occurring about half of the time. In the first presentation, the optic disc has a chalky white color with a surrounding circumpapillary "white" zone. Hemorrhages are usually absent in this type. In the other type, the disc appears edematous and pink but slightly pale. Over time, the edema encroaches on the circumpapillary area, and associated flame-shaped hemorrhages appear. Optic atrophy eventually develops secondary to the infarct. The second eye may become involved within 1 week if the condition is not treated promptly.

Physical diagnosis includes palpation to determine if a hard, nonpulsating, tender temporal artery is present. Other signs useful in the differential diagnosis include an altitudinal or central visual field defect, central retinal vein occlusion, and cranial nerve palsy. If arteritic AION

is suspected, a Westergren ESR should be ordered immediately. Although the normal range for ESRs varies in elderly patients, any patient with a Westergren ESR above 40 mm per hour should be considered to have giant cell arteritis until proven otherwise. Normal values for Westergren ESR are age/2 for males and (age + 10)/2 for females. A temporal artery biopsy should be performed to aid diagnosis in equivocal cases or to confirm the diagnosis of arteritic AION. The biopsy should be performed within 1 week after therapy is initiated.

Plan

Visual acuity rarely improves with arteritic AION. Systemic steroids should be given as soon as AION is suspected to prevent involvement of the contralateral eye. The steroids act to decrease arterial inflammation. In some cases, despite the use of steroid therapy, loss of vision can occur in the second eye.

OPTIC NEURITIS FROM DEMYELINATING DISEASE

Subjective

Demyelination is the most frequent cause of optic neuropathy. Multiple sclerosis is the most frequent cause of demyelination. Usually patients with this condition are 18–45 years of age. Patients with demyelinating optic neuropathy often present with suddenly decreased vision or blurred vision that is exacerbated with physical exertion or increase in body temperature (Uhthoff symptom). They also may complain of pain or tenderness of the globe near the insertion of the superior rectus, especially with gross eye movements. The patient should be questioned about other signs of demyelinating disease, including tingling of the extremities, motor weakness, mobility, problems in balance or gait, and difficulty in urination.

Objective

Visual acuities associated with optic neuritis range from 20/20 to no light perception. Other findings include a positive afferent pupillary defect, color desaturation, variation in light-brightness comparison, abnormal Pulfrich stereo phenomenon, and increased response latency in the visual evoked potential. Visual field defects associated with demyelinating optic neuropathy vary considerably. The majority of defects are cecocentral, but they can be peripheral or generalized depressions. The ophthalmoscopic appearance can also be quite variable. Often there are no noticeable ophthalmoscopic nerve head changes, but optic disc edema secondary to axoplasmic stasis may occur. After the acute process runs its course, some degree of optic atrophy appears.

With demyelinating optic neuritis, the prognosis for regaining visual function is generally good. Visual acuity and visual fields usually begin to improve within 2–3 weeks of the attack and stabilize in 4–5 weeks. However, a washing out or desaturation of perceived colors often remains. Recurrences can occur in up to 20–30% of cases, causing further reduction in acuity, an increase in visual field defects, and further optic atrophy.

Certain tests are helpful in the diagnosis of demyelinating optic neuropathy. Magnetic resonance imaging (MRI) has been proven to be an excellent tool for revealing plaques of demyelination. Up to 80–90% of patients with demyelinating optic neuropathy show plaque formation. A spinal tap with analysis of cerebrospinal fluid can provide additional diagnostic information. Any patient suspected of having demyelinating optic neuropathy should have a neurologic consultation.

Plan

The use of systemic steroids to treat optic neuritis has been controversial. The results of the optic neuritis treatment trial suggest that the initial treatment of choice is intravenous corticosteroids followed by oral prednisone.

OPTIC NEURITIS FROM INFLAMMATORY DISEASE

Subjective

Optic neuritis can be caused by a number of infectious diseases, including herpes simplex, herpes zoster, toxoplasmosis, tuberculosis, syphilis, Behçet's disease, and Reiter's disease. Children and young adults (<20 years) are most susceptible to inflammatory optic neuritis. Symptoms are similar to those of other optic neuropathies and include sudden decrease in vision, pain on eye movement, and color desaturation. In inflammatory optic neuritis the vision reduces rapidly over a course of 2–3 days then stabilizes over the next 7–10 days. A period of gradual improvement follows.

Objective

The changes in inflammatory optic neuritis visible with ophthalmoscopy include optic disc edema, often with accompanying hemorrhage; vitreitis; and circumpapillary choroiditis. In children the neuroretinopathy associated with viral infections is characterized by retinal edema and exudates scattered throughout the papillomacular bundle in a stellate pattern. This type of papillitis may resolve spontaneously. Neuroretinitis involving the ganglion cells is characterized by a yellow, swollen disc with edema that obscures the vessels. Flame hemorrhages may appear adjacent to the disc. In addition, posterior vitreous cells are often present. This form usually results in gliosis, perivascular sheathing, and optic atrophy. Optic atrophy usually occurs 4–8 weeks after the inflammation starts. Poor acuity, red desaturation, and a positive afferent pupillary defect are usually present.

Differential diagnosis includes evaluation for ischemic optic neuropathy, diabetic optic neuropathy, papillophlebitis, malignant hypertension, papilledema from intracranial tumor, pseudotumor cerebri, and toxic optic neuropathy. Diagnostic tests include blood pressure assessment, careful threshold visual field examination, CBC, ESR, fluorescent treponemal antibody absorption test for syphilis, collagen vascular screening including antinuclear antibody test, chest radiography, and computed tomography or MRI.

Plan

Diagnosis of the underlying causative agent or condition is crucial in order to determine the proper therapeutic intervention. The sooner the inflammation is resolved, the better the prognosis for return of visual function. If management of the underlying condition is not sufficient to reduce the inflammation, steroid therapy can be initiated. Steroid therapy must be monitored closely due to the potential side effects of treatment.

RETROBULBAR NEUROPATHY

Subjective

Demyelination is the most frequent cause of retrobulbar optic neuropathy. Multiple sclerosis is the most frequent cause of demyelination. Other causes include syphilis, Guillain-Barré syndrome, carbon monoxide poisoning, optic nerve or orbital tumor, Leber's optic neuropathy, and toxic metabolic factors. The patient with retrobulbar optic neuropathy typically presents with a sudden unilateral loss of vision. The patient may also mention pain and tenderness of the globe near the insertion of the superior rectus. The clinician should question the patient with suspected retrobulbar optic neuropathy about any other symptoms of neurologic disease.

Objective

Retrobulbar optic neuropathy is classically described as a case in which "the patient sees nothing and the doctor sees nothing." Very often no appreciable nerve head changes are visible with ophthalmoscopy, but optic disc edema secondary to axoplasmic stasis may occur. After the acute process runs its course, optic atrophy appears. Patients may present with a visual acuity ranging from 20/20 to severe vision loss, or with visual field defects. Other signs are similar to those described in the section above on optic neuritis from demyelinating disease. Multiple sclerosis is a major cause of the condition and must be ruled out. MRI is the definitive test for detecting demyelinating plaques in the central nervous system.

Plan

Systemic steroids have been used to treat retrobulbar optic neuropathy, but their use is controversial. The results of the optic neuritis treatment trial suggest that the initial treatment of choice is intravenous corticosteroids followed by oral prednisone.

NEOVASCULARIZATION OF THE DISC

Subjective

Neovascularization of the disc is most commonly associated with proliferative diabetic retinopathy or retinal vein occlusion. The new vessels do not cause symptoms, but associated manifestations of retinal vascular disease—including edema, exudation, and hemorrhage of the retina or vitreous—can cause vision loss.

Objective

Neovascularization of the disc is characterized by the presence of a fine network of abnormal blood vessels that can be seen on the optic disc. Other signs of retinal vascular disease include dot-and-blot or flame hemorrhages, exudates, cotton-wool spots, microaneurysms, venous caliber changes, and intraretinal microvascular abnormalities. In addition to neovascularization of the disc, other signs associated with proliferative retinopathy include neovascularization elsewhere (>1 disc diameter away from the optic disc), fibrovascular vitreoretinal membranes, vitreous hemorrhage, and rubeosis iridis.

Plan

If the neovascularization involves at least one-third of the disc, prompt referral for laser photocoagulation is nec-essary, since the patient is at high risk for severe vision loss. Panretinal photocoagulation can decrease the demand for oxygen in the retina and promote regression of the abnormal vessels.

OPTOCILIARY SHUNT VESSELS

Subjective

Optociliary shunt vessels are typically associated with an occlusion that is located in the vicinity of the optic nerve. Other causes include compressive optic nerve tumor and primary open-angle glaucoma. Symptoms are related to the underlying condition. Vision may be reduced during the acute phase of the disease, but often improves with the development of the shunt vessels.

Objective

Optociliary shunt vessels have a dilated, tortuous appearance. There may be hooked or looped vessels that seem to extend from the optic nerve or adjacent retina into the vitreous. They usually connect the arterial and venous circulations, but occasionally involve the choroidal circulation. There may be an associated "ghost vessel" due to a prior occlusion. Other residual signs of occlusive venous disease, such as hemorrhages, exudates, and cotton-wool spots, may also be present.

Plan

Since optociliary shunt vessels are secondary to other ocular or systemic diseases, an evaluation for the underlying cause is indicated. Tonometry and visual field testing aid in the diagnosis of primary open-angle glaucoma. A vascular workup is indicated if the condition appears to be occlusive in origin. If the fundus appears otherwise unremarkable, and yet there is formation of a short vessel, a disease process outside the globe, such as optic nerve glioma or meningioma, must be ruled out with MRI.

PREPAPILLARY VASCULAR LOOPS

Subjective

Prepapillary vascular loops are a unilateral congenital vessel anomaly. Patients with prepapillary vascular loops are usually asymptomatic but may experience amaurosis fugax if the blood flow is disrupted due to elevated intraocular pressure or carotid artery disease. Symptoms are more commonly associated with arterial loops than with venous loops.

Objective

Prepapillary vascular loops appear to protrude into the vitreous. The loops extend from the optic disc and link two branches of the central retinal vessels. Arterial loops usually affect the inferior central retinal vessels, while venous loops usually affect the superior retinal vessels. The loops may be short and have twists resembling a corkscrew. Many loops are surrounded by a white sheath that represents remnants of Bergmeister's papilla, although some are unsupported and float freely in the vitreous.

Plan

No treatment is necessary for prepapillary vascular loops. It is important, however, to differentiate this condition from more serious conditions that have a similar appearance, such as optociliary vessels and neovascularization of the disc.

SUGGESTED READING

Alexander LJ. Primary Care of the Posterior Segment (2nd ed). Norwalk, CT: Appleton & Lange, 1994.

Gurwood AS, Muchnick BG. The Optic Nerve in Clinical Practice. Boston: Butterworth–Heinemann, 1997.

Harkins T. Treating multiple sclerosis. Clinical Eye Vision Care 1994;6(3):133–136.

Haskes C, Haskes LP. Acquired optociliary shunt vessels and their natural occurrences. Clinical Eye Vision Care 1995;7:69–77.

Kritzinger EE, Beaumont HM. A Colour Atlas of Optic Disc Abnormalities. Chicago: Wolfe Medical Publications Ltd., 1987.

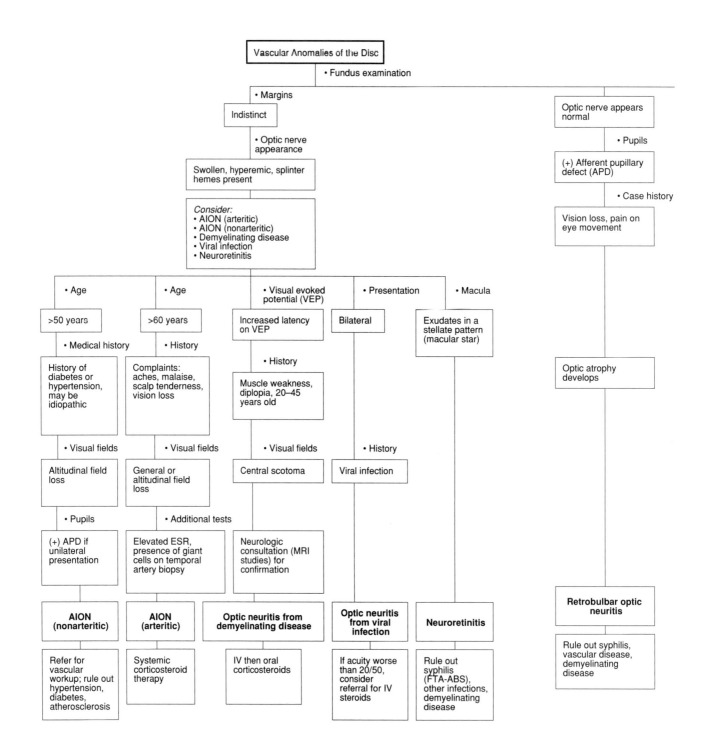

Vascular Anomalies of the Disc
• Fundus examination

• Margins

Indistinct

Optic nerve appears normal

• Optic nerve appearance

• Pupils

Swollen, hyperemic, splinter hemes present

(+) Afferent pupillary defect (APD)

Consider:
• AION (arteritic)
• AION (nonarteritic)
• Demyelinating disease
• Viral infection
• Neuroretinitis

• Case history

Vision loss, pain on eye movement

• Age | • Age | • Visual evoked potential (VEP) | • Presentation | • Macula

>50 years | >60 years | Increased latency on VEP | Bilateral | Exudates in a stellate pattern (macular star)

• Medical history | • History | | |

History of diabetes or hypertension, may be idiopathic | Complaints: aches, malaise, scalp tenderness, vision loss | • History | |

Muscle weakness, diplopia, 20–45 years old

Optic atrophy develops

• Visual fields | • Visual fields | • Visual fields | • History |

Altitudinal field loss | General or altitudinal field loss | Central scotoma | Viral infection |

• Pupils | • Additional tests | |

(+) APD if unilateral presentation | Elevated ESR, presence of giant cells on temporal artery biopsy | Neurologic consultation (MRI studies) for confirmation |

AION (nonarteritic) | **AION (arteritic)** | **Optic neuritis from demyelinating disease** | **Optic neuritis from viral infection** | **Neuroretinitis**

Retrobulbar optic neuritis

Refer for vascular workup; rule out hypertension, diabetes, atherosclerosis | Systemic corticosteroid therapy | IV then oral corticosteroids | If acuity worse than 20/50, consider referral for IV steroids | Rule out syphilis (FTA-ABS), other infections, demyelinating disease

Rule out syphilis, vascular disease, demyelinating disease

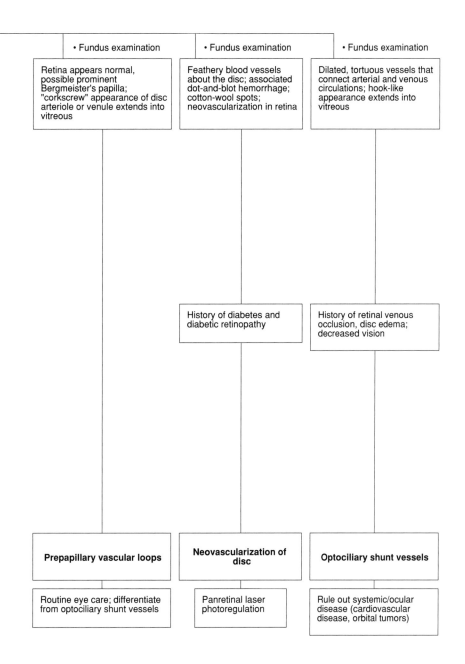

• Fundus examination

Retina appears normal, possible prominent Bergmeister's papilla; "corkscrew" appearance of disc arteriole or venule extends into vitreous

Prepapillary vascular loops

Routine eye care; differentiate from optociliary shunt vessels

• Fundus examination

Feathery blood vessels about the disc; associated dot-and-blot hemorrhage; cotton-wool spots; neovascularization in retina

History of diabetes and diabetic retinopathy

Neovascularization of disc

Panretinal laser photoregulation

• Fundus examination

Dilated, tortuous vessels that connect arterial and venous circulations; hook-like appearance extends into vitreous

History of retinal venous occlusion, disc edema; decreased vision

Optociliary shunt vessels

Rule out systemic/ocular disease (cardiovascular disease, orbital tumors)

52

Anomalies of Globe Size

David P. Sendrowski

ANOMALIES OF GLOBE SIZE AT A GLANCE

Microphthalmos
  Cytomegalovirus infection
  Congenital rubella syndrome
  Congenital toxoplasmosis
  Idiopathic
  Rieger's syndrome
  Patau's syndrome
  Nanophthalmos
  Norrie's disease
  Simple microphthalmos
  Klinefelter's syndrome
  Facial cleft syndrome
Macrophthalmos
  Congenital glaucoma
  Hurler's syndrome
  Neurofibromatosis
  Rieger's syndrome
  Sturge-Weber syndrome
  Hereditary, autosomal recessive
  Pathologic myopia

The position of the globes relative to the orbital rims shows considerable individual and racial variation. Subtle degrees of proptosis are difficult to detect and even more difficult to measure. Some techniques that are useful in determining the presence of relative unilateral proptosis include viewing the position of the globes and lids from above the brows, inserting the fingertips between the inferior orbital rim and globe, and simultaneously palpating the corneal apices through the closed lids.

After taking a history and conducting a thorough orbital examination, the clinician should be able to make at least a tentative diagnosis, even before special diagnostic studies are performed.

NANOPHTHALMOS

Subjective

Nanophthalmos is a rare form of congenital microphthalmos. The condition represents an arrested development of the globe in all directions after the embryonic tissue has closed. The eye is small in its overall dimensions but has no other gross developmental defects. The microphthalmos is not accompanied by other systemic congenital anomalies.

The condition is often bilateral. In unilateral cases, the ipsilateral side of the face or the body is occasionally poorly developed. The majority of cases are sporadic, but there is a strong hereditary factor with both recessive and dominant pedigrees being reported. The incidence of nanophthalmos does not vary by sex or race.

Objective

The condition features severe hyperopia (usually > 10 D), short total axial length, microcornea, marked iris convexity, and a shallow anterior chamber. The shallow anterior chamber combined with a normal lens size predisposes the patient to angle-closure glaucoma in the fourth to sixth decades of life. The sclera is inelastic and thickened, becomes more sclerosed with age, and reduces venous outflow near the vortex veins.

Chronic primary closed-angle glaucoma occurs in middle-aged patients with nanophthalmos. Gonioscopy shows varying degrees of angle closure. Peripheral anterior synechiae may also be present.

A dilated fundus examination may reveal macular hypoplasia in some patients, which results in subnormal vision. In early life, however, most patients have good correctable visual acuity.

Plan

Surgical intervention to treat cataracts and glaucoma usually has very poor results in these cases. Surgery may cause sudden decompression of the globe, worsening the degree of uveal effusion and causing nonrhegmatogenous retinal detachments.

Glaucoma is better controlled with noninvasive laser procedures, such as laser iridotomy and gonioplasty. Early initiation of laser therapy, before peripheral anterior synechiae have formed, is recommended if filtration surgery is to be avoided.

If uveal effusion occurs spontaneously, sclerectomy can be performed to relieve the effusion and prevent other complications, such as intraocular hemorrhage, exudative retinal detachment, and malignant glaucoma.

CONGENITAL RUBELLA SYNDROME

Subjective

Rubella can occur at any time during pregnancy, but the risk for congenital infection declines with increasing gestational age. Congenital rubella should be considered in any child with characteristic eye findings and a known history of maternal exposure, or in infants with significantly low birth weight. Damage to the fetus from prenatally acquired disease can be devastating. Manifestations include mental retardation, deafness, heart disease, and blindness.

Objective

Visual acuity is affected by the formation of nuclear cataracts with a surrounding zone of clear cortex. Gradual progression of the cataract causes the lens to become pearly white. Microphthalmos is closely associated with the presence of the cataract in this syndrome.

The intraocular pressure may be elevated from congenital or infantile glaucoma. A hypermature cataract may cause elevated pressure by producing a condition of relative pupillary block or a phacoanaphylactic inflammation in reaction to lens proteins in the anterior chamber.

The corneas can be hazy without increased intraocular pressure due to a keratitis or to an endothelial dysfunction. Another form of corneal haze is caused by elevated intraocular pressure accompanied by breaks in Descemet's membrane.

Salt-and-pepper retinopathy may be accompanied by the loss of the foveal reflex. The retinopathy alone generally does not interfere significantly with the visual potential of the child. Electrodiagnostic testing may show minimal changes from normal.

Congenital heart disease and neurosensory deafness are also present in congenital rubella syndrome.

Viral cultures for rubella can be performed from conjunctival scrapings, cerebrospinal fluid, urine, or nasopharyngeal samples. Elevated IgM or persistently elevated serum IgG titers for rubella also aid in the diagnosis of the syndrome.

Plan

Ocular care is directed at managing the cataracts and glaucoma. Cataracts, especially when bilateral, should be surgically removed in the first few months of life.

The glaucoma may be treated initially with a topical beta blocker (e.g., timolol) or a topical or oral carbonic anhydrase inhibitor (e.g., dorzolamide hydrochloride or acetazolamide) to bring the pressure under control. A surgical or laser goniotomy or trabeculotomy is very effective for treating the glaucoma.

Comanagement with a pediatric ophthalmologist, pediatrician, and optometrist is very important in these cases.

PATAU'S SYNDROME (TRISOMY 13)

Subjective

Patau's syndrome is present at birth. Most infants with this disorder have normal birth weights but are hypotonic. The life expectancy is only a few months, and therefore ocular intervention is minimal. The incidence of this syndrome increases with maternal age.

Objective

About half the infants born with Patau's syndrome have a cleft lip or palate. These infants have a sloping forehead and bulbous nose. Other systemic findings include polycystic renal cortices, hyperconvex nails, muscular and skeletal abnormalities, cutaneous scalp defects, and microcephaly.

Ocular findings include coloboma, microphthalmos, cyclopia, cataracts, corneal opacities, glaucoma, persistent hyperplastic primary vitreous, and retinal dysplasia.

Plan

There is no treatment for this condition. Life-threatening abnormalities, including cardiovascular and central nervous system malformations, cause perinatal death. Almost all victims die by age 3.

PHTHISIS BULBI

Subjective

Microphthalmos from multiple surgeries, chronic inflammatory disease, or end-stage intraocular disease is termed *phthisis bulbi.* The patient should be questioned about ocular surgeries, prolonged inflammation of the eye, severe ocular trauma, and congenital disorders. The patient's current and past medications should also be reviewed. Symptoms include significantly reduced vision and ocular pain.

Objective

The globe should be inspected for signs of old traumatic injury and sites of surgical incision. If the globe is in the end stages of glaucoma or intraocular inflammatory disease, the intraocular pressure is usually decreased.

Visual acuity is dramatically decreased from macular or optic nerve head involvement. There may be evidence of corneal damage or haze from glaucoma, and the anterior chamber may show signs of old inflammatory disease such as posterior synechiae or keratic precipitates.

Posterior segment involvement is common, and dilation should be performed to view the optic nerve and retina. Exudative retinal detachments, retinal hemorrhaging, and condensed vitreous all may be present from old inflammatory disease. The optic nerve may be cupped out from end-stage glaucoma. Ultimately, fibrous tissue replaces most of the ocular contents, and Bowman's membrane, the lens, retina, and choroid show increased calcification.

Plan

No cure exists for phthisis bulbi. Any ongoing intraocular inflammatory disease should be treated. If the patient has end-stage glaucoma and some visual field remains intact, low vision consultation may be warranted.

If the patient develops pain, a retrobulbar alcohol block may provide relief. Enucleation should also be considered, especially if the eye has no usable vision.

CONGENITAL GLAUCOMA AND PRIMARY INFANTILE GLAUCOMA

Subjective

The terms *congenital glaucoma* and *primary infantile glaucoma* are used synonymously to describe glaucoma that appears soon after birth. The typical infant with congenital glaucoma presents with epiphora, photophobia, and some degree of blepharospasm. However, many symptoms produced by pediatric glaucoma vary in accordance with the age at which the glaucoma develops. The later the onset of the glaucoma, the fewer structural anomalies there are, and the more likely that the glaucoma will respond to therapy.

Parents should be questioned regarding a history of glaucoma in the family, congenital disorders, term of the pregnancy, patient's birth weight, and any abnormalities that were noted after birth.

Objective

The infant should be evaluated for megalocornea, corneal edema, conjunctival injection, optic nerve cupping, and buphthalmos (ocular enlargement). The sclera in an infant is less rigid and more elastic, allowing distention of the globe.

Corneal enlargement (megalocornea) is tolerated well by the epithelium and stroma, but not by the endothelium and Descemet's membrane. Acute breaks in Descemet's membrane can occur. Corneal edema is common in infants with glaucoma in the first months of life, and usually accounts for the symptoms of photophobia and epiphora.

The optic nerve head should be evaluated for cupping changes, since formalized visual field testing cannot be performed. Optic nerve head cupping usually progresses most rapidly in the first few weeks of life. Intraocular pressure can be taken with a hand-held applanation tonometer (e.g., Tono-Pen) or pneumotonometer. Evaluation of the nerve head is difficult; if corneal edema is present, it can be almost impossible. The optic nerve is better evaluated under anesthesia, particularly when corneal edema is present. Intraocular pressure should be measured while the infant is under mild sedation to get a more accurate reading.

Axial myopia induced by buphthalmos is common in congenital glaucoma. Amblyopia secondary to the axial myopia is a common cause of poor vision in infants with the disease. Thus, retinoscopy to assess refractive error should be part of the ocular examination performed while the child is under anesthesia.

Disc photography and A-scan or B-scan ultrasonography are additional procedures that can be helpful in the diagnosis of congenital glaucoma. It should be noted that the diagnosis of congenital glaucoma is derived from the total clinical picture and not from one particular sign or symptom.

Plan

Topical and oral antiglaucoma medications can be of value in the treatment of congenital glaucoma. A nonselective beta blocker (e.g., timolol maleate) may be effective in reducing the pressure in congenital glaucoma before surgery. Oral carbonic anhydrase inhibitors are generally more effective, but should be used with caution. Sympathomimetic agents such as epinephrine and dipivefrin hydrochloride, parasympathomimetics such as pilocarpine, or one of the anticholinesterases are less useful in the early stages of congenital glaucoma.

Surgical intervention is the mainstay of therapy for congenital glaucoma. The procedures of goniotomy, trabeculotomy, trabeculectomy, cyclocryotherapy, and valve implantation are commonly used to reduce the intraocular pressure. Goniotomy is the most widely used procedure. Complications of goniotomy are uncommon but include cataract, hemorrhage, infection, and shallow anterior chamber. The infant should be followed closely after the surgery to check for reduction of corneal edema, intraocular pressure, and optic nerve head cupping, and to monitor for complications.

JUVENILE GLAUCOMA

Subjective

Juvenile glaucoma represents a late onset of primary infantile glaucoma. The disorder usually begins at age 4 years.

The condition has very few symptoms. Unlike congenital glaucoma, there is no photophobia, tearing, or blepharospasm. The disease is very insidious, often with unrecognized intraocular pressure elevations and occult optic nerve head damage.

The parents should be asked about congenital glaucoma in the family and chromosomal abnormalities, since this disease has been linked to chromosome 1q21-31.

Objective

The cornea should be evaluated for edema and Descemet's folds, but they are not usually present in juvenile glaucoma.

The finding of optic nerve head cupping in a young child should alert the examiner to the possibility of juvenile glaucoma. Intraocular pressures can be measured with applanation tonometry (e.g., Tono-Pen) or pneumotonometer. Visual field testing might be accomplished with a very attentive child.

If possible, gonioscopy should be performed to evaluate the anterior chamber angle for abnormalities. Ultrasonography may also be helpful in assessing axial length.

Plan

Topical and oral antiglaucoma medications can be of value in the treatment of juvenile glaucoma. Carbonic anhy-

drase inhibitors (e.g., acetazolamide), as well as beta blockers, are very useful on a temporary basis to lower the intraocular pressure before surgery. Sympathomimetic agents such as epinephrine and dipivefrin hydrochloride, parasympathomimetics such as pilocarpine, or one of the anticholinesterases are less useful in the early stages of juvenile glaucoma.

As with congenital glaucoma, surgical intervention is the mainstay of therapy for juvenile glaucoma. The procedures of goniotomy, trabeculotomy, trabeculectomy, cyclocryotherapy, and valve implantation are commonly used to reduce the intraocular pressure. Goniotomy is the most widely used procedure. Complications of goniotomy are uncommon but include cataract, hemorrhage, infection, and shallow anterior chamber.

The child should be followed closely after the procedure to check for reduction of intraocular pressure and to evaluate the optic nerve head for cupping.

PATHOLOGIC MYOPIA

Subjective

Myopia can be classified into three main categories: physiologic, intermediate, and pathologic. In pathologic myopia, a high refractive error is present from early childhood and is progressive. Difficulty seeing objects at a distance is the most common complaint. Children may report difficulty in seeing the blackboard in school and may squint to improve their distance vision. Vitreous floaters are often reported in high degrees of myopia as well.

Objective

Visual acuity is diminished in accordance with the amount of myopia. Pupillary responses, motilities, and other entrance tests should be normal or at least unrelated to the myopia. Refraction shows a high degree of myopia, usually 10 D or more.

A dilated examination may show localized areas of retinal pigment epithelial attenuation in the posterior pole and an optic nerve head crescent or conus. The crescent and attenuation are usually seen on the same side of the nerve. These changes are the earliest signs and are seen in infancy or early childhood. When these findings are present at this age, they are often a harbinger of a staphyloma. Many types of staphyloma have been described in pathologic myopia. Posterior staphylomas are the most common.

Lacquer cracks may develop in or near the macula. These are linear, whitish lesions representing breaks in Bruch's membrane. They have been associated with blue-yellow color deficiencies. They signal a poor prognosis because of the retinal degeneration, hemorrhaging, and choroidal neovascularization associated with them. Fuchs' spot may occur in the macula in these patients.

Acute hemorrhages are seen in pathologic myopia. These spontaneous bleeds may be related to Valsalva maneuvers or other physical activities, or they may be idiopathic. A second type of hemorrhage is related to the choroidal neovascular nets that form in association with the lacquer cracks.

Large and small areas of chorioretinal atrophy are seen in some eyes. As patients get older, these areas may coalesce into large regions of atrophy with scalloped edges.

Additional testing may include Amsler grid testing to evaluate central field loss, A-scan ultrasonography to assess axial length, and retinal photography to document changes. Fluorescein angiography is performed to detect choroidal neovascular membranes.

Plan

Spectacle and contact lens correction can be helpful for many patients. Keratorefractive surgery of various types can be performed in an attempt to improve acuity without visual aids. These procedures should not be considered in children because the final amount of myopia is not known. Clear lens extraction or anterior chamber minus intraocular lenses are also used to correct high myopia.

Retinal complications are common and sight threatening. Because tears may develop weeks after a posterior vitreous detachment, a dilated fundus examination should be performed again 4–6 weeks after a new posterior vitreous detachment is diagnosed. Symptomatic retinal tears should be referred immediately for repair. All highly myopic children and their parents should know the symptoms of retinal tears and detachments, and should be told whom to call if they should occur.

Extrafoveal choroidal neovascular membranes are often treated with laser photocoagulation. These membranes do not respond to treatment as well as do membranes with other causes.

Annual dilated fundus examinations are necessary for early detection of sight-threatening complications.

SUGGESTED READING

Brockhurst RJ. Nanophthalmos with uveal effusions: a new clinical entity. Trans Am Ophthalmol Soc 1974;72:371.

Franks W, Taylor D. Congenital glaucoma—a preventable cause of blindness. Arch Dis Child 1989;64:649.

Tokorot MT. Macular hemorrhage associated with high myopia. In Proceedings of the Fourth International Conference on Myopia. San Francisco: Myopia International Research Foundation, 1990.

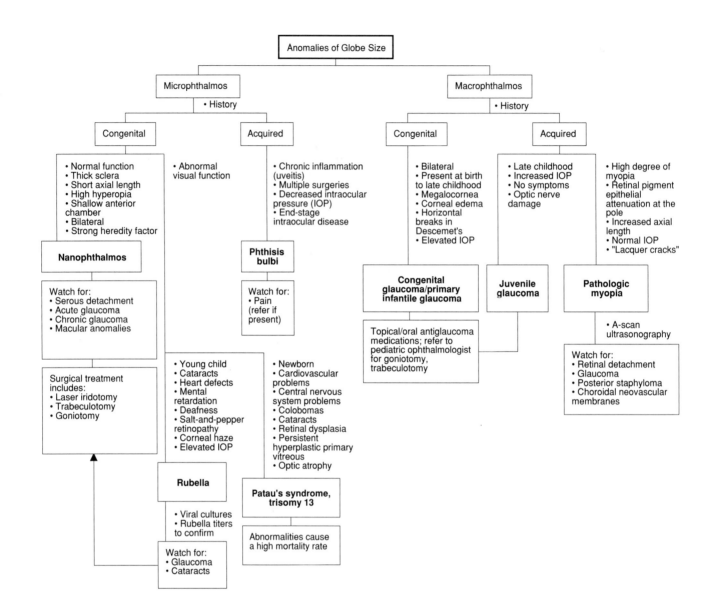

53

Anomalies of Globe Position

David P. Sendrowski

ANOMALIES OF GLOBE POSITION AT A GLANCE

Exophthalmos
  Thyroid eye disease (Graves' disease)
  Orbital pseudotumor
  Orbital cellulitis
  Orbital hemorrhage
  Arteriovenous aneurysm
  Arteriovenous fistula
  Obesity
  Dermoid cyst
  Mucocele
  Cavernous hemangioma
  Capillary hemangioma
  Kaposi's sarcoma
  Neurofibroma
  Optic nerve glioma
  Fibroma
  Osteoma
  Rhabdomyosarcoma
  Lacrimal gland tumor
  Metastatic tumor (breast, prostate, lung)
  Burkitt's lymphoma
  Intraorbital foreign body
  High axial myopia
Enophthalmos
  Age related
  Blow-out fracture
  Wasting diseases
  Superior sulcus deformity
  Cretinism (hypothyroidism)
  Metastatic adenocarcinoma
  Apparent enophthalmos
  Orbital varices
  Sympathetic paresis

Postirradiation
Lipodystrophy
Postinflammation
Post–surgical shortening
Linear scleroderma
Orbital asymmetry
Destruction of the orbital floor
Absence of the sphenoid wing

The etiology of many orbital disorders is not apparent with gross inspection. Therefore, a very thorough history is important in reaching a correct diagnosis.

The orbital examination consists of a routine ophthalmic examination plus some specialized evaluations that are specific to orbital disease, including palpation, exophthalmometry, auscultation, and forced ductions. The examiner should be careful to note subtle changes in globe and lid position as well.

ORBITAL BLOW-OUT FRACTURE

Subjective

Patients with a blow-out fracture have a recent history of blunt trauma to the eye. The trauma is commonly from a nonpenetrating object such as a fist or ball, and is produced by the transmission of forces through the orbital soft tissues.

The patient often complains of pain on eye movement, local tenderness, diplopia, and eyelid swelling after attempting to blow his or her nose. The orbital trauma may also cause a nosebleed, ecchymosis, periorbital edema, ptosis, and subconjunctival hemorrhage.

The patient should be asked about the type of object that caused the trauma, use of protective eyewear, and the time and location of the event.

Objective

The primary concern of the clinician is to rule out perforation of the globe; this is accomplished by performing Seidel's test, measuring intraocular pressure, and assessing the anterior chamber structure.

The extraocular muscles should be tested for restrictions, and the globe should be assessed for displacement. A forced duction test should be performed when a restricted muscle is believed to be trapped in a break in the orbital floor. Commonly, if a blow-out fracture exists, the eye is enophthalmic.

The eyelids should be checked for lacerations and abrasions. The periorbital tissues should be palpated for crepitus (subcutaneous emphysema). Crepitus is a crackling sound made by air escaping the dermal tissues.

A biomicroscope examination should be performed to evaluate the anterior segment for the following: corneal abrasion or laceration, conjunctival laceration, hyphema, iritis, and damage to the structures of the anterior chamber and iris. The intraocular pressure should also be measured, as a low reading suggests globe rupture of the traumatized eye.

The eye should be dilated to allow evaluation of the retina and choroid for tears, breaks, or detachments. The dilated examination may need to be repeated several days later if poor pupil dilation from secondary trauma does not permit a good view of the retina during the initial evaluation.

Orbital blow-out fractures are usually evident on plain-film radiographs. Computed tomography (CT) is more useful in demonstrating damage to or entrapment of the extraocular muscles.

Plan

Surgery is usually performed 1–2 weeks post-trauma and is indicated in those cases with persistent diplopia or when enophthalmos remains. Most fractures, however, do not require surgery.

The patient should be given nasal decongestants for several weeks to reduce the likelihood of blowing his or her nose and forcing the sinus contents into the orbit. The patient should also be advised not to blow his or her nose.

Oral broad-spectrum antibiotics (e.g., cephalexin) reduce the chance of secondary infection of the orbit. Oral analgesics (e.g., acetaminophen) should be given as needed for pain. Cold packs are also helpful in reducing the orbital edema and inflammation.

The patient should be followed every 3–5 days until the inflammation has subsided. Gonioscopy should be performed after several weeks to rule out angle recession from the trauma.

DESTRUCTIVE SINUS DISEASE

Subjective

Chronic sinus infections, mucoceles, and tumors can lead to destruction of the bony wall of the orbit. The destruction of the bony wall causes the globe to become enophthalmic. However, if left untreated, the inflammation can cause the eye to become proptotic as well.

Mucoceles are most common in adults. They occur in the frontal sinus because the sinus drains dependently, and it is therefore more susceptible to inflammatory debris that can accumulate and clog the ostium. The patient presents with inflammatory signs and symptoms of the frontal sinus, including pain that mimics an orbital cellulitis.

Chronic sinusitis may lead to contraction and secondary enophthalmos, but globe elevation and proptosis may also occur.

Sinus tumors that invade the orbit occur primarily in males in their 40s and 50s. Patients with sinus masses often present with proptosis, lid edema with ptosis, visual loss, and tearing. The symptoms relating to the sinus and nose are nasal obstruction, discharge, epistaxis, facial pain, and edema.

Patients often have a history of chronic sinusitis of allergic or infectious origin. Many patients have a history of cigarette smoking, and a history of nasal polyps is not uncommon.

Objective

Entrance testing should include assessment of visual acuities, pupillary responses, and extraocular muscle motility. The lids should be evaluated for signs of inflammatory disease, and the sinuses should be transilluminated to evaluate for infection and neoplasms. Exophthalmometry should be performed to rule out enophthalmos or proptosis of the eye in question.

A dilated fundus examination should be performed to evaluate the optic nerve head for edema and the retina and choroid for folds. Visual field screening may indicate macular or optic nerve head involvement.

Additional testing may include plain film radiography for evaluation of the orbital bones and sinuses. Ultrasonography is an additional technique for evaluating sinus and orbital lesions. CT is the most useful imaging technique for orbital and sinus evaluation. Magnetic resonance imaging (MRI) can also be used to evaluate sinus and skeletal abnormalities.

Plan

Patients with infectious mucoceles should be treated with broad-spectrum antibiotics. Once the infection is under control, surgical intervention is required.

Patients with chronic sinusitis should be treated with broad-spectrum antibiotics and should be followed closely for infectious orbital involvement. The patient should be referred to an ear, nose, and throat specialist for further evaluation and treatment.

Patients with suspected sinus neoplasms should have an incisional biopsy at the site of the suspected tumor. Depending on the test results, the patient should be referred to an ear, nose, and throat specialist.

DEVELOPMENTAL ANOMALIES OF THE ORBIT

Subjective

Patients with minor degrees of facial or orbital asymmetry commonly show pseudoproptosis. Craniofacial dysostosis and other developmental anomalies may result in profound orbital anomalies.

Most patients are either newborns or infants at initial presentation, as these anomalies are noticed very soon after birth. The parents should be asked about congenital or developmental problems in the family and any problems with the pregnancy, delivery, or birth weight of the infant.

Objective

There is limited testing that can be done on these patients because of their age. Testing should be limited to the evaluation of the structural anomaly and assessment of visual acuity.

Plan

Management of the cosmetic and functional disturbances related to the dysostosis and other developmental anomalies is in the domain of a multidisciplinary craniofacial team.

The patient should be followed after craniofacial surgery for visual development and visual rehabilitation, if indicated.

ORBITAL FAT ATROPHY WITH AGING

Subjective

Elderly patients, typically those in their 80s and 90s, may present with an enophthalmos from fat atrophy of the orbit. These patients have few or no ocular complaints related to this condition. The rare complaint is regarding secondary ptosis from the enophthalmos.

The medical history should be investigated for trauma, inflammatory disease, and irradiation procedures involving the orbit. The patient should also be questioned about ocular surgeries, cancer, and distensible orbital varices.

Objective

Entrance tests should include an assessment of visual acuities, pupillary responses, and extraocular motility and should all be normal. Palpation of the bony orbital rim reveals no cracks or notches. Dilated examination reveals a normal posterior segment with expected age-related changes.

Plan

The patient should be reassured about the loss of orbital fat from aging. The patient should be told to watch for signs of diplopia or ptosis, and should be followed on a regular basis.

FAT ATROPHY FROM DISEASE

Subjective

Unlike patients with normal fat atrophy from aging, patients with fat atrophy secondary to a chronic disease state have a past history of pathology involving the orbit. Patients with this type of enophthalmos may present with ptosis and diplopia. The patient should be asked about radiation treatment of the periorbital tissues or face, traumatic injury to the orbit, and severe disease states such as cancer, advanced diabetes, and autoimmune disease.

Objective

Entrance testing results vary depending on the cause of the enophthalmos. Visual acuities, pupillary responses, and extraocular muscle motility should all be assessed.

A dilated fundus examination should be performed to evaluate the posterior segment for optic nerve head disorders and retinal abnormalities. Orbital CT is very helpful in revealing the cause in many of these cases.

Plan

The patient should be referred to the appropriate specialist for continued treatment of the underlying disease. Cosmetically disfiguring enophthalmos is treatable, and orbital repair may be an important contribution to managing the patient's needs. The patient should be followed closely after this procedure.

AXIAL MYOPIA

Subjective

The most common complaint of patients with axial myopia is distance blur. The condition may be worse at night because of a larger pupillary diameter. Near vision is usually good. Patients may complain of floaters as well.

Patients should be asked about myopia in the immediate family. Past medical and ocular history are typically unremarkable.

Objective

Uncorrected visual acuity is diminished for distance and usually good for near. Pinhole testing markedly increases the distance acuity. Additional entrance testing of pupillary responses, color vision, and extraocular muscles is normal.

If keratometry readings are normal, this finding suggests an axial type of myopia.

Globe position may show pseudoexophthalmos along the visual axis. This pseudoexophthalmos is more prominent as the degree of axial myopia increases. Pseudoexophthalmos is an apparent abnormal prominence of the eye that is not caused by an orbital mass, inflammation, or vascular abnormality. Exophthalmometry readings are within normal limits for these patients.

Additional testing might include an A-scan to measure the axial length of the eye. A reading of 26 mm or more is common in these patients. If an orbital disease is still suspected, a CT scan can be ordered.

Plan

Once the diagnosis of axial myopia has been established, the patient's condition is best corrected with either spectacles or contact lenses. Another option is refractive surgery to correct the myopia.

Axial myopes are at greater risk for peripheral retinal degenerations and vitreoretinal traction; therefore, they should be educated about the signs and symptoms of retinal detachment. The myopic patient is also slightly at risk for developing chronic open-angle glaucoma as he or she gets older.

THYROID EYE DISEASE (GRAVES' DISEASE)

Subjective

Patients with thyroid eye disease are most commonly women in their mid-20s to early 40s. They may complain of dry eye, frequent blinking, and photophobia. When questioned, they may also complain of heat intolerance, agitated mood swings, tachycardia, thinning hair and hair loss, dyspnea, increased appetite without weight gain, constipation or diarrhea, and muscle cramps while exercising.

Patients should be asked about thyroid disease in the family and about present medications. Lithium has been shown to sometimes cause thyroid disease.

Objective

Physical examination of the patient with suspected thyroid disease should begin with the practitioner standing behind the patient and palpating the thyroid gland to assess for enlargement and evidence of nodules. The thyroid gland should be auscultated for bruits as well. The hair should be examined for evidence of alopecia and a fine, silky texture. The patient should be asked to extend his or her arm with palm down, and the hand should be observed for fine muscle tremors. The fingernails should be examined for onycholysis, a separation of the nailbed. Finally, the pretibial area of the leg should be examined for evidence of an orange peel–like texture with a scaly surface called *pretibial myxedema.*

The ocular examination should begin with an assessment of the lid position and globe displacement. The lids may be retracted from exaggerated sympathetic tone and may also show mild tremors. There may also be a lid lag on downgaze in these patients.

Exophthalmometry should be performed to evaluate the globe position. Unilateral and bilateral proptosis are common in thyroid eye disease. The globe should be auscultated to rule out a vascular lesion of the orbit. Restriction of the extraocular muscles in upgaze is common and is due to inflammation and fibrosis over time of the inferior rectus muscle. A red lens over the more proptotic eye may help to isolate the restricted muscle. A forced duction test should be done on the isolated muscle to discriminate restriction from paresis.

Biomicroscopy of the cornea with sodium fluorescein may reveal staining of the cornea due to exposure. If there is moderate to severe staining of the central cornea, the clinician should be concerned about the development of a central ulcerative keratitis.

Tonometry reveals normal intraocular pressure in primary gaze. If a hand-held instrument is used, it may be possible to observe a transient elevation in pressure on upgaze of 10–15 degrees. The pressure elevation is secondary to a tethering effect of the inferior rectus muscle on the globe. This increase in intraocular pressure is transient and does not increase the patient's risk for developing glaucoma.

A dilated fundus examination allows evaluation of the posterior segment for choroidal folds. Extended ophthalmoscopy of the optic nerve head helps to rule out disc edema. Threshold visual field testing should also be performed to evaluate the integrity of the optic nerve head.

The extraocular muscles can be further evaluated with A-scan and B-scan ultrasonography to look for muscle belly enlargement. Imaging series (CT or MRI) are very diagnostic for muscle and orbital changes consistent with Graves' orbitopathy.

A thyroid profile should be ordered and should include tests such as free thyroxine, free triiodothyronine, and thyrotropin assay. These three blood tests are the cornerstone of the diagnosis of hyperthyroidism. It should be noted, however, that a few patients with thyroid eye disease have normal laboratory findings and are classified as euthyroid.

Plan

The clinician should refer the patient to an endocrinologist or internist, if the patient has not already been diagnosed with thyroid disease at the time of the examination. The patient should be followed closely during the early stages of treatment of the systemic disease because the ocular disease tends to accelerate after systemic treatment and then comes under control.

Ocular therapy consists of keeping the cornea hydrated with ocular lubricants during the day and bland ophthalmic ointment at night. If lagophthalmos is present, the patient may tape the lids shut at night or use swimming goggles or a plastic wrap to keep the cornea moist during sleep.

Oral corticosteroids (e.g., prednisone) are extremely helpful in reducing the orbital inflammation in the early stages of the disease. If oral steroids are not well tolerated, orbital radiation (which has an anti-inflammatory effect on the orbital tissues) may be attempted. Diplopia and proptosis may also be improved to some extent by the use of corticosteroids, radiation, or a combination of both.

If diplopia from muscle involvement is present, Fresnel prisms or patching may be necessary for several months until the condition has stabilized, and strabismus surgery may be attempted.

If the patient demonstrates visual field loss, disc edema, visual acuity loss, or multiple keratic infections from exposure keratotomy, the patient should be referred for orbital decompression surgery. In extreme cases of exophthalmos, decompression surgery may be considered for cosmetic purposes.

CAVERNOUS HEMANGIOMA

Subjective

Patients presenting with cavernous hemangioma are commonly adult women in the second to fourth decade of life. The hemangiomas are rarely clinically evident in childhood. They are very slow growing, and the symptoms are insidious.

The patient may complain of diplopia, lagophthalmos, proptosis, or cosmesis, or may be asymptomatic. Cavernous hemangioma may cause a hyperopic shift by compression of the posterior globe forward. Patients may therefore complain of decreased distance and near acuities in the affected eye from the hyperopic shift.

Patients should be questioned about the rate of progression of visual symptoms, as well as headaches, sinusitis, and any history of cancer or trauma. Old photographs can be helpful in documenting the slow change in the proptosis.

Objective

The ocular examination should include a refraction to test for a hyperopic shift. Pupillary response, ocular motility, and color vision are unaffected by the cavernous hemangioma.

Exophthalmometry should be performed to evaluate the extent of the proptosis. It is commonly of an axial type, because the hemangioma is usually located inside the muscle cone.

Retropulsion can be performed by pushing on the globe through the closed upper lid with two fingers; when this maneuver is attempted on cavernous hemangiomas, the globe moves backward without resistance because of the vascular nature of the tumor.

Biomicroscopy with sodium fluorescein staining can be used to check for exposure keratopathy caused by the proptosis.

A dilated fundus examination should be performed to check for choroidal folds. These are a common finding in the affected eye of these patients. The optic nerve head should be evaluated for signs of disc edema. Threshold visual field testing is also helpful in determining nerve head involvement.

Additional testing should include ultrasonography and CT of the brain and orbit.

Plan

If the patient is asymptomatic and there is no evidence of abnormal pupillary responses, color vision, or visual field loss, then the patient can be followed every 6–12 months.

If the patient is symptomatic or complains of the cosmetic appearance of the proptosis, referral for surgical excision is warranted. Complete surgical excision by a lateral orbitotomy is usually performed and is very successful. The tumor generally does not recur.

ARTERIOVENOUS MALFORMATION

Subjective

Carotid cavernous sinus fistula is the most common arteriovenous malformation affecting the orbit. This condition represents an abnormal communication between the arterial and venous systems within the cavernous sinus.

Young, male patients with carotid cavernous fistula usually present after severe head trauma. This history is very important. Trauma to the orbit may also be associated with complaints of pain, throbbing, diplopia, eyelid swelling, restricted eye movements, and ptosis. Spontaneous development of a cavernous sinus fistula usually occurs in older adults, usually females, and commonly involves the meningohypophyseal artery. These patients have very few symptoms.

Objective

Patients usually show severe congestion and chemosis of the conjunctiva. These may be so severe that the conjunctiva is brick red and extrudes over the lower lid. The affected eye is pulsatile, a very important diagnostic finding. The pulsating proptosis is coincident with the heartbeat. When a stethoscope is placed over the eye, an audible bruit is present.

Evaluation of ocular motility may reveal limited movement or a total ophthalmoplegia in the more severe cases.

The intraocular pressure is elevated in the affected eye. Dilation should be attempted and may reveal disc edema, choroidal folds, and retinal edema. Additional testing should include fluorescein angiography and MRI scans of the orbit and brain to show the extent of the malformation or traumatic injury.

Plan

Carotid cavernous sinus fistula of traumatic origin is best managed with surgical repair. The prognosis for these cases is guarded.

Carotid cavernous sinus fistula of spontaneous origin (which occurs primarily in elderly females) may spontaneously resolve and require no surgical intervention.

RHABDOMYOSARCOMA

Subjective

Rhabdomyosarcoma is the most common primary malignant tumor of the orbit in childhood. It usually manifests around age 7 but may occur from infancy to adulthood. It is commonly misdiagnosed as orbital or preseptal cellulitis, especially if it occurs near the eyelid region.

The parent usually brings in the child with a swollen lid. The progression of the proptosis typically occurs over days to weeks, similar to the progression in an infection. However, a somewhat more indolent progression does not exclude the diagnosis of rhabdomyosarcoma. The child should be asked about diplopia, trauma, sinus infection, insect bites, recent upper respiratory tract infections, and nosebleeds. The parents should be asked about a family history of collagen vascular diseases, rheumatoid diseases, blood-borne disorders, and neoplastic diseases.

Objective

The ocular evaluation should include a careful examination of the lids. In rhabdomyosarcoma, the lids have a bluish appearance, whereas in infections they have a reddish appearance. Rhabdomyosarcoma can occur in the periorbital region; thus, the lids should be palpated for a possible supranasal or subconjunctival mass. If the rhabdomyosarcoma is in the supranasal region, the globe is displaced downward and outward. Evaluation of the Hirschberg reflexes may reveal a lack of symmetric positions on the cornea. Exophthalmometry should be performed with a Luedde exophthalmometer to evaluate the extent of proptosis. The neck area should be examined for elevated lesions suggestive of lymph node metastasis.

Dilation may reveal choroidal folds if the tumor is located within the orbit. Disc edema may also be present; if it is, there may also be associated pupillary, color vision, and visual field defects.

Additional testing should include a biopsy of the orbital mass as soon as possible. A- and B-scan ultrasonography show a relatively well circumscribed mass with low- to medium-amplitude echoes. CT or MRI imaging series should be done to evaluate the extent and location of the mass. With rhabdomyosarcoma, bone destruction is also a common finding on CT or MRI. Chest radiography and bone marrow aspiration should be performed to rule out distant metastasis.

Plan

The patient should be referred immediately to a pediatric oncologist or ophthalmologist. Treatment includes a combination of high-dose radiation and chemotherapy. These two treatment modalities have replaced enucleation and are associated with much lower mortality and morbidity rates.

Patients should be followed closely for signs of distant metastasis and ocular complications of the radiation and chemotherapy.

DERMOID CYST

Subjective

Patients can present with dermoid cysts from birth to young adulthood. The cysts occur in the orbit and periorbital region. There are several different categories, including dermoids, epidermoids, and lipodermoids. Dermoids contain hair follicles and sebaceous glands, and commonly occur in the supratemporal quadrant. Epidermoids are cystic lesions without adnexal structures such as hair. They usually occur near the superior orbital rim. Lipodermoids are solid tumors composed of fatty tissue. They occur below the conjunctiva near the superior temporal area of the globe.

The patient may be asymptomatic or may be symptomatic from movement of the globe due to growth of the dermoid. The patient may also complain of the cosmetic appearance of the globe or proptosis. Proptosis may develop spontaneously as a result of hormonal influence on the dermoid. Such hormonally induced proptosis occurs in puberty and pregnancy.

The patient should be asked about age of onset of the cyst, rate of progression, systemic illnesses, and present medications.

Objective

The ocular examination should include palpation of the orbital or paraorbital mass. Hirschberg reflexes should be measured for symmetry. Exophthalmometry should be performed to assess the degree of proptosis. Pupillary responses, color vision, ocular motility, and visual fields are unaffected by dermoids. Dilated fundus examination shows a normal posterior segment.

Additional testing should include B-scan ultrasonography for visible dermoids. These show a cystic lesion with good transmission of echoes. If the lesion is deeper in the orbit, CT and MRI scans should be considered. They usually reveal a well-defined lesion that may mold to the bone of the involved orbital wall.

Plan

Patients with dermoids or epidermoids should be referred for surgical removal. The prognosis is excellent. Lipodermoids can be monitored and should be followed for growth over time. Surgical removal of these lesions under the conjunctiva can result in postsurgical complications of ptosis, restricted ocular motility, and damage to the globe.

ORBITAL PSEUDOTUMOR

Subjective

Orbital pseudotumor is an idiopathic inflammation of the orbit. It occurs in both adults and children. It may be acute, recurrent, or chronic. In children, orbital pseudotumors can occur with fever, myalgia, and other constitutional complaints. These associated systemic symptoms do not occur in the adult population. In the acute form, patients complain of a prominent eye redness, diplopia, pain, and decreased visual acuity. An asymptomatic proptosis may occur in the chronic form of the disorder.

The patient should be asked about the onset of the condition, occurrence of previous episodes, associated ocular pain, and systemic symptoms. Patients should also be questioned about a history of trauma or systemic diseases such as cancer, diabetes, pulmonary and renal diseases, and dermatologic disorders.

Objective

The examination should start with the evaluation of the proptosis. Exophthalmometric readings should be taken to assess the degree of proptosis. The eyelids may show erythema as well as edema. The eyes should be tested for restrictions in ocular motility. The lacrimal gland should be palpated for enlargement. A stethoscope can be used to rule out orbital bruits.

Intraocular pressure should be evaluated and may be elevated from ocular venous congestion. Biomicroscopy of the anterior segment may reveal conjunctival injection and chemosis. The anterior chamber should be evaluated to rule out uveitis. Dilation should be performed to evaluate the retina, choroid, and optic nerve head. Retinal edema, choroidal folds, and disc edema may all be present from the orbital inflammation.

The patient's oral temperature, blood pressure, and other vital signs should also be assessed. Such assessment is especially important for children with orbital pseudotumor because they are usually febrile at the time of presentation.

Additional testing should include orbital CT scans of axial and coronal views. The CT scan shows a thickened posterior sclera, orbital fat, and lacrimal gland involvement. It also shows a thickening of the extraocular muscles, including the tendons; thickening of the tendons is not seen in thyroid eye disease. Blood testing can be helpful in bilateral or atypical cases. The testing may include, but should not be limited to, erythrocyte sedimentation rate, antinuclear antibody level, complete blood count (CBC), serum urea nitrogen level, and creatinine level to help rule out an inflammatory vasculitis such as temporal arteritis.

Measurement of fasting blood sugar level should be considered to rule out mucormycosis in patients with diabetes. An orbital biopsy can be performed in those cases in which the diagnosis is still uncertain.

Plan

Orbital pseudotumor responds very well to administration of oral steroids (e.g., prednisone). The steroids should be given with an antiulcer medication (e.g., ranitidine). If steroid therapy is not successful or the patient has complications, low-dose orbital radiation therapy may be helpful.

The patient should be followed closely while on the oral steroids. Intraocular pressure assessment and exophthalmometry should be performed at every visit. Recovery takes several weeks.

ORBITAL CELLULITIS

Subjective

Orbital cellulitis occurs in both children and adults. It is a very common orbital infection in children. Orbital cellulitis is a result of trauma or an extension of a concurrent sinus infection. The microbes that are most commonly associated with orbital cellulitis in children are *Haemophilus influenzae*, *Streptococcus*, and *Staphylococcus aureus*. *Staphylococcus aureus* is the most common cause in adults.

Patients with orbital cellulitis complain of fever, pain, swollen eyelids, and diplopia or restriction of gaze. Other complaints include eye redness, blurred vision, and headache.

The patient should be asked about trauma; concurrent infection of the sinuses, ear, nose, or throat; stiff neck; and changes in mental status. The patient should also be questioned about a history of diabetes or immunosuppressive disease and about recent dental work, specifically tooth extractions.

Objective

Visual acuity may be diminished depending on the severity of the disease. Pupils, color vision, and visual fields may be affected if there is associated optic nerve involvement. Ocular motility may show mild restriction, and, in the more severe cases, a complete ophthalmoplegia may be present. Pain upon eye movement is very common in these patients.

Proptosis should be assessed visually and with an exophthalmometer. If the trigeminal nerve is involved, there may be an associated decreased skin sensation around the eye. Transillumination of the sinuses may be performed to help rule out sinus involvement. The light source should be very bright (i.e., a transilluminator), and the room should be made as dark as possible. Fluid from cellular debris may be noted inside an infected sinus.

A dilated fundus examination should be performed to rule out disc edema, choroidal folds, retinal edema, and retinal vessel engorgement.

Blood pressure, pulse, and oral temperature should also be assessed.

Additional testing should include CT or MRI scans of the orbit and sinuses. Since the sinuses, especially the ethmoid sinus, are commonly involved, they should be investigated as well. Axial and coronal views of the orbit should be ordered in the imaging series. The imaging series also helps to rule out foreign body, orbital abscess, and sinus neoplasms.

Blood testing should be ordered to rule out systemic involvement. A CBC with differential and blood cultures should be performed. If there is discharge from the eye, Gram's stain and culture results should be obtained.

If spinal meningitis is suspected, a lumbar puncture should be ordered. The clinician should be suspicious of meningitis if the patient has signs of an orbital cellulitis, stiff neck, and mental status changes.

Plan

Orbital cellulitis should be treated as a sight- and life-threatening situation. The adult or child should be admitted to the hospital, where intravenous administration of broad-spectrum antibiotics (e.g., vancomycin, ceftriaxone sodium) should be initiated, and additional laboratory testing should be performed. The patient should be monitored on a daily basis until the infection and the patient's symptoms have subsided.

If the sinuses are the site of the infection, a consult with an ear, nose, and throat specialist should be considered.

If there is corneal exposure keratopathy from the proptosis, a topical broad-spectrum antibiotic (e.g., ciprofloxacin) may be started to reduce the chance of ulcerative keratitis.

ORBITAL METASTATIC TUMOR

Subjective

Orbital metastasis is usually from the breast in women and from the lung in men. In children, neuroblastoma and Ewing's sarcoma are the most common distant tumors that metastasize to the orbit. Metastatic tumors are much more common in the choroid than in the orbit, probably because of the nature of the blood supply.

The symptoms of orbital metastatic disease have a very rapid onset. Commonly, patients develop diplopia, vision loss, lid edema, and ptosis over a very short time span of days to weeks. The ophthalmoplegia and diplopia are more marked in the early stages of metastatic disease than with primary tumors of the orbit. Orbital pain is another distinctive and persistent complaint in these patients.

Patients do not complain of proptosis, since this is not a common feature of metastatic disease. In fact, women with breast carcinoma can develop enophthalmos, which makes the normal eye look proptotic.

The patient should be asked about a history of cancer, orbital trauma, and sinus disease. A history of cigarette smoking is significant. If there is a positive history of smoking, the patient should be asked about the number of packs smoked per day.

Objective

Since metastatic disease may affect the macula, patients may show varying degrees of visual acuity loss. Pupils may be sluggish, and, if the optic nerve head is involved, the involved eye may show a relative pupillary defect. Motility testing reveals varying degrees of restriction.

Color vision and visual fields are also affected if there is concurrent optic nerve head involvement.

Exophthalmometry should be performed to assess the degree of proptosis, if present. The sinuses may be transilluminated to help rule out secondary involvement. Intraocular pressure should be measured, but it is usually unaffected unless there is orbital swelling, which can cause an increase in the pressure. A dilated fundus examination may reveal choroidal folding, disc and macular edema, and retinal vessel engorgement. The choroid should be examined for evidence of metastatic lesions.

CT or MRI scans of the orbit, sinus, and brain should be performed. Axial and coronal views of the orbit are usually preferred. The scans may show a poorly defined, diffuse tumor, which may conform to the shape of the adjacent structures of the orbit. It is not uncommon to see bone destruction near the tumor as well. Fine-needle biopsy of the orbital tumor to confirm the diagnosis is highly recommended.

Additional testing is dictated by the results of the scan and biopsy. The patient should be referred for a breast examination and mammogram if carcinoma of the breast is suspected. Chest radiography should be ordered to rule out lung cancer.

Plan

Children with suspected Ewing's sarcoma or neuroblastoma should be referred to a pediatric oncologist and ophthalmologist. A combination of local orbital radiation and systemic chemotherapy is used to reduce both orbital and primary site disease.

Adults should be referred to an oncologist and ophthalmologist as well. Systemic chemotherapy and radionucleotide therapy may be used on the primary site of the tumor. The orbital disease is treated with local radiotherapy. The ocular structures hold up very well to this type of treatment.

Both adults and children should have a dilated fundus examination every few months to rule out secondary retinal occlusive disease from the radiotherapy.

The prognosis varies depending on the extent and degree of malignancy of the primary tumor.

SUGGESTED READING

Glaser JS. Neuro-Ophthalmology (2nd ed). Philadelphia: Lippincott, 1990.

Rootman J. Diseases of the Orbit. Philadelphia: Lippincott, 1988.

Taylor D. Pediatric Ophthalmology. London: Blackwell, 1990.

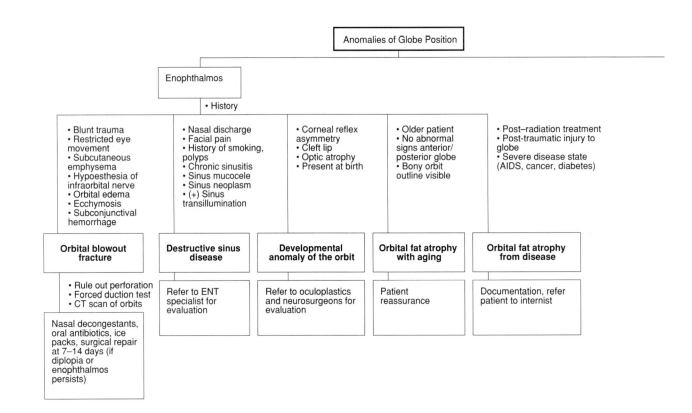

Anomalies of Globe Position

Enophthalmos

• History

• Blunt trauma
• Restricted eye movement
• Subcutaneous emphysema
• Hypoesthesia of infraorbital nerve
• Orbital edema
• Ecchymosis
• Subconjunctival hemorrhage

• Nasal discharge
• Facial pain
• History of smoking, polyps
• Chronic sinusitis
• Sinus mucocele
• Sinus neoplasm
• (+) Sinus transillumination

• Corneal reflex asymmetry
• Cleft lip
• Optic atrophy
• Present at birth

• Older patient
• No abnormal signs anterior/posterior globe
• Bony orbit outline visible

• Post–radiation treatment
• Post-traumatic injury to globe
• Severe disease state (AIDS, cancer, diabetes)

Orbital blowout fracture

Destructive sinus disease

Developmental anomaly of the orbit

Orbital fat atrophy with aging

Orbital fat atrophy from disease

• Rule out perforation
• Forced duction test
• CT scan of orbits

Refer to ENT specialist for evaluation

Refer to oculoplastics and neurosurgeons for evaluation

Patient reassurance

Documentation, refer patient to internist

Nasal decongestants, oral antibiotics, ice packs, surgical repair at 7–14 days (if diplopia or enophthalmos persists)

Exophthalmos
• History

Axial myopia	Thyroid eye disease	Cavernous hemangioma	Orbital metastatic tumor	Orbital cellulitis

Top branch clinical features:

- **Axial myopia:** • Myopic • Normal keratometry • Axial proptosis • Normal exophthalmometry readings
- **Thyroid eye disease:** • Bilateral/unilateral • Lid retraction • Lid lag • Heat intolerant • More common in women aged 20–40 • Thyroid bruit/enlargement • Pretibial myxedema
- **Cavernous hemangioma:** • Middle-aged women • Slow growing • (+) Retropulsion • Axial proptosis • Increased hyperopia • Unilateral
- **Orbital metastatic tumor:** • Rapid onset of proptosis • Primary tumor (breast, lung) • Motility problems • Orbital pain • Diplopia
- **Orbital cellulitis:** • Lid edema • Sinus disease • (+) Restricted motility with pain • Tenderness • (±) Lid trauma • Fever

Tests:

- Axial myopia: • A-scan ultrasonography
- Thyroid eye disease: • Thyroid panel • CT/MRI • Ultrasonography
- Cavernous hemangioma: • CT/MRI • A/B ultrasound
- Orbital metastatic tumor: • MRI/CT • Biopsy
- Orbital cellulitis: • MRI/CT • Blood testing

Management:

- Axial myopia: Watch for: • Retinal detachment • Glaucoma
- Thyroid eye disease: Refer to endocrinologist. Watch for: • Cornea • Extraocular movements • Optic nerve
- Cavernous hemangioma: Refer for surgical evaluation or monitor
- Orbital metastatic tumor: Consultation with oncologist, radiotherapy of the orbit
- Orbital cellulitis: Hospitalization and surgical evaluation

Orbital pseudotumor	Dermoid cyst	Rhabdomyosarcoma	Arteriovenous malformation

Bottom branch clinical features:

- **Orbital pseudotumor:** • Inflammation of orbit • Sudden onset/chronic • Adults/children • Prominent red eye • Diplopia/pain • Trigeminal involvement
- **Dermoid cyst:** • Little/no inflammation • Orbital lesion with small cilia • Young child/adult • Slow growing • Located near bone sutures of orbit
- **Rhabdomyosarcoma:** • Young child (average age 7–8) • History of nosebleeds • Bluish color to lids • Unilateral proptosis • Superonasal mass • Lymph node involvement
- **Arteriovenous malformation:** • History of trauma (young males) • Pulsatile proptosis • Severe conjunctival chemosis/injection • Orbital bruit • Also older females

Tests:

- Orbital pseudotumor: • CT/MRI • Blood testing
- Dermoid cyst: • Ultrasound • CT/MRI
- Rhabdomyosarcoma: • Ultrasound • CT/MRI
- Arteriovenous malformation: • Arteriography • MRI

Management:

- Orbital pseudotumor: Oral steroids and antiulcer medication; low-dose orbital radiation, if steroids fail
- Dermoid cyst: Surgical removal
- Rhabdomyosarcoma: Immediate referral to oncologist
- Arteriovenous malformation: Refer for surgical repair

54

Esodeviation

JOHN H. NISHIMOTO

ESODEVIATION AT A GLANCE

True esodeviation
  Sixth nerve palsy
  Accommodative esotropia
  Congenital (infantile) esotropia
  V-type esodeviation (overaction of the inferior obliques)
  A-type esodeviation (overaction of the superior obliques)
Pseudoesodeviation
  Enophthalmos
  Prominent epicanthal fold
  Hypotelorism
  Telecanthus

There are many causes of esodeviation, including binocular vision anomalies, vascular pathologies, and orbital conditions. This chapter reviews the common conditions causing esodeviation. In addition, it discusses some of the pseudoesodeviations that may be mistaken for a true esodeviation.

TRUE ESODEVIATION

Sixth Nerve Palsy

Subjective
The sixth cranial nerve (CN VI) supplies the lateral rectus muscle. The major function of the lateral rectus is to provide abduction. Patients with a sixth nerve palsy often complain of diplopia and may adopt a head turn to the side of the weak muscle. Headache may accompany the diplopia. Single vision is achieved when one eye is occluded. The patient may have a history of a vascular disease such as diabetes or hypertension. Since the sixth nerve has the longest course at the base of the brain, it is susceptible to damage from trauma, inflammation (such as meningitis), tumor, and increased intracranial pressure. In general, neoplasm is a more common cause of sixth nerve palsy in young people, and ischemia is a more common cause in older people. Thus, a careful systemic history taking and evaluation are important when a patient presents with this condition.

Objective
Evaluation of ocular motility reveals a restriction in abduction to the affected side. Associated findings can help determine the cause for sixth nerve palsy. In adults, the most common causes are vascular diseases such as diabetes, hypertension, and atherosclerosis. Evaluation for elevated blood pressure, fasting blood sugar level, and erythrocyte sedimentation rate is helpful for determining vascular pathology. In children, a sixth nerve palsy can be caused by a viral infection, which can also affect the seventh and eighth nerves (Gradenigo's syndrome). In addition, since the facial nerve (CN VII) loops around the sixth nerve nucleus, there can be an associated facial weakness. Brain stem gliomas, small metastatic lesions, and arteriovenous malformations are other causes of nucleus sixth nerve palsy. In the subarachnoid space, especially as the sixth nerve crosses over the petrous apex and under the petroclinoid ligament, the abducens nerve is subject to trauma and inflammation. Traumatic sixth nerve palsies may be associated with basilar skull fractures. There may be facial pain and decreased hearing secondary to petrositis. If there is pain or associated neurologic signs and symptoms associated with a sixth nerve palsy, a magnetic resonance imaging (MRI) scan should be obtained.

Plan

As mentioned earlier, in older adults, an evaluation to rule out microvascular diseases such as diabetes, hypertension, and atherosclerosis is indicated. If other neurologic signs are present on physical examination, a complete imaging workup (computed tomography [CT], MRI, cerebral angiography) is required. To manage diplopia, either eye patching or prisms can be used to provide relief. In children, it may be best to alternate the patching according to a schedule based on the child's age to prevent amblyopia. A re-examination is required approximately every 6 weeks following the onset until the condition resolves. CT or MRI of the head is required if the isolated sixth nerve palsy does not resolve in 3–6 months.

Accommodative Esotropia

Subjective

Patients with accommodative esotropia usually have a noticeable inward eye turn. They may also complain of diplopia, asthenopia, headache, and blurred vision, especially at near viewing distances.

Objective

Accommodative esotropia is typically of the convergence-excess type. Convergence excess is a type of heterophoria or heterotropia in which the esodeviation is larger at near distances than at far distances. In addition to a high accommodative convergence/accommodation ratio, many of these patients have a significant amount of hyperphoria. Measuring the amount of deviation with prism neutralization at different viewing distances and through different corrective lenses can provide useful diagnostic information.

Plan

In cases of accommodative esotropia, the deviation can be reduced significantly with the use of plus lenses. Refractive errors should be corrected as soon as possible to prevent an excessive amount of esodeviation from being manifest. Orthoptics and vision therapy may also be needed in the treatment.

Congenital (Infantile) Esotropia

Subjective

Congenital (infantile) esotropia usually becomes apparent by the age of 6 months. Parents may notice that one eye is turning inward and bring the child to the eye doctor for cosmetic reasons. Patients with congenital esotropia may have no symptoms, since in many esotropes the deviation angle is constant and the tropic eye is suppressed.

However, some esotropia is intermittent, so that the patient experiences diplopia. Asthenopia and excessive blinking also can occur.

Objective

Congenital (infantile) esotropia is typically a comitant deviation; that is, the angle of deviation is approximately the same in all directions of gaze when a distant fixation target is used. The deviation can be measured by performing a unilateral and alternating cover test with prism neutralization. Amblyopia may be present, especially if there is anisometropia in which the greater refractive error is in the strabismic eye. In Bruchner's test, the patient fixates the ophthalmoscope light at a distance of approximately 1 m, and the beam of light is large enough to illuminate both eyes at the same time. Binocular alignment can be evaluated by measuring the Hirschberg reflex, and the amblyopia can be evaluated by observing the relative whiteness and brightness of each pupillary reflex. If amblyopia is present, the pupil of the turned eye appears brighter and whiter than the pupil of the fixating eye. A dilated fundus examination should be performed to rule out pathologies such as retinoblastoma that may be associated with the esotropia.

Plan

The intended outcome of a particular management plan for congenital esotropia may vary considerably, but the plan should be designed to address the individual patient's entering signs and symptoms, the visual anomalies diagnosed, and the interests and outcome expectations of the patient or parents. Depending on the amount and type of deviation, strabismus surgery, orthoptic training, or a combination of the two can be used to treat strabismus. If cosmetic improvement alone is the goal, then only surgery may be needed. If efficient binocular vision is desired, a combination of surgery and vision therapy often provides the best result. Once a binocular treatment plan is prescribed, multiple steps within the plan must be accomplished to achieve the final goal of efficient binocular vision.

PSEUDOESODEVIATION

Enophthalmos

Subjective

Patients with enophthalmos often have a history of trauma to the orbit or face, since this condition occurs most frequently with blow-out fracture. Other causes include inflammation, neoplasms, and age-related loss of orbital fat. The patient with enophthalmos may notice that the eye seems to be smaller or that the eye appears sunken in.

The patient may complain of diplopia if the extraocular muscles are entrapped within the fractured orbital floor.

Objective

With some fractures of the orbital floor, the globe and adjacent structures move inward and downward, producing a sunken, enophthalmic appearance. Exophthalmometry may reveal a difference of 2 mm or more in the locations of the two corneal apices relative to the lateral orbital rims. Lacrimal fossa lesions from inflammation, neoplasm, or metastasis can also displace the globe inward. Forced duction testing can aid in the classification of eye movement disorders. If the forced duction test is negative and the globe can be moved freely up or down, yet clinically the patient shows limited vertical gaze motility, the possibility of intraocular hematoma or traumatic nerve injury must be considered.

Radiographic imaging with plain-film radiography, CT, or MRI is very useful in determining the cause of the enophthalmos. CT is the ideal technique for assessing most cases of orbital trauma because it provides excellent visualization of bone fractures. MRI, though a poor choice for visualization of bone fractures, can demonstrate soft-tissue detail and is helpful if there is orbital tumor involvement.

Plan

Blow-out fractures that do not affect the patient functionally or cosmetically may be left alone without surgical intervention. Indications for surgical repair by an oculoplastic or maxillofacial surgeon after orbital blow-out fracture include severe disruption of the orbital floor, 3 mm or more of enophthalmos, and diplopia within 30 degrees of primary gaze. Surgery is also indicated in cases where daily work-related activity is compromised by restricted motility. If trauma or aging is not the apparent cause of enophthalmos, an evaluation to rule out neoplasia and metaplasia is indicated.

Epicanthal Fold

Subjective

An epicanthal fold is a fold of the upper lid that partially covers the inner canthus, caruncle, and plica semilunaris.

It is found in Asians and in some patients with congenital abnormalities such as Down syndrome, fetal alcohol syndrome, hypotelorism, and telecanthus. Patients with epicanthal folds do not have any visual symptoms related to this condition; however, the patient or parent may express concern about an "eye turn" due to the anatomic positioning of the lid and the bridge of the nose.

Objective

The examiner should rule out true strabismus, as well as characteristics that might conceal or exacerbate the appearance of strabismus. This objective can be accomplished using procedures such as the cover test, Krimsky reflex position test, Bruchner's test, and Hirschberg test. Characteristics that may result in pseudoesotropia include a wide, broad nasal bridge and epicanthal folds, a small interpupillary distance, and wide face. The examiner may need to actually pinch the bridge of the nose, pulling the epicanthal folds up and away, to convince the parent that no strabismus is present.

Plan

No treatment is necessary for pseudoesotropia. Reassurance to the patient and parent concerning the absence of any eye turn can comfort all parties. If the patient is suspected of having a pathologic syndrome of which pseudoesotropia is just one manifestation, the patient should be referred to a pediatrician or other appropriate specialist for further evaluation.

SUGGESTED READING

Caloroso EE, Rouse MW. *Clinical Management of Strabismus.* Boston: Butterworth–Heinemann, 1993.

Casper DS. *Orbital Disease Imaging and Analysis.* New York: Thieme Medical Publishers, 1993.

Kanski JJ. *Clinical Ophthalmology* (3rd ed). Oxford, UK: Butterworth–Heinemann, 1994.

Milukas AT. *Diagnosis and Management of Blowout Fractures of the Orbit with Clinical, Radiological and Surgical Aspects.* Springfield, IL: Charles C Thomas, 1969.

Roy FH. *Ocular Differential Diagnosis.* Baltimore: Williams & Wilkins, 1996.

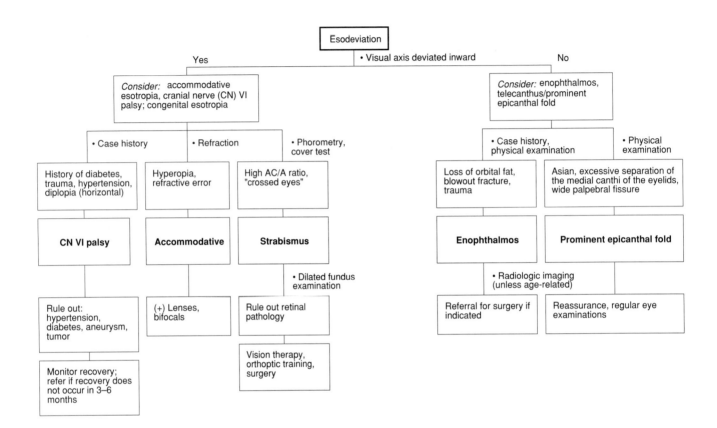

55

Exodeviation

JOHN H. NISHIMOTO

EXODEVIATION AT A GLANCE

True exodeviation
  Exotropia
    V-type exodeviation (overaction of the inferior obliques)
    A-type exodeviation (overaction of the superior obliques)
    Internuclear ophthalmoplegia
    Exophthalmos
Pseudoexodeviation
    Retinopathy of prematurity (dragged disc)
    Pseudoexotropia (narrow lateral canthus)

There are several causes for exodeviation, including binocular vision anomalies, retinal anomalies, and ocular conditions involving the orbit. This chapter reviews common conditions that result in exodeviation.

TRUE EXODEVIATION

Exotropia

Subjective

Exotropia is characterized by an outward turning of the eye, either constantly or intermittently. In children, exotropia may become apparent between early infancy and 4 years of age. Parents or teachers may notice that the child has a head turn, squints one eye, or blinks excessively. Symptoms associated with exotropia can be due to recent onset of strabismus or to a change in the deviation frequency or magnitude of a long-standing strabismus. Symptoms include diplopia, asthenopia, and poor visual acuity.

Objective

The clinician should note the position of the head of the patient with suspected exotropia. The head-turning response occurs to prevent diplopia in certain fields of gaze. Amblyopia may be noted in a constant exotrope, with visual acuity ranging from 20/20 to 20/200; however, most alternating or intermittent exotropes have normal acuity. The angle of turn can be measured using the cover test and prism neutralization. A dilated fundus examination is also indicated to rule out maculopathy, intraocular tumor, or other lesions that may be causing the strabismus.

Plan

Exotropia not associated with retinal pathology is managed with vision therapy and, in some cases, with surgery. The goal is for the patient to achieve clear, single binocular vision. One strategy for treating a patient with exotropia is to (1) stimulate an accommodative-convergence response, (2) teach eye movement awareness, (3) stabilize voluntary convergence control, (4) establish sensory fusion at the ortho position, (5) teach awareness of diplopia that occurs when the eye drifts out, (6) teach fast voluntary convergence recovery, (7) teach accommodative accuracy, (8) teach fusional convergence accuracy, and (9) stabilize efficient binocular vision in open visual space.

Internuclear Ophthalmoplegia

Subjective

Internuclear ophthalmoplegia (INO) is caused by lesions of the medial longitudinal fasciculus (MLF) between the third and sixth nerve nuclei. INO is characterized by muscle weakness and may be secondary to multiple sclerosis, brain stem infarction, brain stem and fourth ventricular tumor, or drug toxicity (e.g., from phenothiazines and tricyclic antidepressants). Patients with INO may complain of diplopia, especially upon lateral gaze, but may not experience it in the primary position. Other significant history includes previous or concurrent episodes of optic neuritis, urinary incontinence, numbness or paralysis of an extremity, or other unexplained neurologic events.

Objective

INO may be unilateral or bilateral. An upbeat nystagmus in upgaze may be noted in bilateral INO. The typical MLF syndrome consists of medial rectus paresis in the eye on the side of the lesion, nystagmus of the abducting eye on lateral gaze to the side opposite the lesion, and normal medial rectus activity on convergence. An MLF lesion produces disconjugate eye movement and diplopia on lateral gaze. Ocular motility can appear full, but a muscle weakness is indicated by slower saccadic eye movements in the affected eye as the patient shifts fixation from the examiner's laterally positioned finger to the examiner's nose.

Plan

If the patient with INO is less than 50 years of age, it is imperative to rule out multiple sclerosis as an underlying cause. Magnetic resonance imaging (MRI) scans are particularly helpful in the diagnosis of multiple sclerosis. INO in patients older than 50 years is more commonly due to brain stem vascular disease. Fasting blood sugar level, erythrocyte sedimentation rate, computed tomographic (CT) scan, angiogram, or MRI for local midbrain infarct can be helpful in determining the diagnosis. If stroke is suspected, it is recommended that the patient be admitted to the hospital within 72 hours of the onset of symptoms for further neurologic evaluation and observation.

Exophthalmos (Proptosis)

Subjective

Exophthalmos is characterized by a bulging or protruding appearance of the globe. It can be unilateral or bilateral. Thyroid eye disease is the most frequent cause of both unilateral and bilateral exophthalmos. Orbital tumors such as lymphoma, hemangioma, and venous vascular malformation can also lead to exophthalmos. Patients with exophthalmos may complain of diplopia due to a restriction myopathy. Occasionally, the orbital contents displace the eye outward, leading to exotropia. In advanced cases, the patient may experience vision loss from optic nerve compression. In addition, the exophthalmic patient may complain of dry-eye symptoms due

to exposure keratitis or may express concern about the cosmetic appearance of the eyes.

Objective

Thyroid ophthalmopathy is one of the most frequent causes of both unilateral and bilateral exophthalmos and acquired diplopia in adulthood. Lid position changes offer important clues in the differential diagnosis of orbital diseases. Lid retraction is an important sign of thyroid orbitopathy, but it can also occur in cirrhosis. Exophthalmometry is useful in measuring the amount of exophthalmos and monitoring changes over time. Patients with a clinical presentation suggestive of thyroid orbitopathy should be evaluated for thyroid disease. Thyroid function tests such as measurement of free triiodothyronine, thyroxine, and thyrotropin can give an accurate assessment of thyroid function. It is important to note, however, that the results of these tests can be normal even in the presence of thyroid eye disease. If orbital tumor is suspected, CT and MRI and, in some cases, tissue biopsies can provide important diagnostic information.

Plan

Applying artificial lubricants or moisture chambers, or taping the lids shut at night can provide relief from the symptoms of exposure keratitis secondary to exophthalmos. Diplopia can be treated effectively using prisms. Surgery may be indicated when optic nerve compression or an orbital tumor causes the exophthalmos.

PSEUDOEXODEVIATION

Retinopathy of Prematurity (Dragged Disc)

Subjective

The patient with retinopathy of prematurity (ROP) typically has a history of premature birth (less than 36 weeks' gestation), low birth weight (under 4 lb 6 oz), and supplemental oxygen therapy. The manifestations of ROP depend on the stage of the condition. Vision loss can be due to tractional displacement of the macula, strabismus, or retinal detachment.

Objective

The clinical manifestations of ROP occur in three stages: primary vaso-obliteration, secondary fibrovascular proliferation, and tertiary scarring. The changes are classified according to location, extent, and severity. In the early phases, there is a demarcation line between the vascular and avascular peripheral retina that develops into a ridge. Later, in the proliferative stage, peripheral fibrovascular bands can cause traction on the retina, which results in macular heterotopia (dragged disc) and retinal detachment. In the advanced cicatricial stage, the detached retina may form a white retrolental mass. It is important to note that, in many patients, ROP does not progress to the more advanced stages.

Plan
Because ROP can progress to blindness during the first 3 months of life and because treatment such as cryopexy and laser photocoagulation has been proved effective in controlling the condition, for very low-birth-weight infants (i.e., less than or equal to 1,500 g), a dilated fundus examination should be performed between 4 and 6 weeks' chronologic age or between 31 and 33 weeks' postconception age. Follow-up examinations depend on the initial examination. According to the International Classification of Retinopathy of Prematurity, follow-up examinations should be planned at approximately 2- to 4-week intervals until evidence is found of normal vascularization of the retina. Other patients at risk for retinal damage (i.e., retinal detachment and tears) from ROP should be evaluated at 3 months of age at a minimum and then regularly thereafter (approximately every 6–12 months).

Pseudoexotropia

Subjective
Patients with pseudoexotropia do not have strabismus and are not symptomatic. On occasion, the patient or parent may express concern about the possibility of an "eye turn" due to the anatomic positioning of the lids and bridge of the nose.

Objective
Direct observation is critical to evaluate the patient's eye movements and facial characteristics. Characteristics that may mimic the appearance of exotropia include a narrow bridge of the nose, the absence of an epicanthus, a large interpupillary distance, and a narrow face. An evaluation should be performed to rule out true strabismus (e.g., cover test, Krimsky reflex test, Bruchner's test).

Plan
No treatment is needed other than reassuring the patient and parents about the absence of a true eye turn.

SUGGESTED READING

Bartlett JD, Jaanus SD. Clinical Ocular Pharmacology (3rd ed). Boston: Butterworth–Heinemann, 1995.

Caloroso EE, Rouse MW. Clinical Management of Strabismus. Boston: Butterworth–Heinemann, 1993.

Char DH. Thyroid Eye Disease (2nd ed). New York: Churchill Livingstone, 1990.

Mauriello JA, Flanagan JC. Management of Orbital and Ocular Adenexal Tumors and Inflammations. New York: Field and Wood Medical Publishers, 1990.

Roy FH. Ocular Differential Diagnosis. Baltimore: Williams & Wilkins, 1996.

Ryan SJ. Retina. Vol. 2. St. Louis: Mosby, 1994.

American Academy of Pediatrics. Screening examination of premature infants for retinopathy of prematurity. Pediatrics 1997;100:273.

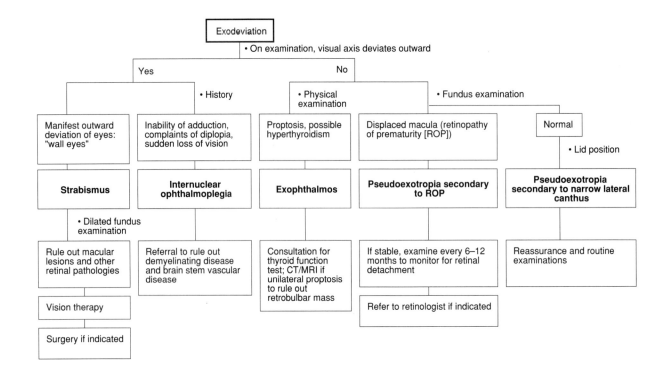

56

Extraocular Muscle Paresis

CARL H. SPEAR AND TAMMY P. THAN

EXTRAOCULAR MUSCLE PARESIS AT A GLANCE

Third nerve palsy
  Partial
    Microvascular disease
  Complete
    Pupillary involvement
      Aneurysm
      Tumor
      Vasculitis
      Syphilis
      Trauma
    No pupillary involvement
      Microvascular disease
Fourth nerve palsy
  Trauma
  Microvascular disease
  Surgically induced
Sixth nerve palsy
Multiple nerve palsy
Conditions that mimic extraocular muscle paresis
  Myasthenia gravis
  Thyroid eye disease (Graves' disease)
  Orbital inflammatory pseudotumor
  Chronic progressive external ophthalmoplegia
  Muscle entrapment secondary to trauma
  Duane's retraction syndrome
  Brown's superior oblique tendon syndrome
  Möbius syndrome
  Internuclear ophthalmoplegia

Patients with a recent onset of extraocular muscle paresis often present complaining of double vision. Other symptoms may include drooping eyelid, blurred vision, and unequal pupil size, depending on the nerve or nerves involved. Taking a thorough case history is important to differentiate congenital from acquired conditions. Additional tests useful in the diagnosis of extraocular muscle paresis are ocular motility assessment, Park's three-step test, and forced duction testing.

PARTIAL THIRD NERVE PALSY (SUPERIOR DIVISION)

Subjective

Patients with a partial third nerve palsy (superior division) report a recent onset of double vision that is present with binocular viewing. They may also complain of eyelid droop. Typically these patients have a positive history of microvascular disease.

Objective

A hypotropia of the involved eye and unilateral restricted upgaze of recent onset are hallmarks of this condition. The patient also generally has a unilateral ptosis. A normal pupillary response is a critical sign in deciding how to manage these patients. All other ocular findings are normal.

Plan

Patients with suspected third nerve palsy of unknown origin should be referred for systemic evaluation to rule out undiagnosed microvascular conditions. Laboratory work or notification of the primary care physician is indicated for patients with a known microvascular disease. Occlusion of the involved eye is beneficial in relieving the diplopia. The patient should be monitored for pupillary involvement and progression of the paresis. If either occurs, the patient should be referred for a neurologic evaluation and diagnostic imaging (computed tomography [CT] or magnetic resonance imaging [MRI]).

PARTIAL THIRD NERVE PALSY (INFERIOR DIVISION)

Subjective

Patients with a partial third nerve palsy (inferior division) complain of a recent onset of double vision that is present with binocular viewing. Typically, these patients have a positive history of microvascular disease.

Objective

Exotropia or hypertropia (or both) of the involved eye is characteristic of this paresis. A unilateral restriction of downgaze is also present. A normal pupillary response is a critical sign in determining how to manage these patients. All other ocular findings are normal.

Plan

Patients with suspected third nerve palsy of unknown origin should be referred for systemic evaluation to rule out undiagnosed microvascular conditions. Laboratory work or notification of the primary care physician is indicated in patients with known microvascular disease. Occlusion of the involved eye is beneficial in relieving the diplopia. The patient should be monitored for pupillary involvement or progression of the paresis. If either occurs, the patient should be referred for a neurologic evaluation and diagnostic imaging (CT or MRI).

COMPLETE THIRD NERVE PALSY (PUPILLARY INVOLVEMENT)

Subjective

Patients complain of a recent onset of double vision that is present with binocular viewing. The involved eye turns downward and outward, the eyelid droops, and one pupil is larger than the other. Patients are also sensitive to light and may have varying degrees of blurred vision (especially at near distances). Patients may also complain of headache. A detailed history to rule out episodes of blackout, trauma, and other possible causes is mandatory.

Objective

Unilateral dilatation of the pupil and inferotemporal deviation of the eye are the classic presentation of a complete third nerve palsy. A unilateral ptosis and inability of the patient to elevate or adduct the involved eye are also observed. Vision decrease is variable but may be more pronounced at near distances due to reduced accommodation.

Plan

Immediate referral to a neurologist for diagnostic imaging and possible cerebral angiography is indicated, since the most likely cause is an aneurysm. Other possible causes include syphilis, trauma, and tumor. Diagnostic imaging is indicated in all instances of third nerve paresis in which the pupil is involved.

COMPLETE THIRD NERVE PALSY (NO PUPILLARY INVOLVEMENT)

Subjective

Patients complain of a recent onset of double vision that is present with binocular viewing. The involved eye turns downward and outward, and the eyelid droops. Patients may also report varying degrees of blurred vision. Systemic history is often positive for microvascular disease (diabetes or hypertension).

Objective

Normal pupillary response of the involved eye, which is deviated inferotemporally, is the critical sign. A unilateral ptosis and inability of the patient to elevate or adduct the eye are also observed.

Plan

Occlusion therapy may be used to relieve the diplopia. Referral for treatment of the underlying microvascular disorder is also indicated. Referral to a neurologist is indicated if the paresis is not resolved within 3 months; referral should be immediate if the patient is less than 50 years of age, regardless of pupillary findings. Surgical intervention to relieve diplopia is not indicated prior to 6 months after onset.

Twenty-five percent of all isolated third nerve palsies are idiopathic.

FOURTH NERVE PALSY

Subjective

Patients present with a recent onset of double vision with binocular viewing. One eye appears higher than the other. A detailed patient history to elicit information regarding any recent trauma, recent surgery, or microvascular disorders is critical.

Objective

The patient's diplopia is relieved with head tilt to the shoulder opposite the involved eye. A hypertropia and inability to depress the eye on adduction are also observed. An increase in diplopia is noted on downgaze. The patient may or may not have signs of trauma.

Plan

Occlusion therapy can be used to relieve the diplopia. Laboratory work to rule out systemic causes and referral for treatment of any underlying systemic disorder may also be indicated. If the palsy is unresolved in 3 months, the patient should be referred for a neurologic evaluation and diagnostic imaging (CT or MRI). Correction of the diplopia with prism use or surgery may be indicated if the condition is not resolved within 6 months.

SIXTH NERVE PALSY

Subjective

Patients report with a recent onset of double vision with binocular viewing. One eye turns inward. The patient often has a positive history of microvascular disease or trauma.

Objective

An esotropia is observed. The diplopia is decreased or relieved with head turn toward the affected side.

Plan

If there is no known history of a microvascular disorder, referral to a neurologist for diagnostic imaging is indi-
cated. If the cause is a known microvascular disorder, occlusion therapy may be used for relief of the diplopia, and monitoring is the appropriate plan. However, if the diplopia has not resolved within 3 months, then the patient should be referred for neurologic evaluation and laboratory work. Prism or surgical treatment for relief of diplopia may be considered after 6 months.

MULTIPLE NERVE PALSY

Subjective

Patients report with one or more of the following symptoms: diplopia, eyelid droop, facial pain or numbness, pupils of different sizes, and a varying degree of decreased vision.

Objective

The patient's eye deviation cannot be attributed to an isolated nerve palsy. Other signs that may or may not be present include ptosis, miosis or dilatation of the pupil, decreased corneal sensitivity, orbital pain, and other neurologic deficits based on the underlying cause.

Plan

When the diagnosis of an isolated nerve palsy cannot be made, an immediate neurologic consult is indicated. Possible causes include orbital pseudotumor, arteriovenous fistula, disorders of the cavernous sinus, and Tolosa-Hunt syndrome.

SUGGESTED READING

Alexander LA. Primary Care of the Posterior Segment (2nd ed). Norwalk, CT: Appleton & Lange, 1994.
Fraunfelder FT, Roy FH. Current Ocular Therapy 4. Philadelphia: Saunders, 1995.
Kanski JJ. Clinical Ophthalmology (3rd ed). Oxford: Butterworth–Heinemann, 1994.
Spalton DJ. Atlas of Clinical Ophthalmology. Philadelphia: Lippincott, 1991.
Walsh TJ. Neuro-Ophthalmology: Clinical Signs and Symptoms (3rd ed). Philadelphia: Lea & Febiger, 1992.

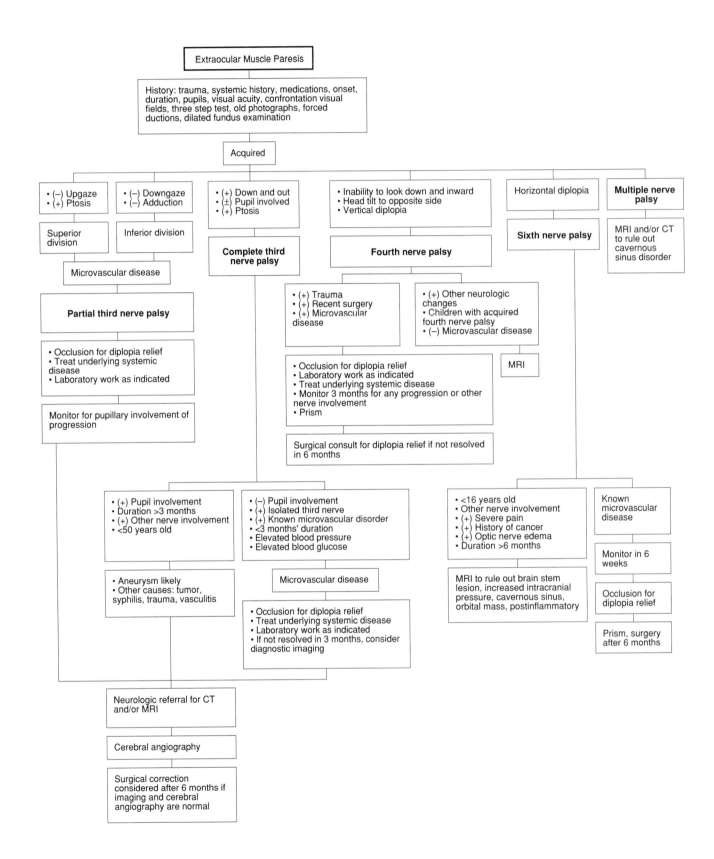

57

Nystagmus

TAMMY P. THAN

Patients presenting with nystagmus may be asymptomatic or may complain of oscillating vision (oscillopsia) or blurred vision. It is important to obtain a careful history to determine the onset of the nystagmus. Characterization of the eye movements (i.e., direction, type of nystagmus, speed) is essential to help identify the specific type of nystagmus.

CONGENITAL NYSTAGMUS

Subjective

The patient typically presents with a horizontal, pendular nystagmus in primary gaze that has been present since birth or infancy. Oscillopsia is not an associated symptom.

Objective

The nystagmus is typically horizontal and pendular, and is present in primary and vertical gazes. The nystagmus usually changes to jerk nystagmus upon lateral gaze. There is an area of fixation, called the *null point*, in which the nystagmus disappears or dampens, and the patient may acquire a head tilt to position the eyes at this point. Convergence causes the nystagmus to decrease, and anxiety causes it to increase. The majority of these patients show an inversion of the optokinetic response in which the fast phase is in the direction of the moving target. Pathology of the visual system is present if the congenital nystagmus is sensory in origin.

Plan

Diagnostic testing such as electroretinography and measurement of visual evoked potential should be performed to rule out underlying pathology. A base-out prism can be prescribed to dampen the nystagmus by inducing convergence. A referral can be made for surgery in which muscle resection procedures are used to position the eyes at the null point.

SPASMUS NUTANS

Subjective

Patients with spasmus nutans typically are between the ages of 4 and 18 months. In addition to the fast asymmetric eye movements, head nodding and torticollis are reported.

Objective

The nystagmus is usually bilateral but is often asymmetric. The movements are of small amplitude with varying direction. Head and neck movements are present but do not appear to be compensatory for the eye movements.

Plan

Spasmus nutans is usually a self-limiting condition that resolves by the age of 3 years. However, all patients should be referred for diagnostic imaging to rule out a pathologic cause, that is, a tumor.

LATENT NYSTAGMUS

Subjective

Patients with latent nystagmus are often asymptomatic but may report rapid eye movements when one eye is occluded.

Objective

When one eye is occluded, nystagmus is noted in the unoccluded eye. The fast phase is toward the uncovered eye.

Plan

Latent nystagmus is a benign condition for which no treatment is indicated.

GAZE-EVOKED NYSTAGMUS

Subjective

Patients with gaze-evoked nystagmus may report rapid eye movements in horizontal and vertical gaze; the eyes are steady in primary gaze. A history of cerebellar disease, myasthenia gravis, or orbital restrictive muscle disease may be elicited. Several medications—including anticonvulsants, sedatives, alcohol, and recreational drugs—may also induce gaze-evoked nystagmus.

Objective

When the patient looks in the affected direction, jerk nystagmus may be observed. The fast, corrective movement is in the direction of gaze.

Plan

Treatment should be directed toward the underlying cause.

VESTIBULAR NYSTAGMUS

Subjective

Patients with vestibular nystagmus, in addition to reporting rapid eye movements, often complain of dizziness and vertigo. Nausea may or may not be present.

Objective

Two types of vestibular nystagmus exist: peripheral and central. The salient feature of peripheral vestibular nystagmus is the inhibition of nystagmus in the primary gaze. The nystagmus is usually a combination of horizontal and torsional nystagmus. The duration is brief, but the nystagmus may be recurrent. Tinnitus and deafness are often associated with this condition. Other neurologic symptoms are usually absent.

Unlike peripheral nystagmus, central vestibular nystagmus is uniplanar, is not inhibited with fixation, and is chronic. Auditory symptoms are rare, but other neurologic symptoms are frequently present.

Plan

Timely referral to a neurologist is indicated due to the multitude and severity of the possible causes, which include cerebellopontine angle tumor, brain stem ischemia, demyelinating disease, and brain stem lesions.

SEESAW NYSTAGMUS

Subjective

Patients with seesaw nystagmus may present complaining of rapid eye movements. History may include head trauma.

Objective

In seesaw nystagmus, one eye moves upward with an associated intorsion, while the other eye moves downward with extorsion.

Plan

Visual fields should be tested to rule out chiasmal lesions. A neurologic consult is also indicated.

UPBEAT NYSTAGMUS

Subjective

Patients with upbeat nystagmus may report rapid eye movements.

Objective

In primary gaze, jerk nystagmus is observed with the fast phase upward.

Plan

Because upbeat nystagmus is usually associated with posterior fossa disease, a neurologic consult is indicated. In rare cases, upbeat nystagmus may be congenital or drug induced; these conditions can be ruled out with a careful case history.

DOWNBEAT NYSTAGMUS

Subjective

Patients with downbeat nystagmus may present reporting rapid eye movements that are more noticeable when looking downward.

Objective

Nystagmus is observed in primary gaze with the fast phase downward. This type of nystagmus typically increases when the patient changes gaze to an inferior position.

Plan

The most common cause of downbeat nystagmus is an Arnold-Chiari malformation. Therefore, the patient should be referred to a neurologist for diagnostic imaging.

CONVERGENCE-RETRACTION NYSTAGMUS

Subjective

Patients with convergence-retraction syndrome may report rapid eye movements. In addition, these patients may also report difficulty with upgaze eye movements.

Objective

The nystagmus may be spontaneous or may be elicited when the patient attempts to look up. The fast phase is accompanied by convergence of the eyes and lid retraction. Absent or limited upgaze and light-near dissociation are often associated with convergence-retraction syndrome.

Plan

The patient should be referred to a neurologist for diagnostic imaging.

VISUAL-DEPRIVATION NYSTAGMUS

Subjective

Patients with visual-deprivation nystagmus are usually unaware of the onset of nystagmus. History includes either a unilateral or bilateral acquired vision loss.

Objective

If the vision loss is unilateral, the blind eye may exhibit vertical nystagmus. If the visual deprivation is bilateral, nystagmus is observed in primary gaze and is typically pendular.

Plan

The cause of vision loss should be determined and treated as indicated.

PERIODIC ALTERNATING NYSTAGMUS

Subjective

Patients with periodic alternating nystagmus typically report rapid eye movements.

Objective

A jerk horizontal nystagmus is observed for a short period (<2 minutes). An absence of nystagmus follows. The nystagmus then switches direction for another 2 minutes.

Plan

The patient should be referred to a neurologist for diagnostic imaging. Baclofen has been used successfully to treat cases of acquired periodic alternating nystagmus.

REBOUND NYSTAGMUS

Subjective

Patients with rebound nystagmus may report rapid eye movements when changing fixation. History may include cerebellar disease, ataxia, or alcohol abuse.

Objective

A reversal of gaze-evoked nystagmus is observed when patients look eccentrically. In addition, refixation to primary gaze induces a transient nystagmus in the direction opposite to the eye movements.

Plan

A neurologic referral is indicated.

VOLUNTARY NYSTAGMUS

Subjective

Patients with voluntary nystagmus may report the ability to induce small, rapid eye movements.

Objective

A small-amplitude, rapid horizontal nystagmus is noted. This nystagmus can be sustained only for a brief period of approximately 25 seconds.

Plan

No treatment is indicated. However, the astute clinician should be aware that some patients may attempt to use this ability for financial gain.

ACQUIRED PENDULAR NYSTAGMUS

Subjective

Patients with acquired pendular nystagmus may present reporting a recent onset of rapid eye movements.

Objective

The nystagmus is bilateral but is often asymmetric. The movement is pendular and may occur in any direction.

Plan

Given that the most common cause of this type of nystagmus is multiple sclerosis, a neurologic consult is indicated.

PHYSIOLOGIC NYSTAGMUS

Subjective

Patients with physiologic nystagmus may report that they are aware of rapid eye movements when their eyes are positioned in extreme gazes, or they may be asymptomatic.

Objective

A small-amplitude jerk horizontal nystagmus is noted in extreme lateral gaze, that is, with gaze angles in excess of 30 degrees. The nystagmus is of equal amplitude in both right and left directions of gaze.

Plan

No treatment is required. The patient may need to be reassured that this is a normal physiologic finding.

SUGGESTED READING

Amos J. Diagnosis and Management in Vision Care. Stoneham, MA: Butterworth, 1987.

Dell'Osso L, Daroff R, Troost B. Nystagmus and Saccadic Intrusions and Oscillations. In TD Duane, EA Jaeger (eds), Clinical Ophthalmology. Philadelphia: Lippincott, 1995.

Kanski JJ. Clinical Ophthalmology (3rd ed). Oxford: Butterworth–Heinemann, 1994.

Marks E, Adamczyk D, Thomann K. Primary Eyecare in Systemic Disease. Norwalk, CT: Appleton & Lange, 1995.

Vaughan D, Asbury T, Riordan-Eva P. General Ophthalmology (14th ed). Norwalk, CT: Appleton & Lange, 1995.

Walsh T. Neuro-Ophthalmology: Clinical Signs and Symptoms (3rd ed). Philadelphia: Lea & Febiger, 1992.

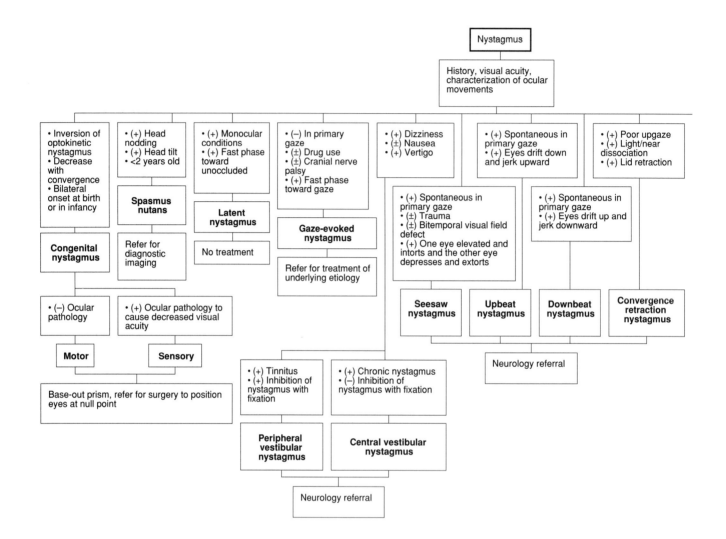

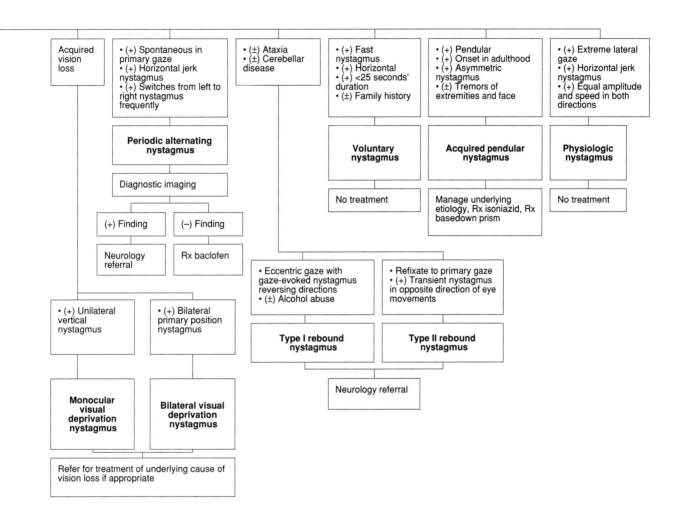

Acquired vision loss

- (+) Spontaneous in primary gaze
- (+) Horizontal jerk nystagmus
- (+) Switches from left to right nystagmus frequently

Periodic alternating nystagmus

Diagnostic imaging

(+) Finding

(−) Finding

Neurology referral

Rx baclofen

- (+) Unilateral vertical nystagmus

- (+) Bilateral primary position nystagmus

Monocular visual deprivation nystagmus

Bilateral visual deprivation nystagmus

Refer for treatment of underlying cause of vision loss if appropriate

- (±) Ataxia
- (±) Cerebellar disease

- (+) Fast nystagmus
- (+) Horizontal
- (+) <25 seconds' duration
- (±) Family history

Voluntary nystagmus

No treatment

- (+) Pendular
- (+) Onset in adulthood
- (+) Asymmetric nystagmus
- (±) Tremors of extremities and face

Acquired pendular nystagmus

Manage underlying etiology, Rx isoniazid, Rx basedown prism

- (+) Extreme lateral gaze
- (+) Horizontal jerk nystagmus
- (+) Equal amplitude and speed in both directions

Physiologic nystagmus

No treatment

- Eccentric gaze with gaze-evoked nystagmus reversing directions
- (±) Alcohol abuse

- Refixate to primary gaze
- (+) Transient nystagmus in opposite direction of eye movements

Type I rebound nystagmus

Type II rebound nystagmus

Neurology referral

58

Anisocoria

FRANK P. LaRUSSA

ANISOCORIA AT A GLANCE

Physiologic anisocoria
Anisocoria with miosis of the affected pupil
  Horner's syndrome
  Iritis
  Argyll-Robertson pupil
  Pharmacologic miosis
  Long-standing Adie's tonic pupil
Anisocoria with a fixed, dilated pupil
  Traumatic anisocoria
  Adie's tonic pupil
  Acute angle-closure glaucoma
  Pharmacologic mydriasis
  Third nerve palsy

A patient presenting with anisocoria is a cause of concern for any clinician. The vast majority of cases are benign; however, some patients with anisocoria have sight- or life-threatening conditions. It is the job of the prudent clinician to sort out the former and attend diligently and rapidly to the latter. The first step is to determine if the pupillary response in each eye is normal. This initial determination is key to the diagnostic process.

PHYSIOLOGIC ANISOCORIA

Subjective

The overwhelming majority of patients with anisocoria have a physiologic difference in the sizes of the two pupils. The patient with physiologic anisocoria has no symptoms and may or may not be aware of the size difference between the two pupils.

Objective

Both pupils respond normally to light and near testing. The anisocoria is equal under photopic and scotopic conditions. There is generally less than 1 mm of difference pupil size between the two eyes. Old photographs of the patient may be useful in determining the long-term status of the condition.

Plan

The patient should be educated that this condition is benign.

ANISOCORIA WITH MIOSIS OF THE AFFECTED PUPIL

Horner's Syndrome

Subjective

Horner's syndrome can be either congenital or acquired. The clinician should carefully question the patient with suspected acquired Horner's syndrome about a history of trauma or surgery involving the neck. Questions about the presence of associated systemic conditions such as migraine, stroke, lung tumors, and demyelinating diseases should also be included in the history taking. The patient with Horner's syndrome usually has no symptoms but may complain of monocular lid droop. Raeder's syndrome is a painful variant of Horner's syndrome.

Objective

In congenital Horner's syndrome, the iris on the affected side is lighter in color, so that there is heterochromia. In both congenital and acquired Horner's syndrome, one pupil is miotic, and there is an ipsilateral ptosis. The pupillary reactions to light and a near stimulus are intact; however, the anisocoria is greater in dim than in bright illumination. Facial anhydrosis on the affected side also may be present. To confirm the diagnosis the clinician may instill topical 10% cocaine in each eye. Horner's pupil dilates less vigorously. Instillation of 1% hydroxyamphetamine is used to determine the location of the lesion causing Horner's pupil. Failure of Horner's pupil to dilate to the same extent as the normal pupil strongly indicates a third-order neuron lesion. The hydroxyamphetamine test should not be performed within 24 hours of the cocaine test. Phenylephrine 1% may be used as an alternative drug to hydroxyamphetamine.

Plan
If the third-order neuron is the lesion site, the condition is often due to an extracranial lesion or is related to a headache syndrome. A referral to a neurologist is recommended if further evaluation is indicated. If the first- or second-order neuron is the probable lesion site, the clinician should suspect an underlying serious systemic condition such as Pancoast's tumor of the lung apex. Referral to an internist is in order in this situation. Radiologic studies of the chest, cervical spine, or skull are typically performed at this stage in the diagnostic evaluation. If these tests are negative, then a neurologic referral is indicated, and the most likely diagnosis is cerebrovascular accident.

Iritis

Subjective
Iritis can be secondary to trauma, can be associated with systemic disease, or can be idiopathic. Patients with acute iritis often present with an associated miotic pupil. The patient usually complains of pain in the eye and sensitivity to light.

Objective
Cells and flare in the anterior chamber and circumlimbal injection of the affected eye are common signs of iritis. In acute iritis, the pupil is typically round and miotic; however, the presence of posterior synechiae can cause the pupil to have an irregular shape.

Plan
Initially iritis should be treated with a topical steroid such as 1% prednisolone acetate and a cycloplegic agent such as 1% cyclopentolate or 5% homatropine. If the iritis is bilateral, recurrent or chronic, or granulomatous, or is associated with suggestive systemic symptoms, laboratory and radiologic testing are indicated to rule out underlying systemic disease.

Argyll-Robertson Pupil

Subjective
Argyll-Robertson pupil is a light-near dissociative response most commonly associated with neurosyphilis. It is usually bilateral but may be asymmetric. Patients with this condition generally do not experience symptoms directly related to the abnormal pupillary response.

Objective
Pupillary testing reveals pupils that are irregular and react poorly to light but constrict normally to a near stimulus.

Plan
Laboratory tests should be performed to rule out syphilis (rapid plasma reagin or VDRL test, fluorescent treponemal antibody absorption test, *Treponema pallidum*-microhemagglutination assay). If the resultant clinical picture suggests syphilis, referral to an internal medicine practitioner or neurologist is indicated for further evaluation and treatment.

Pharmacologic Miosis

Subjective
The most common cause of pharmacologic anisocoria with miosis of the affected eye is unilateral instillation of a miotic drop for the treatment of glaucoma. Patients with this condition may complain of blurred vision or brow ache on the affected side.

Objective
The pupil on the affected side reacts poorly to light and pharmacologic dilation. Other signs of glaucoma such as advanced optic nerve cupping and visual field loss are usually present.

Plan
If the miotic drop causes significant side effects for the patient, alternative topical, oral, or surgical glaucoma therapies should be considered.

ANISOCORIA WITH A FIXED, DILATED PUPIL

Anisocoria Related to Previous Trauma

Subjective
The patient with this type of anisocoria usually has no symptoms; however, the patient may complain of light sensitivity. There is a history of trauma.

Objective

Biomicroscopy reveals iris atrophy, sphincter rupture, or synechiae in the affected eye.

Plan

The patient should be educated about the benign nature of the condition. Sun protection should be recommended. An opaque contact lens may be used to improve cosmetic appearance and reduce photophobia. Gonioscopy and dilated fundus examination should be performed on any patient with recent trauma to rule out other damage to the eye.

Adie's Tonic Pupil

Subjective

Adie's tonic pupil is more common in females than in males. Most cases are idiopathic; however, in some instances the condition is associated with viral infections, systemic neuropathies, or trauma. Patients with this condition usually have no symptoms but occasionally may complain of blurred vision through the affected pupil.

Objective

The pupil is fixed and dilated, and may be slightly irregular in shape. The pupillary response to light is poor and response to a near stimulus is slow. Vermiform (worm-like) movements at the pupil margin may be noted during slit-lamp evaluation. A solution of 0.125% pilocarpine may be instilled in each eye to confirm the diagnosis. The Adie's tonic pupil constricts to the weak pilocarpine. Reduced deep-tendon reflexes are sometimes associated with Adie's tonic pupil. It is important to note that an Adie's tonic pupil may become more miotic with time and may actually become smaller than the normal pupil.

Plan

The patient should be educated about the benign nature of the condition and should be followed on a routine basis. If the patient desires, 0.125% pilocarpine may be instilled for cosmetic purposes.

Acute Angle-Closure Glaucoma

Subjective

Patients with acute angle-closure glaucoma usually complain of eye pain or brow pain on the affected side. They also often complain of blurred vision and haloes around lights. In addition they may be nauseated.

Objective

Slit-lamp biomicroscopy usually reveals a steamy, edematous cornea. The conjunctiva is often mildly injected, and the pupil is fixed in a mid-dilated position. The intraocular pressure is elevated and is usually above 40 mm Hg. Gonioscopy reveals a closed angle.

Plan

The initial management of acute pupillary-block angle-closure glaucoma involves reducing the intraocular pressure through medical means. If the intraocular pressure is above 50 mm Hg, a topical beta blocker or apraclonidine hydrochloride should be tried initially. Concurrent therapy with oral acetazolamide or isosorbide is often needed to reduce the pressure. An antiemetic may be needed prior to initiating oral therapy if the patient is nauseated. Once the intraocular pressure is below 50 mm Hg, topical 2% pilocarpine is effective in lowering intraocular pressure. Pilocarpine should be avoided if the patient is aphakic or pseudophakic, or has mechanical closure of the angle. In some cases, corneal indentation can be effective in breaking an angle-closure attack. Once the intraocular pressure is brought under reasonable control, a peripheral iridotomy is indicated for long-term management of acute angle closure.

Pharmacologic Mydriasis

Subjective

Patients with pharmacologic anisocoria typically complain of photophobia and blurring of near vision in the affected eye, and are aware of the sudden onset of anisocoria. The patient may have a recent history of instilling eye drops, going on a cruise, or handling plants. Common causes are the accidental use of mydriatic/cycloplegic drops, use of a scopolamine patch to prevent motion sickness, or contact with a vegetative agent like the belladonna plant.

Objective

The examination reveals a fixed, dilated pupil with no associated ptosis or extraocular muscle motility abnormalities. The pupil does not constrict to 0.5% pilocarpine.

Plan

Once the causative agent has been confirmed, no treatment is indicated other than reassurance.

Third Nerve Palsy with Pupillary Involvement

Subjective

Third nerve palsy without pupillary involvement is most commonly associated with a microvascular disease such as diabetes. A third nerve palsy with pupillary involvement is more often due to an aneurysm. Patients with third nerve palsy complain of a sudden lid droop, diplopia, and possibly pain.

Objective
The clinical signs of this condition include a fixed, dilated pupil and ipsilateral ptosis. With a complete palsy, extraocular motility will be restricted except temporally.

Plan
Radiologic imaging of the brain must be performed immediately to rule out an aneurysm or mass. A cerebral angiogram may be needed to provide additional information.

SUGGESTED READING

Bajandas FJ, Kline LB. Neuro-Ophthalmology Review Manual (3rd ed). Thorofare, NJ: Slack, 1988.

Bartlett JD, Jaanus SD. Clinical Ocular Pharmacology (3rd ed). Boston: Butterworth–Heinemann, 1995.

Cullom RD, Chang B. The Wills Eye Manual: Office and Emergency Room Diagnosis and Treatment of Eye Disease (2nd ed). Philadelphia: Lippincott, 1994.

London R, Eskridge JB. Clinical Procedures in Optometry. Philadelphia: Lippincott, 1991.

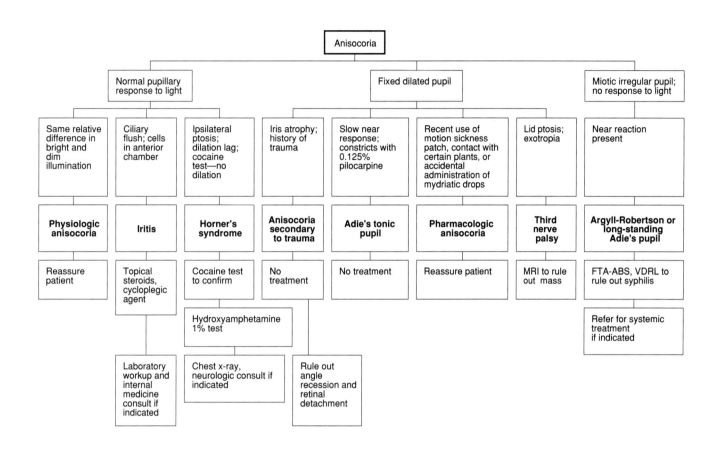

Appendices

A

Some Common Laboratory and Adjunct Tests Used in Primary Eye Care

Note: The reference range for some of these tests may vary slightly among clinical laboratories.

Suspected Disease or Condition	Tests	Reference Range
Diabetes mellitus	Fasting blood sugar	65–115 mg/dl
	Random blood sugar	<200 mg/dl
	2-Hour postprandial glucose	<120 mg/dl
	Glycosylated hemoglobin (Hgb A_{1c})	3.9–6.7%
	Oral glucose tolerance test	
	30 minutes	<200 mg/dl
	1 hour	95–177 mg/dl
	2 hour	80–160 mg/dl
	3 hour	65–135 mg/dl
Thyroid disease	Thyroid profile	
	Triiodothyronine uptake	25–35% uptake
	Free thyroxine index	4.0–13.2
	Thyroxine	4.5–11.5 μg/ml
	Thyroid stimulating hormone	0.6–4.6 μU/ml
Hyperlipidemia	Lipid profile	
	Total cholesterol	133–199 mg/dl
	High-density lipoprotein	30–90 mg/dl
	Low-density lipoprotein	0–130 mg/dl
	Very low-density lipoprotein	5–40 mg/dl
	Triglycerides	35–150 mg/dl
	Blood pressure assessment	<130 mm Hg systolic
		<85 mm Hg diastolic
Collagen vascular disease	Erythrocyte sedimentation rate (Westergren)	0–15 mm/hr or ≤ age/2 (males)
		0–20 mm/hr or ≤ (age + 10)/2 (females)
	Antinuclear antibody	Negative (<1:20)
	HLA (e.g., HLA-B27)	Negative
	Rheumatoid factor	Negative (<1:20)
	Sjögren's antibody	Negative
	Antiscleroderma antibody	Negative
	Joint x-ray	Negative (no anomalies)
Sarcoidosis	Angiotensin-converting enzyme	10–50 U/liter
	Serum lysozyme	2.8–15.8 μg/ml
	Chest x-ray	Negative (no anomalies)
	Gallium scan	Negative
	Tissue biopsy	Negative
Myasthenia gravis	Acetylcholinesterase receptor antibody	Negative (≤0.03)
	Edrophonium (Tensilon) test	Negative

Suspected Disease or Condition	Tests	Reference Range
Hematologic disease	Complete blood cell count (CBC with differential)	
	White blood cell count (WBC)	$4.0–11.0 \times 10$ cells/mm
	WBC differential	
	Neutrophils	47–75%
	Lymphocytes	18–46%
	Monocytes	0–12%
	Eosinophils	0–6%
	Basophils	0–2%
	Red blood cell count (RBC)	$3.8–5.4 \times 10$ cells/mm
	Hematocrit	35–48%
	Hemoglobin (Hgb)	11.5–16.0 g/dl
	RBC indices	
	Mean corpuscular volume	75–100 μm
	Mean corpuscular hemoglobin	27–35 pg
	Mean corpuscular hemoglobin concentration	31–37%
	Platelet count	$140–450 \times 10$ cells/mm
	Clotting indices	
	Prothrombin time	10.3–13.3 secs
	Partial thromboplastin time	22.9–34.9 secs
	Sickle cell test (Sickledex)	Negative
	Hemoglobin electrophoresis	
	Hgb A_1	96–98%
	Hgb A_2	0–4%
	Hgb F	0–2%
	Hgb S	0%
	Hgb C	0%
Cardiovascular or cerebro-vascular disease	CBC (See above)	
	Blood chemistry	
	Glucose	65–115 mg/dl
	Blood urea nitrogen	7–25 mg/dl
	Creatinine	0.6–145.0 mEq/liter
	Uric acid	3.0–8.0 mg/dl
	Cholesterol	133–199 mg/dl
	Triglycerides	35–150 mg/dl
	SGOT (AST)	5–40 IU/liter
	SGPT (ALT)	7–56 IU/liter
	Lactate dehydrogenase	0–240 IU/liter
	Alkaline phosphatase	38–126 IU/liter
	Total bilirubin	0–1.2 mg/dl
	Total protein	6.0–8.5 g/dl
	Albumin	3.5–5.0 g/dl
	Calcium	8.5–10.8 mg/dl
	Phosphorus	2.5–4.5 mg/dl
	Sodium	135–145 mEq/liter
	Potassium	3.5–5.3 mEq/liter
	Chloride	96–109 mEq/liter
	Carbon dioxide	22–31 mmol/liter
	Iron	42–135 mg/dl
	Blood pressure assessment	(See above)
	Carotid bruits assessment	Negative
	Duplex scan	Negative
Systemic infection with ocular manifestations		
Syphilis	Rapid plasma reagin	Nonreactive
	VDRL	Nonreactive
	Fluorescent treponemal antibody absorption	Nonreactive
	Microhemagglutination–*Treponema pallidum*	Nonreactive

Suspected Disease or Condition	Tests	Reference Range
Tuberculosis	Purified protein derivative	Negative (<5 mm)
	Chest x-ray	Negative
Lyme disease	ELISA (IgG, IgM) for Lyme disease	Negative (<0.8)
Human immunodeficiency	ELISA for HIV	Negative
virus (HIV)	Western blot	Negative
Chlamydia	Chlamydiazyme	Negative
Toxoplasmosis	ELISA (IgG) for toxoplasmosis	0–0.79 or <1:1
Toxocara	ELISA for *Toxocara*	<1:8
Primary ocular infection	Culture and sensitivity	No growth
	Gram's stain	Negative for pathogens

RESOURCES AND SUGGESTED READING

Burden G, Bryant SA. Laboratory and Radiologic Tests for Primary Eye Care. Boston: Butterworth–Heinemann, 1997.

Marks ES, Adamczyk DT, Thomann KH. Primary Eyecare in Systemic Disease. Norwalk, CT: Appleton & Lange, 1995.

Sowka J, Gurwood A, Kabat A. The Handbook of Ocular Disease Management (2nd ed). Supplement to Rev Optom, March 1998:66A–67A.

B

Commonly Used Ophthalmic Pharmaceuticals

Generic name	Some Common Trade Names	Manufacturer	How Supplied	Common Dosage
Topical ophthalmic dyes				
Sodium fluorescein*	Fluorets	Akorn	Strips	Apply moistened strip to conjunctiva
	Fluor-i-Strip	Storz		
	Ful-Glo	PBH Wesley Jessen		
Rose bengal	Rosets	Akorn	Strips	Apply moistened strip to conjunctiva
	Rose Bengal	PBH Wesley Jessen		
Lissamine green	Lissamine Green (0.1%, 0.5%, 1.0%)	Dakryon	5 ml	Instill 1 drop into eye
Injectable ophthalmic dyes				
Sodium fluorescein	AK-Fluor (10%, 25%)	Akorn	2, 5 ml amps or vials	Inject one vial into vein
	Fluorescite (10%, 25%)	Alcon		
	Funduscein (10%, 25%)	Ciba Vision		
Indocyanine green	Cardio-Green	Becton Dickinson	25, 50 mg in 10 ml solvent	Inject 10 ml solution into vein
Topical anesthetics				
Proparacaine HCl*	Alcaine	Alcon	15 ml	Instill 1–2 gtt
	Ophthaine	Apothecon		
	Ophthetic	Allergan		
Tetracaine HCl*	Pontocaine	Sanofi Winthrop	15 ml	Instill 1–2 gtt
	AK-T-Caine	Akorn		
Proparacaine with sodium fluorescein*	Fluoracaine	Akorn	5 ml	Instill 1 drop
Benoxinate HCl with sodium fluorescein	Fluress	PBH Wesley Jessen	5 ml	Instill 1 drop
	Flurate	Bausch & Lomb		
	Fluoxinate	Taylor		
Lidocaine HCl*	Xylocaine-MPF (4%)	Astra USA	5 ml ampule	Inject amount desired for specific tissue
Lidocaine HCl with epinephrine*	Xylocaine (1%) with epinephrine (1:100,000)	Astra USA	10, 20, 50 ml vials	
Mepivacaine HCl*	Carbocaine (1%, 2%)	Sanofi Winthrop	20, 30, 50 ml vials	
	Polocaine (1.0%, 1.5%, 2.0%)	Astra USA		
Bupivacaine HCl	Marcaine (0.75% and 0.75% with epinephrine)	Sanofi Winthrop	10, 30 ml vials	
	Sensorcaine (0.75%)	Astra USA	10, 30 ml vials	
Etidocaine HCl	Duranest-MPF (1.0%, 1.0% with epinephrine, 1.5% with epinephrine)	Astra USA	30 ml vials, 20 ml amps	
Topical mydriatics				
Phenylephrine HCl*	Neo-Synephrine (2.5%, 10.0%)	Sanofi Winthrop	15 ml	Instill 1 drop

Generic name	Some Common Trade Names	Manufacturer	How Supplied	Common Dosage
	Mydfrin (2.5%)	Alcon	3, 5 ml	
	AK-Dilate (2.5%, 10.0%)	Akorn	2, 15 ml	
Topical mydriatics and cycloplegics				
Atropine Sulfate*	Isopto Atropine (0.5%, 1.0%)	Alcon	2, 5, 15 ml	Instill 1 drop 1–3 times/day
	Atropine Sulfate (2%)	Alcon	2 ml	
	Atropisol (1%)	Ciba Vision	1 ml	
	Atropine Care (1%)	Akorn	2, 5, 15 ml	
	Atropine Sulfate Ointment (1%)	Bausch & Lomb, Pharmafair, etc.	3.5 g	Instill ½ in. strip in fornix/day
Homatropine HBr*	Isopto Homatropine (2%; 5%)	Alcon	5, 15 ml; 1, 2, 5 ml	Instill 1 drop 1–3 times/day
	AK-Homatropine (5%)	Akorn	5 ml	
Scopolamine HBr	Isopto Hyoscine (0.25%)	Alcon	5, 15 ml	Instill 1 drop 1–3 times/day
Cyclopentolate HCl*	Cyclogyl (0.5%, 2.0%)	Alcon	2, 5, 15 ml	Instill 1 drop 1–3 times/day
	AK-Pentolate (1%)	Akorn	2, 15 ml	
	Pentolair (1%)	Bausch & Lomb	2, 15 ml	
Tropicamide*	Mydriacyl (0.5%, 1%)	Alcon	15 ml	Instill 1–2 drops
	Tropicacyl (0.5%, 1%)	Akorn	2, 15 ml	
	Opticyl (0.5%, 1.0%)	Optopics	2, 15 ml	
Cyclopentolate HCl (0.2%) and phenylephrine HCl (1%)	Cyclomydril	Alcon	2, 5 ml	Instill 1–2 drops
Scopolamine HBr (0.3%) and phenylephrine HCl (10%)	Murocoll-2	Bausch & Lomb	5 ml	Instill 1 drop
Topical hyperosmotic agents				
Hypertonic sodium chloride*	Muro 128 Solution (2%, 5%)	Bausch & Lomb	15, 30 ml	Instill 1 drop 1–4 times/day
	Adsorbonac (2%, 5% solution)	Alcon	15 ml	
	Muroptic-5 (5% solution)	Optopics	15 ml	
	AK-NaCl (5% solution)	Akorn	15 ml	
	Muro 128 Ointment (5%)	Bausch & Lomb	3.5 g	Instill ¼ in. strip in fornix 1–4 times/day
Glucose	Glucose-40 (40%; ointment)	Ciba Vision	3.5 g	Instill ¼ in. strip in fornix 2–6 times/day
Glycerin	Ophthalgan (0.55%)	Storz	7.5 ml	1–2 drops before examination
Topical antihistamines and mast cell stabilizers				
Levocabastine HCl	Livostin (0.05% susp.)	Ciba Vision	5, 10 ml	Instill 1 drop 4 times/day
Cromolyn sodium	Crolom (4%)	Bausch & Lomb	2.5, 10 ml	Instill 1 drop 4–6 times/day
Lodoxamide tromethamine	Alomide (0.1%)	Alcon	10 ml	Instill 1 drop 4 times/day
Olopatadine HCl	Patanol (0.1%)	Alcon	5 ml	Instill 1 drop q6–8h
Emedastine difumarate	Emadine (0.05%)	Alcon	5 ml	Instill 1 drop 4 times/day
Topical decongestants				
Naphazoline HCl*	Naphcon (0.012%)	Alcon	15 ml	Instill 1 drop q4h
	Clear Eyes (0.012%)	Ross	15, 30 ml	
	Degest 2 (0.012%)	Akorn	15 ml	
	VasoClear (0.012%)	Ciba Vision	15 ml	
	Allergy Drops (0.12%)	Bausch & Lomb	15 ml	
	Comfort Eye Drops (0.03%)	PBH Wesley Jessen	15 ml	
	Maximum Strength Allergy Drops (0.03%)	Bausch & Lomb	15 ml	

Generic name	Some Common Trade Names	Manufacturer	How Supplied	Common Dosage
	Albalon (0.1%)	Allergan	15 ml	
	AK-Con (0.1%)	Akorn	15 ml	
	Naphcon Forte (0.1%)	Alcon	15 ml	
	Nafazair (0.1%)	Bausch & Lomb	15 ml	
	Vasocon Regular (0.1%)	Ciba Vision	15 ml	
Phenylephrine HCl	Prefrin Liquifilm (0.12%)	Allergan	20 ml	Instill 1 drop q4h
	Relief (0.12%)	Allergan	0.3 ml UD	
	AK-nephrin (0.12%)	Akorn	15 ml	
	Zincfrin (0.12%)	Alcon	15, 30 ml	
Tetrahydrozoline HCl*	Collyrium Fresh (0.05%)	Storz	15 ml	Instill 1 drop q4h
	Eye Drops (0.05%)	Bausch & Lomb	15 ml	
	Eyesine (0.05%)	Akorn	15 ml	
	Murine Plus (0.05%)	Ross	15, 30 ml	
	Tetrasine (0.05%)	Optopics	15, 22.5 ml	
	Visine (0.05%)	Pfizer	15, 22.5, 30 ml	
Oxymetazoline	OcuClear (0.025%)	Schering-Plough	30 ml	Instill 1 drop q4h
	Visine LR (0.025%)	Pfizer	15, 30 ml	
Topical decongestant/antihistamine combinations				
Naphazoline HCl (0.025%) and pheniramine maleate (0.3%)*	Naphcon-A	Alcon	5, 15 ml	Instill 1 drop q4h
	Naphazoline Plus	Parmed	15 ml	
Naphazoline HCl (0.027%) and pheniramine maleate (0.315%)*	Opcon-A	Bausch & Lomb	15 ml	
Naphazoline HCl (0.05%) and antazoline phosphate (0.5%)*	Vasocon-A	Ciba Vision	15 ml	
Oral antihistamines				
Diphenhydramine HCl* (OTC)	Benadryl	Parke-Davis	50 mg tablets	1 tablet orally 3–4 times/day
Chlorpheniramine maleate (OTC)	Chlor-Trimeton	Schering-Plough	4 mg tablets	1 tablet q4–6h
			8 mg tablets	1 tablet q8–12h
			12 mg tablets	1 tablet q12h
Loratadine	Claritin	Schering-Plough	10 mg	1 tablet/day
Fexofenadine	Allegra	Marion Merrill Dow	60 mg	1 tablet 2 times/day
Astemizole	Hismanal	Janssen	10 mg	1 tablet/day
Cetirizine	Zyrtec	Pfizer	5, 10 mg tablets	1 tablet/day
Topical corticosteroid solutions and suspensions				
Medrysone	HMS Suspension (1%)	Allergan	5, 10 ml	Instill 1 drop q1–4h, depending on severity of inflammation
Fluorometholone	FML Suspension (0.1%)	Allergan	1, 5, 10, 15 ml	
	Fluor-Op Suspension (0.1%)	Ciba Vision	5, 10, 15 ml	
Fluorometholone acetate	Flarex Suspension (0.1%)	Alcon	2.5, 5, 10 ml	
	Eflone Suspension (0.1%)	Ciba Vision	5, 10 ml	
	FML Forte Suspension (0.25%)	Allergan	2, 5, 10, 15 ml	
Prednisolone acetate	Pred Mild Suspension (0.12%)	Allergan	5, 10 ml	
	Econopred Suspension (0.125%)	Alcon	5, 10 ml	
	Pred Forte Suspension (1%)	Allergan	1, 5, 10, 15 ml	
	Econopred Plus Suspension (1%)	Alcon	5, 10 ml	
Prednisolone sodium phosphate*	Inflamase Mild (0.125%)	Ciba Vision	3, 5, 10 ml	
	AK-Pred (0.125%, 1.0%)	Akorn	5, 15 ml	
	Inflamase Forte (1%)	Ciba Vision	3, 5, 10, 15 ml	

Generic name	Some Common Trade Names	Manufacturer	How Supplied	Common Dosage
Rimexolone	Vexol (1% susp.)	Alcon	5, 10 ml	
Loteprednol	Alrex (0.2% susp.)	Bausch & Lomb	5, 10 ml	
Etabonate	Lotemax (0.5% susp.)	Bausch & Lomb	5, 10, 15 ml	
Oral corticosteroids				
Prednisone*	Deltasone	Upjohn	2.5, 5, 10, 20, 50 mg tablets	5–60 mg/day orally, depending on condition
Methylprednisolone*	Medrol	Upjohn	2, 4, 8, 16, 24, 32 mg tablets	4–48 mg/day orally, depending on condition
Topical nonsteroidal anti-inflammatory agents (NSAIDs)				
Diclofenac sodium	Voltaren (0.1%)	Ciba Vision	2.5, 5 ml	Instill 1 drop 4
Ketorolac tromethamine	Acular (0.5%)	Allergan	5 ml	times/day
Oral NSAIDs				
Ibuprofen* (OTC)	Advil Motrin IB Nuprin	Whitehall-Robins Pharmacia & Upjohn Bristol-Meyers Squibb	200 mg tablets	1–2 tablets orally q4–6h
Naproxen sodium* (OTC)	Aleve	Bayer	220 mg tablets	1 tablet orally q8–12h
Ketoprofen (OTC)	Orudis KT	Whitehall-Robins	12.5 mg tablets	1 tablet orally q4–6h
Topical antibacterial agents				
Bacitracin*	AK-Tracin Ointment (500 μ/g)	Akorn	3.5 g	Apply ½ in. strip in inferior fornix 1–3
Erythromycin*	Ilotycin (5 mg/g; ointment)	Dista	3.5 g	times/day
Gentamicin sulfate*	Garamycin (3 mg/ml)	Schering-Plough	5 ml	Instill 1 drop 4
	Genoptic (3 mg/ml)	Allergan	1, 5 ml	times/day
	Gentacidin (3 mg/ml)	Ciba Vision	5 ml	
	Gentak	Akorn	5, 15 ml	
	Garamycin Ointment (3 mg/g)	Schering-Plough	3.5 g	Apply ½ in. strip in inferior fornix 1–3
	Genoptic Ointment (3 mg/g)	Allergan	3.5 g	times/day
	Gentacidin Ointment (3 mg/g)	Ciba Vision	3.5 g	
	Gentak Ointment (3 mg/g)	Akorn	3.5 g	
Tobramycin*	Tobrex (0.3%)	Alcon	5 ml	Instill 1 drop 4
	AKTob, Defy (0.3%)	Akorn	5 ml	times/day
	Tobrex Ointment	Alcon	3.5 g	Apply ½ in. strip in inferior fornix 1–3 times/day
Ciprofloxacin	Ciloxan (0.3%)	Alcon	2.5, 5 ml	Instill 1 drop 4 times/day (dosage is more frequent for initial treatment of corneal ulcer)
	Ciloxan Ointment (0.3%)	Alcon	3.5 g	Instill ½ in. strip in inferior fornix 1–3 times/day
Ofloxacin	Ocuflox (0.3%)	Allergan	1, 5, 10 ml	
Norfloxacin	Chibroxin (3 mg/ml)	Merck	5 ml	
Sulfacetamide sodium*	Bleph-10 (10%)	Allergan	2.5, 5, 15 ml	Instill 1 drop 4 times/day
	Sodium Sulamyd (10%)	Schering-Plough	5, 15 ml	
	Sulf-10 (10%)	Ciba Vision	1, 15 ml	
	Ocusulf-10 (10%)	Optopics	2, 5, 15 ml	
	AK-Sulf (10%)	Akorn	2, 5, 15 ml	

Generic name	Some Common Trade Names	Manufacturer	How Supplied	Common Dosage
	Isopto Cetamide (15%)	Alcon	5, 15 ml	
	Bleph-10 Ointment (10%)	Allergan	3.5 g	Instill ½ in. strip in
	Sodium Sulamyd Ointment (10%)	Schering-Plough	3.5 g	inferior fornix 1–3 times/day
	Cetamide Ointment (10%)	Alcon	3.5 g	
	AK-Sulf Ointment (10%)	Akorn	3.5 g	
Chloramphenicol*	Chloroptic (5 mg/ml)	Allergan	2.5, 7.5 ml	Instill 1 drop 4
	AK-Chlor (5 mg/ml)	Akorn	7.5, 15 ml	times/day
	Chloroptic S.O.P. Ointment (10 mg/g)	Allergan	3.5 g	Instill ½ in. strip in inferior fornix 1–3
	Chloromycetin Ointment (10 mg/g)	Parke-Davis	3.5 g	times/day
	AK-Chlor Ointment (10 mg/g)	Akorn	3.5 g	

Topical combination antibiotics

Generic name	Some Common Trade Names	Manufacturer	How Supplied	Common Dosage
Trimethoprim sulfate/ polymyxin B sulfate*	Polytrim Ophthalmic Solution	Allergan	10 ml	Instill 1 drop 4 times/day
Bacitracin zinc/polymyxin B sulfate*	Polysporin Ophthalmic Ointment	Glaxo Wellcome	3.5 g	Instill ½ in. strip in inferior fornix 1–3
	AK-Poly-Bac Ointment	Akorn	3.5 g	times/day
Neomycin sulfate/ polymyxin B sulfate/gramicidin*	Neosporin Ophthalmic Solution	Glaxo Wellcome	10 ml	Instill 1 drop 4 times/day
	AK-Spore Solution	Akorn	2, 10 ml	
Neomycin sulfate/ polymyxin B sulfate/ bacitracin zinc*	Neosporin Ophthalmic Ointment	Glaxo Wellcome	3.5 g	Instill ½ in. strip in inferior fornix 1–3
	Ocutricin Ointment	Bausch & Lomb	3.5 g	times/day
	AK-Spore Ointment	Akorn	3.5 g	
Polymyxin B sulfate/ oxytetracycline	Terramycin with Polymyxin B Ointment	Roerig	3.5 g	
	Terak Ointment	Akorn	3.5 g	

Topical corticosteroid/antibiotic combinations

Generic name	Some Common Trade Names	Manufacturer	How Supplied	Common Dosage
Dexamethasone phosphate 0.1%/ tobramycin 0.3%	TobraDex Suspension	Alcon	2.5, 5 ml	Instill 1 drop 4 times/day
	TobraDex Ointment	Alcon	3.5 g	Instill ½ in. in inferior fornix 3 times/day
Prednisolone acetate 1%/gentamicin sulfate 0.3%	Pred-G Suspension	Allergan	2, 5, 10 ml	Instill 1 drop 4 times/day
	Pred-G S.O.P. Ointment	Allergan	3.5 g	Instill ½ in. in inferior fornix 3 times/day
Prednisolone acetate 0.5%/neomycin 0.35%/polymyxin B sulfate	Poly-Pred Suspension	Allergan	5, 10 ml	Instill 1 drop 4 times/day
Dexamethasone phosphate 0.1%/ neomycin sulfate 0.35%*	NeoDecadron (susp.)	Merck	5 ml	
	AK-Neo-Dex (susp.)	Akorn	5 ml	
	NeoDecadron Ointment	Merck	3.5 g	Instill ½ in. in inferior fornix 3 times/day
Dexamethasone phosphate 0.1%/neomycin sulfate 0.35%/polymyxin B sulfate*	Maxitrol Suspension	Alcon	5 ml	Instill 1 drop 4 times/day
	Dexacidin Suspension	Ciba Vision	5 ml	
	AK-Trol	Akorn	5 ml	
	Maxitrol Ointment	Alcon	3.5 g	Instill ½ in. in inferior fornix 3 times/day
	Dexacidin Ointment	Ciba Vision	3.5 g	
	Dexasporin Ointment	Bausch & Lomb	3.5 g	
	AK-Trol Ointment	Akorn	3.5 g	
Hydrocortisone 1%/ neomycin sulfate 0.35%/polymyxin B sulfate*	Cortisporin (susp.)	Glaxo Wellcome	7.5 ml	Instill 1 drop 4 times/day
	AK-Spore (susp.)	Akorn	7.5 ml	

Generic name	Some Common Trade Names	Manufacturer	How Supplied	Common Dosage
Hydrocortisone 1%/ neomycin sulfate 0.35%/polymyxin B sulfate/bacitracin zinc*	Cortisporin (ointment) AK-Spore HC Ointment	Glaxo Wellcome Akorn	3.5 g 3.5 g	Instill ½ in. in inferior fornix 3 times/day
Hydrocortisone acetate 1.5%/oxy-tetracycline 0.5%	Terra-Cortril (susp.)	Roerig	5 ml	Instill 1 drop 4 times/day
Hydrocortisone acetate 0.5%/chlor-amphenicol 0.25%	Chloromycetin/Hydro-cortisone (susp.)	Parke-Davis	5 ml	
Prednisolone acetate 0.2%/sodium sulfacetamide 10%	Blephamide Suspension Blephamide Ointment	Allergan Allergan	2.5, 5, 10 ml 3.5 g	Instill 1 drop q4h Instill ½ in. strip in inferior fornix 3 times/day
Prednisolone acetate 0.25%/sodium sulfacetamide 10%	Isopto Cetapred (susp.) Cetapred (ointment)	Alcon Alcon	5, 15 ml 3.5 g	Instill 1 drop q4h Instill ½ in. strip in inferior fornix 3 times/day
Prednisolone acetate 0.5%/sodium sulfacetamide 10%	Metimyd (susp.) AK-Cide Metimyd (ointment) AK-Cide Ointment	Schering-Plough Akorn Schering-Plough Akorn	5 ml 5 ml 3.5 g 3.5 g	Instill 1 drop q4h Instill ½ in. strip in inferior fornix 3 times/day
Prednisolone sodium phosphate 0.25%/ sodium sulfaceta-mide 10%*	Vasocidin Sulster Solution	Ciba Vision Akorn	5, 10 ml 5, 10 ml	Instill 1 drop q4h
Fluorometholone 0.1%/sodium sulfacetamide 10%	FML-S Suspension	Allergan	5, 10 ml	
Oral antibacterial agents				
Tetracycline HCl*	Achromycin V (250, 500 mg)	Lederle	Capsules	250–500 mg orally q6h
Doxycycline hyclate*	Doryx (100 mg) Vibramycin Hyclate (50 mg) Vibra-Tabs (100 mg)	Warner Chilcott Pfizer Pfizer	Pellets Capsules Tablets	50–100 mg 1–2 times/day
Erythromycin*	Ery-Tabs (250, 333, 500 mg) Erythromycin Base Filmtab (250, 500 mg)	Abbott Abbott	Enteric coated tablets Tablets	250–500 mg orally four times/day
Erythromycin ethylsuccinate	EES (400 mg)	Abbott	Tablets	400 mg orally 4 times/day
Erythromycin estolate	Ilosone (250, 500 mg)	Dista	250 mg pulvules; 500 mg tablets	250 mg orally 4 times/day
Azithromycin	Zithromax	Pfizer	250 mg capsules; 250, 600 mg tablets	1 g orally once/day
Dicloxacillin*	Dicloxacillin	Teva	250, 500 mg	250 mg capsules orally 4 times/day
Cephalexin*	Keflex Keftab Keftab	Dista Dura Lily	250, 500 mg pulvules; 125, 250 mg susp. 500 mg tablets 500 mg tablets	250 mg orally 4 times/day
Cefadroxil*	Duricef	Bristol-Myers Squibb	500 mg capsules; 125, 250, 500 mg oral susp.	1 g orally/day

Generic name	Some Common Trade Names	Manufacturer	How Supplied	Common Dosage
Amoxicillin/ clavulanate	Augmentin	SmithKline Beecham	250, 500, 875 mg tablets; 125, 200, 250, 400 mg/5 ml oral susp.; 125, 200, 250, 400 mg chewable tablets	500 mg orally 2–3 times/day
Topical Antiviral Agents				
Trifluridine*	Viroptic (1%)	Monarch	7.5 ml	Instill 1 drop 9 times/day initially
Vidarabine	Vira-A Ointment (3%)	Parke-Davis	3.5 g	Instill ½ in. strip in inferior fornix 5 times/day
Oral antiviral agents				
Acyclovir*	Zovirax	Glaxo Wellcome	200, 800 mg capsules	800 mg orally 5 times/day
Valacyclovir HCl	Valtrex	Glaxo Wellcome	500 mg, 1 g capsules	1 g orally 3 times/day
Famciclovir	Famvir	SmithKline Beecham	125, 250, 500 mg tablets	500 mg orally 3 times/day
Topical antifungal agents				
Natamycin	Natacyn Suspension (5%)	Alcon	15 ml	Instill 1 drop q1–2h
Topical antiglaucoma agents—beta blockers				
Timolol maleate*	Timoptic (0.25, 0.5%)	Merck	2.5, 5.0, 10.0, 15.0 ml	Instill 1 drop 2 times/day
	Timoptic XE (0.25%, 0.5%) (gel-forming solution)	Merck	2.5, 5.0 ml	Instill 1 drop in morning
Timolol hemihydrate	Betimol (0.25%, 0.5%)	Ciba Vision	2.5, 5.0, 10.0, 15.0 ml	Instill 1 drop 2 times/day
Betaxolol (selective beta blocker)	Betoptic (0.5%)	Alcon	2.5, 5.0, 10.0, 15.0 ml	Instill 1 drop 2 times/day
	Betoptic S (0.25%)	Alcon	2.5, 5.0, 10.0, 15.0 ml	
Levobunolol* (susp.)	Betagan (0.25%, 0.5%)	Allergan	2, 5, 10 ml	Instill 1 drop 1–2 times/day
	AKBeta (0.25%, 0.5%)	Akorn	5, 10, 15 ml	
Metipranolol HCl	OptiPranolol (0.3%)	Bausch & Lomb	5, 10 ml	Instill 1 drop 2 times/day
Carteolol	Ocupress (1%)	Otsuka America	5, 10 ml	Instill 1 drop 2 times/day
Topical antiglaucoma agents—alpha$_2$-adrenergic agonists				
Brimonidine tartrate	Alphagan (0.2%)	Allergan	5, 10 ml	Instill 1 drop 3 times/day
Apraclonidine HCl	Iopidine (0.5%)	Alcon	5, 10 ml	Instill 1 drop 3 times/day
Topical antiglaucoma agents—prostaglandins				
Latanoprost	Xalatan (0.005%)	Pharmacia & Upjohn	2.5 ml	Instill 1 drop in the evening
Topical antiglaucoma agents—carbonic anhydrase inhibitors				
Dorzolamide HCl	Trusopt (2%)	Merck	5, 10 ml	Instill 1 drop 3 times/day
Brinzolamide HCl	Azopt (1%)	Alcon	5, 10, 15 ml	
Topical antiglaucoma agents—epinephrines				
Epinephrine HCl*	Epifrin (0.5%, 1.0%, 2.0%)	Allergan	15 ml	Instill 1 drop 2 times/day
	Glaucon (1%, 2%)	Alcon	10 ml	
Epinephryl borate	Epinal (0.5%, 1.0%)	Alcon	7.5 ml	Instill 1 drop 2 times/day
Dipivefrin HCl*	Propine (0.1%)	Allergan	5, 10, 15 ml	Instill 1 drop 2 times/day
	AKPro (0.1%)	Akorn	2, 5, 10, 15 ml	

Generic name	Some Common Trade Names	Manufacturer	How Supplied	Common Dosage
Topical antiglaucoma agents—direct-acting miotics				
Pilocarpine HCl*	Isopto Carpine (0.25%, 0.5%, 1.0%, 2.0%, 3.0%, 4.0%, 5.0%, 6.0%, 8.0%, 10.0%)	Alcon	15, 30 ml	Instill 1 drop 4 times/day
	Pilocar (0.5%, 1%, 2%, 3%, 4%, 6%)	Ciba Vision	15 ml	
	Pilostat (0.5%, 1.0%, 2.0%, 3.0%, 4.0%, 6.0%)	Bausch & Lomb	15 ml	
	Piloptic (0.5%, 1.0%, 2.0%, 3.0%, 4.0%, 6.0%)	Optopics	15 ml	
	Akarpine (1%, 2%, 4%)	Akorn	15 ml	
	Ocusert Pilo-20, -40	Alza	20 μg/hr	Instill 1 insert/week
	Pilopine HS Gel (4%)	Alcon	3.5 g	Apply ¼ in. strip in inferior fornix at bedtime
Pilocarpine nitrate	Pilagan (1%, 2%, 4%)	Allergan	15 ml	Instill 2 drop 4 times/day
Carbachol	Isopto Carbachol (0.75%, 1.5%, 2.25%, 3%)	Alcon	15, 30 ml	Instill 1 drop 3 times/day
	Carboptic (3%)	Optopics	15 ml	
Topical antiglaucoma agents—combinations				
Timoptic maleate and dorzolamide	Cosopt (0.5%, 2.0%)	Merck	5, 10 ml	Instill 1 drop 2 times/day
Pilocarpine and epinephrine bitartrate 1%	E-Pilo (1%, 2%, 4%, 6% pilocarpine)	IOLAB	10 ml	
	P1E-P4E1 (1%, 2%, 3%, 4% pilocarpine)	Alcon	15 ml	
Oral antiglaucoma agents—carbonic anhydrase inhibitors				
Acetazoloamide*	Diamox (125, 250 mg)	Lederle	Tablets	1 tablet 1–4 times/day
	Dazamide (250 mg)	Major	Tablets	
	Diamox Sequels (500 mg sustained release capsules)	Lederle	Capsules	1 tablet 1–2 times/day
Methazolamide*	Neptazane (25, 50 mg)	Lederle	Tablets	1 tablet 2 times/day
	MZM (25, 50 mg)	Ciba Vision	Tablets	
	GlaucTabs (25, 50 mg)	Akorn	Tablets	
Oral antiglaucoma agents—hyperosmotics				
Glycerin	Osmoglyn (50% solution)	Alcon	220 ml	2–3 ml/kg body weight (4–6 oz)
Isosorbide	Ismotic 45% w/v Solution	Alcon	220 ml	1.5g/kg body weight (one 220-ml bottle)
Oral analgesics				
Acetylsalicylic acid* (OTC)	Bayer Aspirin	Bayer	325 mg tablets	1–2 tablets q4–6h (≤3,900 mg/day)
	Bufferin (buffered)	Bristol-Meyers Squibb		
	Ascriptin (buffered)	Ciba		
	Ecotrin (enteric coated)	SmithKline Beecham		
Acetaminophen* (OTC)	Tylenol	McNeil	325, 650 mg tablets	1–2 tablets q4–6h (≤3,900 mg/day)
Tramadol HCl	Ultram	McNeil	50 mg tablets	1–2 tablets q4–6h
Acetaminophen/ codeine phosphate (300 mg)* (schedule III)	Tylenol with Codeine	Ortho-McNeil	15 mg (#2), 30 mg (#3), 60 mg (#4) tablets	1 tablet orally q4h (max. 24-hr dose is 360 mg codeine, 4,000 mg acetaminophen)

Generic name	Some Common Trade Names	Manufacturer	How Supplied	Common Dosage
Acetaminophen (500 mg)/hydro-codone bitartrate (schedule III)	Lortab	UCB Pharma	2.5, 5.0, 7.5 mg tablets 10 mg tablets	1–2 tablets orally every 4–6 hrs 1 tablet orally every 4–6 hrs
Acetylsalicylic acid (500 mg)/hydro-codone bitartrate (5 mg) (schedule III)	Lortab ASA	UCB Pharma	Tablets	1–2 tablets orally every 4–6 hrs
Acetaminophen (500 mg)/hydro-codone bitartrate (5 mg) (schedule III)	Vicodin	Knoll	Tablets	1–2 tablets orally q4–6h
Acetaminophen (660 mg)/hydro-codone bitartrate (10 mg) (schedule III)	Vicodin HP	Knoll	Tablets	1 tablet orally q4–6h
Acetaminophen (750 mg)/hydro-codone bitartrate (7.5 mg) (schedule III)	Vicodin ES	Knoll	Tablets	1 tablet orally q4–6h
Ibuprofen (200 mg)/hydrocodone bitartrate (7.5 mg) (schedule III)	Vicoprofen	Knoll	Tablets	1 tablet orally q4–6h

OTC = over the counter.
Notes: The dosages listed are for adults. For many of these medications, the dosage may vary with the type, severity, and duration of the condition being treated. All topical medications are solutions unless otherwise specified. An asterisk (*) indicates that this drug is available under its generic name from one or more manufacturers.

RESOURCES AND SUGGESTED READING

Bartlett JD, Fiscella RG, Ghormley NR, et al. (eds). Ophthalmic Drug Facts 1998. St. Louis: Facts and Comparisons, 1998.
Melton R, Thomas R. The 1998 Clinical Guide to Ophthalmic Drugs. Supplement to Review of Optometry, May 1998.
Physicians' Desk Reference 1998 (52nd ed). Montvale, NJ: Medical Economics Data Production, 1998.

Index